全国医学英语水平考试教研中心学术著作基金支持

卓越医师外语能力提升系列教材

临床诊疗英语

English for Clinical Doctors

主　编　胡　涛
副主编　杜笑秋　郭钟庆　胡行超
编　委　饶　辉　顾　萍　李　敏
　　　　施荣根　丁海燕　李晓梅
　　　　薛　勤　徐　畅　曹　华

 南京大学出版社

医学专家顾问

内　　科　张定国（江苏省人民医院）
　　　　　桑华超（南京医科大学附属逸夫医院）
　　　　　吴远帆（江苏省人民医院）
　　　　　刘　静（无锡市第一人民医院）
　　　　　吴文君（无锡市第一人民医院）
外　　科　秦晓东（江苏省人民医院）
　　　　　张殿彩（江苏省人民医院）
　　　　　崔维顶（江苏省人民医院）
　　　　　黄华兴（南京医科大学第一临床医学院）
　　　　　鲁　振（江苏省肿瘤医院）
妇 产 科　曹　郡（江苏省妇幼保健院）
　　　　　殷　茵（江苏省人民医院）
儿　　科　方拥军（南京市儿童医院）
　　　　　薛　瑶（南京市儿童医院）
　　　　　刘　峰（南京市儿童医院）
　　　　　程卫霞（南京市儿童医院）
眼　　科　林小俊（江苏省人民医院）
口 腔 科　王羽立（江苏省口腔医院）
　　　　　钱雅婧（江苏省口腔医院）
　　　　　孙　辉（南京医科大学附属逸夫医院）
耳鼻喉科　陈　曦（江苏省人民医院）
　　　　　张　勇（南京医科大学第二附属医院）
传 染 科　杨永峰（南京市第二医院/江苏省传染病医院）
检 验 科　刘惠敏（江苏省中医院）
影 像 科　丁重阳（江苏省人民医院）
　　　　　张　伟（江苏省人民医院）
中 医 科　胡　赟（南京医科大学附属逸夫医院）
　　　　　戴德纯（昆山市中医医院）

外籍医学顾问
Shan Hemachandra
Nitish Beharee

前　言

中国对外医疗援助最早可追溯至20世纪60年代。近年来,全球公共卫生事件频发,给中国援外医疗队带来更多的挑战。熟练掌握临床英语沟通技巧是每位援外医生的必备条件。

《临床诊疗英语》是一本供中国援外医疗队使用的综合诊疗英语培训特色教材,如何引导临床医生基于共情原则,灵活使用英语与病人交流,避免医患失语,是本书编写的基本理念。本书编写团队共十二人,主要来自南京医科大学外国语学院研究生英语部,他们不仅具有丰富的临床诊疗英语教学经验,而且谙熟医患沟通有效性在临床诊疗过程中的重要地位。主编胡涛曾任1997年江苏省第17期援外医疗队专职翻译,赴桑给巴尔工作两年,归国后承担江苏省援外医疗队医生英语培训工作至今。

《临床诊疗英语》涉及十一个医学临床科室,通过听、说、读、写、译五个维度,为临床诊疗提供基础性和框架性用语,旨在提高医患基本沟通的有效性。科室下分三十个章节,以各临床科室常见疾病为基础,以具体临床病例为背景,通过阅读相关疾病前沿诊疗材料、模拟医患交流经典对话等练习手段,强化相关疾病的高频词汇使用,帮助医生进一步熟练应用英语有效开展具体的临床工作。另外,本书还精心设计了单元练习,并配有答案,供使用者参考。二维码标记处是对相关疾病的最新视听材料补充,内容丰富,话题生动,涵盖患者主诉、询问病史、检验检测、治疗方案等。

《临床诊疗英语》是医学专门用途英语教材的一个新尝试,建议灵活使用。对于即将进入见习与实习阶段的医学院校高年级学生,本书可作为医学英语的延伸材料。对于医疗行业第一线的从业人员,本书可以帮助他们与外籍病人完成基本沟通。对于医科院校国际学生临床带教老师,本书亦可提供备课参考。简言之,这本书是编者们在多年援外英语教学中积累和研究的成果,希望对大家有所帮助。

《临床诊疗英语》的顺利出版得益于各方的合作与努力。在构思初期,我们得到了江苏省卫生健康委员会对外合作交流处的肯定和鼓励;在编写过程中,我们得到了南京医科大学外国语学院、国际教育学院各位同行的支持和帮助;在校对过程中,我们得到了江苏省内多家医院专家的指导和建议。特别感谢与我亦师亦友的原江苏省卫生厅国际交流与合作处陆文民处长,正是他最初的提议和设想,敦促我这些年来积累了大量的临床诊疗教学素材。致谢!

本书根据党的二十大精神编写。书中有不足之处,敬希广大读者和同行专家给予指正。

编者
2023年5月

Table of Contents

Ophthalmology
眼科篇

Stomatology
口腔篇

E.N.T.
耳鼻咽喉篇

Infectious Diseases
传染病篇

Clinical Laboratory Examination
医学检验篇

Medical Imaging and Ultrasound
医学影像及超声篇

Traditional Chinese Medicine
中医篇

Unit 1

Pneumonia

I Warming-up

A. Match the following words and phrases with their Chinese translations.

A	alveolus	1	痰
B	non-invasive ventilation	2	并发症
C	community-acquired	3	氧饱和
D	mucus	4	社区获得性
E	respiratory failure	5	喘息
F	complication	6	无创通气
G	wheezing	7	呼吸衰竭
H	sputum	8	肺泡
I	oxygen saturation	9	胸片
J	chest radiograph	10	粘液

B. Complete the sentences with the following words or phrases in their proper forms.

underlie	hospital	general	inflammation
severe	treat	linger	build up

1. Chronic illnesses like COPD，cardiovascular disease，and diabetes，may put you at greater risk for a more severe case of pneumonia and may put you at risk for having a

trigger of a worsening of your _____ condition.

2. Immunohistochemical studies have shown that the IgG cell fraction is increased up to 30 times, depending on the _____ of the lesion.

3. Copper helps to guard against the bone loss that occurs with ageing, and also against _____ conditions such as arthritis.

4. Apparently, mental illness is one of the few diseases requiring _____ where those afflicted are released before they are cured.

5. Pneumonia is _____. If you have symptoms, talk to your doctor right away.

6. The disease can also cause a _____ of pressure in the inner ear leading to severe earache.

7. An _____ cough can result from many conditions, including bronchitis, asthma, acid reflux, or chronic allergies. Natural remedies, such as drinking tea with honey or inhaling essential oils, can help.

8. Symptoms of pneumonia can be different for each person, but it typically includes fever, cough, chills, loss of appetite, and _____ weakness.

C. Watch the video *Pneumonia—A Serious Condition to Be Taken Seriously* and answer the questions.

扫码获取视频

1. What is the most common kind of pneumonia?

2. Why is it not true that people have to be elderly and in the hospital to get pneumonia?

3. What are risk factors for pneumonia?

4. What are common symptoms of pneumonia?

5. How can people tell the difference between flu and pneumonia?

扫码获取
音频及文本

Ⅱ Dialogue

A. Listen to the dialogue for the first time and try to get the general idea.

B. Listen to the dialogue for the second time and try to answer the following questions.

1. What brings Wang Hai to see Doctor Wang?

2. What does Doctor Wang say after the physical examination on Wang Hai is done?

3. What does the result of the chest X-ray test indicate?

4. How does Doctor Wang explain Wang Hai's symptoms of headaches and an upset stomach?

5. What advice does Doctor Wang give Wang Hai in the end?

C. Choose the following words and/or expressions to complete the sentences in their proper forms.

on top of that	除此之外	auscultation	听诊
upset	不适	audible	听得见的
persist	持续存在	moist rale	湿啰音
bring up	咳出	to my knowledge	据我所知
overtime	加班	vital sign	生命体征
bilateral	双侧的	stress	压力

1. Leaving your comfort zone, as uncomfortable and _____ as that can be sometimes, is a must if you want to grow as a person.

2. There were, of course, rumors that it was haunted, but _____ no one ever saw or heard anything there.

3. What a day! First I woke up late, then the hot water heater burst, and _____ I got a flat tire.

4. During the operation, the airway peak pressure and SPO_2 were monitored, and lung respiratory sound was _____.

5. Distribution of the lesion were diffuse _____ and symmetrical.

6. Since the 2016 event, BMA House has improved the sound system in the Great Hall, which enhanced the _____ of presenters and questioners, and in the last year a larger screen has been installed.

7. Because the muscles in their bellies haven't fully developed yet, babies need to be burped until they can _____ wind on their own, which is typically around 7—9 months.

8. _____ are generated in bronchi and cavities in the lungs in the presence of liquid secretions (sputum, congestive fluid, and blood).

9. The babies in this unit have various devices attached to them that monitor the _____.

10. Typical symptoms of the illness include severe headaches, a high temperature and a _____ dry cough.

D. Read the dialogue and try to make a conversation with your classmates.

扫码获取
提示

E. Translate the following Chinese into English.

WH—Wang Hai   DW—Doctor Wang

DW：Good Morning，Wang Hai.

WH：Good Morning，Doctor Wang.

DW：I see here that you started feeling tired two months ago，and then you started having bad headaches. 1. 你还有胃部不适并持续咳嗽。Did you run a fever?

　　1. _____

WH：No，doctor.

DW：I'll listen to your heart and lungs. 2. 深呼吸，屏住呼吸，呼气。Do it again please. Were there any changes in your diet or your weight lately?

　　2. _____

WH：3. 我就是常规饮食,不过最近两个月体重减了5公斤。

　　3. _____
　　_____

DW：4. 咳嗽时有痰吗?

　　4. _____

WH：Yes，some thick sputum.

DW：What color was it，yellow or white? Any bloody sputum? 5. 容易咳出痰来吗?

　　5. _____

WH：The sputum is yellow colored，but it's easy to cough up.

DW：Do you have hypertension or diabetes?
　　6. 以前有没有得过肺结核?

　　6. _____

WH：No.

DW：Do you drink? Do you smoke?

WH：No，doctor.

DW：How are things at work?

WH：Got a new job and a lot of stress，7. 需要经常加班,甚至周末也得工作。

　　7. _____

DW：Mmm，your heart seems to be normal. Coarse breath sounds are heard bilaterally on auscultation of the lungs. 8. 左下肺闻及少许湿啰音。Take these two slips and go to the lab for blood tests and then X-ray room for the chest film. I'll wait here for the reports.

　　8. _____

Ⅲ　Further Reading：Pneumonia

Overview

Pneumonia is a form of acute respiratory infection that is most commonly caused by viruses or bacteria. It can cause mild to life-threatening illness in people of all ages，however it is the single largest infectious cause of death in children worldwide.

The lungs are made up of small sacs called alveoli, which fill with air when a healthy person breathes. When an individual has pneumonia, the alveoli are filled with pus and fluid, which makes breathing painful and limits oxygen intake. These infections are generally spread by direct contact with infected people.

Signs and symptoms

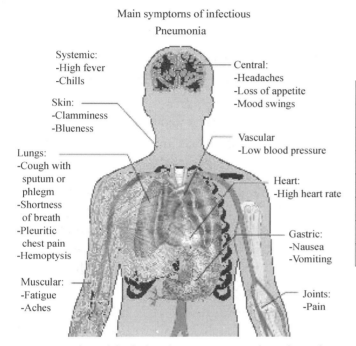

Main symptoms of infectious Pneumonia

Systemic:
-High fever
-Chills

Skin:
-Clamminess
-Blueness

Lungs:
-Cough with sputum or phlegm
-Shortness of breath
-Pleuritic chest pain
-Hemoptysis

Muscular:
-Fatigue
-Aches

Central:
-Headaches
-Loss of appetite
-Mood swings

Vascular
-Low blood pressure

Heart:
-High heart rate

Gastric:
-Nausea
-Vomiting

Joints:
-Pain

Symptoms frequency	
Symptom	Frequency
Cough	79%—91%
Fatigue	90%
Fever	71%—75%
Shortness of breath	67%—75%
Sputum	60%—65%
Chest pain	39%—49%

People with infectious pneumonia often have a productive cough, fever accompanied by shaking chills, shortness of breath, sharp or stabbing chest pain during deep breaths, and an increased rate of breathing. In elderly people, confusion may be the most prominent sign.

The typical signs and symptoms in children under five years old are fever, cough, and fast or difficult breathing. Fever is not very specific, as it occurs in many other common illnesses and may be absent in those with severe disease, malnutrition or in the elderly. In addition, a cough is frequently absent in children less than 2 months old. More severe signs and symptoms in children may include blue-tinged skin, unwillingness to drink, convulsions, ongoing vomiting, extremes of temperature, or a decreased level of consciousness.

Bacterial and viral cases of pneumonia usually result in similar symptoms. Some causes are associated with classic, but non-specific, clinical characteristics. Pneumonia caused by **Legionella** may occur with abdominal pain, diarrhea, or confusion. Pneumonia caused by **Streptococcus pneumoniae** is associated with rusty colored sputum. Pneumonia caused by **Klebsiella** may have bloody sputum often described as "currant jelly". Bloody sputum (known as hemoptysis) may also occur with tuberculosis. Pneumonia caused by **Mycoplasma pneumoniae** may occur in association with swelling of the lymph nodes in the neck, joint pain or a middle ear infection. Viral pneumonia presents more commonly with wheezing than bacterial pneumonia. Pneumonia was historically divided into "typical" and "atypical" based on the belief that the presentation predicted the underlying cause. However, evidence has not supported this distinction, therefore it is no longer emphasized.

Cause

Pneumonia is due to infections caused primarily by bacteria or viruses and less commonly by fungi and parasites. Although more than 100 strains of infectious agents have been identified, only a few are responsible for the majority of cases. Mixed infections with both viruses and bacteria may occur in roughly 45% of infections in children and 15% of infections in adults. A causative agent may not be isolated in about half of cases despite careful testing. In an active population-based surveillance for community-acquired pneumonia requiring hospitalization in five hospitals in Chicago and Nashville from January 2010 through June 2012, 2259 patients were identified who had radiographic evidence of pneumonia and specimens that could be tested for the responsible pathogen. Most patients (62%) had no detectable pathogens in their sample, and unexpectedly, respiratory viruses were detected more frequently than bacteria. Specifically, 23% had one or more viruses, 11% had one or more bacteria, 3% had both bacterial and viral pathogens, and 1% had a fungal or mycobacterial infection. "The most common pathogens were human rhinovirus (in 9% of patients), influenza virus (in 6%), and **Streptococcus pneumoniae** (in 5%)."

Diagnosis

Pneumonia is typically diagnosed based on a combination of physical signs and often a chest X-ray. In adults with normal vital signs and a normal lung examination, the diagnosis is unlikely. However, the underlying cause can be difficult to confirm, as there is no definitive test able to distinguish between bacterial and non-bacterial cause. The overall impression of a physician appears to be at least as good as decision rules for making or excluding the diagnosis.

Physical exam

Physical examination may sometimes reveal low blood pressure, high heart rate, or low oxygen saturation. The respiratory rate may be faster than normal, and this may occur a day or two before other signs. Examination of the chest may be normal, but it may show decreased expansion on the affected side. Harsh breath sounds from the larger airways that are transmitted through the inflamed lung are termed bronchial breathing and are heard on auscultation with a stethoscope. Crackles (rales) may be heard over the affected area during inspiration. Percussion may be dulled over the affected lung, and increased, rather than decreased, vocal resonance distinguishes pneumonia from a pleural effusion.

Imaging

A chest radiograph is frequently used in diagnosis. In people with mild disease, imaging is needed only in those with potential complications, those not having improved with treatment, or those in which the cause is uncertain. If a person is sufficiently sick to require hospitalization, a chest radiograph is recommended. Findings do not always match the severity of disease and do not reliably separate between bacterial and viral infection.

X-ray presentations of pneumonia may be classified as lobar pneumonia, bronchopneumonia, lobular pneumonia, and interstitial pneumonia. Bacterial, community-acquired pneumonia classically show lung consolidation of one lung segmental lobe, which is known as lobar pneumonia. However, findings may vary, and other patterns are common in other types of pneumonia. Aspiration pneumonia may present with bilateral opacities primarily in the bases of the lungs and on the right side. Radiographs of viral pneumonia may appear normal, appear hyper-inflated, have bilateral patchy areas, or present similar to bacterial pneumonia with lobar consolidation. Radiologic findings may not be present in the early stages of the disease, especially in the presence of dehydration, or may be difficult to interpret in the obese or those with a history of lung disease. Complications such as pleural effusion may also be found on chest radiographs. Latero-lateral chest radiographs can increase the diagnostic accuracy of lung consolidation and pleural effusion.

A CT scan can give additional information in indeterminate cases. CT scans can also provide more details in those with an unclear chest radiograph (for example occult pneumonia in chronic obstructive pulmonary disease) and can exclude pulmonary embolism and fungal pneumonia and detect lung abscess in those who are not responding to treatments. However, CT scans are more expensive, have a higher dose of radiation, and cannot be done at bedside.

Lung ultrasound may also be useful in helping to make the diagnosis. Ultrasound is radiation free and can be done at bedside. However, ultrasound requires specific skills to operate the machine and interpret the findings. It may be more accurate than chest X-ray.

Prevention

Prevention includes vaccination, environmental measures, and appropriate treatment of other health problems. It is believed that, if appropriate preventive measures were instituted globally, mortality among children could be reduced by 400,000; and, if proper treatment were universally available, childhood deaths could be decreased by another 600,000.

Vaccination prevents against certain bacterial and viral pneumonias both in children and adults. Influenza vaccines are modestly effective at preventing symptoms of influenza. The Center for Disease Control and Prevention (CDC) recommends yearly influenza vaccination for every person 6 months and older. Immunizing health care workers decreases the risk of viral pneumonia among their patients.

Vaccinations against **Haemophilus influenza** and **Streptococcus pneumonia** have good evidence to support their use. There is strong evidence for vaccinating children under the age of 2 against **Streptococcus pneumoniae** (pneumococcal conjugate vaccine). Vaccinating children against **Streptococcus pneumoniae** has led to a decreased rate of these infections in adults, because many adults acquire infections from children. A **Streptococcus pneumoniae** vaccine is available for adults, and has been found to decrease the risk of invasive pneumococcal disease by 74%, but there is insufficient evidence to suggest using the pneumococcal vaccine to prevent pneumonia or death in the general adult population. The CDC recommends that young children and adults over the age of 65 receive the pneumococcal vaccine, as well as older children or younger adults who have an increased risk of getting pneumococcal disease. The pneumococcal vaccine has been shown to reduce the risk of community acquired pneumonia in people with chronic obstructive pulmonary disease, but does not reduce mortality or the risk of hospitalization for people with this condition. People with COPD are recommended by a number of guidelines to have a pneumococcal vaccination. Other vaccines for which there is support for a protective effect against pneumonia include pertussis, varicella, and measles.

Management

Antibiotics by mouth, rest, simple analgesics, and fluids usually suffice for complete resolution. However, those with other medical conditions, the elderly, or those with significant trouble breathing may require more advanced care. If the symptoms worsen, the pneumonia does not improve with home treatment, or complications occur, hospitalization may be required. Worldwide, approximately 7%—13% of cases in children result in hospitalization, whereas in the developed world between 22% and 42% of adults with community-acquired pneumonia are admitted. The CURB-65 score is useful for determining the need for admission in adults. If the score is 0 or 1, people can typically be managed at home; if it is 2, a short hospital stay or close follow-up is needed; if it is 3—5, hospitalization is recommended. In children those with respiratory distress or oxygen saturations of less than 90% should be hospitalized. The utility of chest physiotherapy in pneumonia has not yet been determined. Over-the-counter cough medicine has not been found to be effective, nor has the use of zinc in children. There is insufficient evidence for mucolytics. There is no strong evidence to recommend that children who have non-measles related pneumonia take vitamin A supplements. Vitamin D, as of 2018 is of unclear benefit in children. Vitamin C administration in pneumonia needs further research, although it can be given to patient of low plasma vitamin C because it is not expensive and low risk.

Pneumonia can cause severe illness in a number of ways, and pneumonia with evidence of organ dysfunction may require intensive care unit admission for observation and specific treatment. The main impact is on the respiratory and the circulatory system. Respiratory failure not responding to normal oxygen therapy may require heated humidified high-flow therapy delivered through nasal cannulae, non-invasive ventilation, or in severe cases invasive ventilation through an endotracheal tube. Regarding circulatory problems as part of sepsis, evidence of poor blood flow or low blood pressure is initially treated with 30 mL/kg of crystalloid infused intravenously. In situations where fluids alone are ineffective, vasopressor medication may be required.

For adults with moderate or severe acute respiratory distress syndrome (ARDS) undergoing mechanical ventilation, there is a reduction in mortality when people lie on their front for at least 12 hours a day. However, this increases the risk of endotracheal tube obstruction and pressure sores.

Prognosis

With treatment, most types of bacterial pneumonia will stabilize in 3—6 days. It often takes a few weeks before most symptoms resolve. X-ray findings typically clear within four weeks and mortality is low (less than 1%). In the elderly or people with other lung problems, recovery may take more than 12 weeks. In persons requiring hospitalization, mortality may be as high as 10%, and in those requiring intensive care it may reach 30%—50%. Pneumonia is the most common hospital-acquired infection that causes death.

Complications may occur in particular in the elderly and those with underlying health problems. This may include, among others: empyema, lung abscess, bronchiolitis obliterans, acute respiratory distress syndrome, sepsis, and worsening of underlying health problems.

A. Translate the following sentences into Chinese.

1. The lungs are made up of small sacs called alveoli, which fill with air when a healthy

person breathes. When an individual has pneumonia, the alveoli are filled with pus and fluid, which makes breathing painful and limits oxygen intake. These infections are generally spread by direct contact with infected people.

2. The typical signs and symptoms in children under five years old are fever, cough, and fast or difficult breathing. Fever is not very specific, as it occurs in many other common illnesses and may be absent in those with severe disease, malnutrition or in the elderly.

3. Antibiotics by mouth, rest, simple analgesics, and fluids usually suffice for complete resolution. However, those with other medical conditions, the elderly, or those with significant trouble breathing may require more advanced care.

4. Pneumonia was historically divided into "typical" and "atypical" based on the belief that the presentation predicted the underlying cause. However, evidence has not supported this distinction, therefore it is no longer emphasized.

5. The pneumococcal vaccine has been shown to reduce the risk of community acquired pneumonia in people with chronic obstructive pulmonary disease, but does not reduce mortality or the risk of hospitalization for people with this condition. People with COPD are recommended by a number of guidelines to have a pneumococcal vaccination.

B. Prepare a lecture on pneumonia after doing the further reading above.

扫码获取
提示

Unit 2

Diabetes

I Warming-up

A. Match the following words and phrases with their Chinese translations.

A	glucose	1	肠胃炎
B	pre-diabetic	2	内分泌学
C	overwhelming thirst	3	空腹血糖
D	insulin resistance	4	葡萄糖
E	endocrinology	5	视力模糊
F	genetic predisposition	6	极度口渴
G	stomach flu	7	糖尿病前期的
H	sedentary	8	胰岛素抵抗
I	fasting blood sugar	9	久坐不动的
J	blurry vision	10	遗传倾向

B. Complete the sentences with the following words or phrases in their proper forms.

creep up	shrug off	couple with	to an extent
accomplish	off the charts	struggle with	absorb

1. As teachers observe their students _____ writing, it is natural for them to think the problem may be physical.

2. The following are some of the diseases that _____ as you age: hearing loss, cataracts and refractive errors, back and neck pain and osteoarthritis, chronic obstructive pulmonary disease, diabetes, depression and dementia.

3. Garrison would finally _____ his depressions, and put his energies back where they belonged, organizing the family business.

4. It's an amazing _____ and one we cannot achieve without generous support from individuals, corporations, and other social organizations.

5. His blood pressure was _____.

6. Overuse of those drugs, _____ poor diet, leads to physical degeneration.

7. Some poisonous gases can enter the body by _____ through the skin.

8. Smoking cessation therapies have improved _____ that some have a 70% success rate.

 C. Watch the video *Diabetes* and answer the questions.

扫码获取视频

1. What was Lolly experiencing before ending up in urgent care?

2. How did she feel when she learned that her blood sugar was off the charts?

3. According to Doctor Earl, what is really frightening for patients

diagnosed with diabetes?

4. What happens to their body when someone gets type 2 diabetes?

5. According to Doctor Earl, what kind of people are at greater risk for developing diabetes?

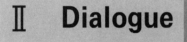 **Ⅱ Dialogue**

扫码获取
音频及文本

 A. Listen to the dialogue for the first time and try to get the general idea.

 B. Listen to the dialogue for the second time and try to answer the following questions.

1. What seems to be the problem with this patient?

2. According to the doctor, what causes

diabetes?

3. Can people with diabetes smoke and drink alcohol? Why?

4. What does DASH stand for? In what way is DASH diet beneficial for diabetic people?

5. Aside from diet, what other lifestyle modifications should diabetics implement to manage their condition?

C. **Choose the following words and/or expressions to complete the sentences in their proper forms.**

scratch	抓伤,刮擦	to name a few	仅举几例
sustain	持续的	depend on	依据
as well	也	benefit from	得益于……
moderate	适度的	incur	造成,引起
set up	制定	energy intake	热量摄入
regime	计划,方案	modify	调整

1. Most treatment programs include behavioral _____ techniques, making the patient's access to pleasurable activities contingent on weight gain.

2. We look forward very much to seeing you again and to meeting your wife _____.

3. Examples of extraordinary measures include those procedures that _____ excessive cost, pain, or burden or lack substantial benefit to the patient.

4. _____ is required to fuel many different body processes, including keeping the heart beating and organs functioning, maintenance of body temperature, muscle contraction and growth.

5. People experience differences in physical and mental capability _____ the time of day.

6. A strict _____ of wheat-free diet in the hospital had a favorable effect.

7. Ingredients used in this homemade soap recipe are drawn from nature—avocado, lemongrass, and chamomile, _____.

8. Developing environmentally _____ products and services requires significant research.

9. The two professors hope to refute that idea, claiming that just as when kids walk themselves through a process, adults can _____ using language not just to communicate, but also to help augment thinking.

10. You don't have to deny yourself everything that's nice when you're pregnant. _____ is the watchword.

D. **Read the dialogue and try to make a conversation with your classmates.**

扫码获取
提示

E. Translate the following Chinese into English.

P—Patient   D—Doctor

D：What has brought you here?

P：1. 最近我总觉得口渴，小便很多。I also feel itchy all over. Look at the scratches here. Is there anything wrong with me?

1. _____

D：How long has this been going on? How is your appetite? 2. 还有什么其他不舒服？

2. _____

P：3. 尽管我的食欲很好，但最近一年体重减轻了10公斤。And I feel weak all the time.

3. _____
_____

D：4. 我给你做个空腹血糖和糖化血红蛋白检查。You may have diabetes.

4. _____
_____

P：What is that? 5. 能够治愈吗？

5. _____

D：Diabetes is a common endocrine disease characterized by sustained high blood sugar levels. Due to insulin deficiency or insulin resistance, diabetic patients have abnormal metabolism of sugars, fats and proteins. Right now, there is no cure for diabetes，6. 但是通过药物和调整生活方式可以使其得到控制，so that you can enjoy life and feel well. You should stick to a healthy diet, do some exercise, and maintain a normal weight.

6. _____
_____

P：Can I smoke?

D：7. 吸烟对任何人都有害。Better give it up.

7. _____

P：Can I drink alcohol?

D：In moderation. As you know alcohol contains calories and must be counted in your meal plan. Come back to me with the results. Once diabetes is confirmed，8. 我会为你制定药物治疗方案以控制你的血糖。

8. _____
_____

Ⅲ Further Reading：Diabetes

Overview

Diabetes，also known as diabetes mellitus, is a group of common endocrine diseases characterized by sustained high blood sugar levels. Diabetes is caused by either a lack of insulin-secreting beta-cells in the pancreas due to an autoimmune response (type 1 diabetes)，an imbalance between blood sugar level and insulin production (type 2 diabetes)，and can be precipitated by pregnancy (gestational diabetes). Symptoms of diabetes can vary, and if untreated, can have a range of acute and chronic complications. Untreated or poorly treated diabetes accounts for approximately 1.5 million deaths per year.

There is no widely-accepted cure for most cases of diabetes. The most common treatment for type 1 diabetes is insulin replacement therapy. Anti-diabetic medications as well as lifestyle modifications, can be used to prevent or respond to type 2 diabetes. Gestational diabetes normally resolves shortly after delivery.

As of 2019, an estimated 463 million people had diabetes worldwide accounting for 8.8% of the adult population. Type 2 diabetes makes up about 90% of all diabetes cases. The prevalence of the disease continues to increase, most dramatically in low- and middle-income nations. Rates are similar in women and men, with diabetes being the 7th-leading cause of death globally. By 2030, it is forecast that global expenditure on diabetes-related healthcare will exceed US $ 1 trillion.

Signs and symptoms

The classic symptoms of untreated diabetes are unintended weight loss, polyuria (increased urination), polydipsia (increased thirst), and polyphagia (increased hunger). Symptoms may develop rapidly (weeks or months) in type 1 diabetes, while they usually develop much more slowly and may be subtle or absent in type 2 diabetes.

Several other signs and symptoms can mark the onset of diabetes although they are not specific to the disease. In addition to the known symptoms listed above, they include blurred vision, headache, fatigue, slow healing of cuts, and itchy skin. Prolonged high blood glucose can cause glucose absorption in the lens of the eye, which leads to changes in its shape, resulting in vision changes. Long-term vision loss can also be caused by diabetic retinopathy. A number of skin rashes that can occur in diabetes are collectively known as diabetic dermadromes.

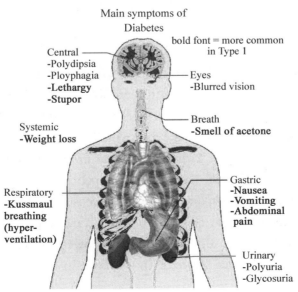

Main symptoms of Diabetes

bold font = more common in Type 1

Central
-Polydipsia
-Ployphagia
-**Lethargy**
-**Stupor**

Eyes
-Blurred vision

Breath
-**Smell of acetone**

Systemic
-**Weight loss**

Gastric
-**Nausea**
-**Vomiting**
-**Abdominal pain**

Respiratory
-**Kussmaul breathing (hyperventilation)**

Urinary
-Polyuria
-Glycosuria

Causes

Diabetes mellitus is classified into six categories: type 1 diabetes, type 2 diabetes, hybrid forms of diabetes, hyperglycemia first detected during pregnancy, "unclassified diabetes", and "other specific types". "Hybrid forms of diabetes" include slowly evolving, immune-mediated diabetes of adults and ketosis-prone type 2 diabetes. "Hyperglycemia first detected during pregnancy" includes gestational diabetes mellitus and diabetes mellitus in pregnancy (type 1 or type 2 diabetes first diagnosed during pregnancy). The "other specific types" are a collection of a few dozen individual causes. Diabetes is a more variable disease than once thought and people may have combinations of forms.

Type 1

Type 1 diabetes is characterized by loss of the insulin-producing beta cells of the pancreatic islets, leading to insulin deficiency. This type can be further classified as immune-mediated or idiopathic. The majority of type 1 diabetes is of an immune-mediated nature, in which a T cell-mediated autoimmune attack leads to the loss of beta cells and thus insulin. It causes approximately 10% of diabetes mellitus cases in North America and Europe. Most affected people are otherwise healthy and of a healthy weight when onset occurs. Sensitivity and responsiveness to insulin are usually normal, especially in the early stages. Although it has been called "juvenile diabetes" due to the frequent onset in children, the majority of individuals living with type 1 diabetes are now adults.

Type 1 diabetes can occur at any age, and a significant proportion is diagnosed during adulthood. Latent autoimmune diabetes of adults (LADA) is the diagnostic term applied when type 1 diabetes develops in adults; it has a slower onset than the same condition in children. Given this difference, some use the unofficial term "type 1.5 diabetes" for this condition. Adults with LADA are frequently initially misdiagnosed as having type 2 diabetes, based on age rather than a cause.

Type 2

Type 2 diabetes is characterized by insulin resistance, which may be combined with relatively reduced insulin secretion. The defective responsiveness of body tissues to insulin is believed to involve the insulin receptor. However, the specific defects are not known. Diabetes mellitus cases due to a known defect are classified separately. Type 2 diabetes is the most common type of diabetes mellitus accounting for 95% of diabetes. Many people with type 2 diabetes have evidence of prediabetes (impaired fasting glucose and/or impaired glucose tolerance) before meeting the criteria for type 2 diabetes. The progression of prediabetes to overt type 2 diabetes can be slowed or reversed by lifestyle changes or medications that improve insulin sensitivity or reduce the liver's glucose production.

Type 2 diabetes is primarily due to lifestyle factors and genetics. A number of lifestyle factors are known to be important to the development of type 2 diabetes, including obesity (defined by a body mass index of greater than 30), lack of physical activity, poor diet, stress, and urbanization. Excess body fat is associated with 30% of cases in people of Chinese and Japanese descent, 60%—80% of cases in those of European and African descent, and 100% of Pima Indians and Pacific Islanders. Even those who are not obese may have a high waist-hip ratio.

Dietary factors such as sugar-sweetened drinks are associated with an increased risk. The type of fats in the diet is also important, with saturated fat and trans fats increasing the risk and polyunsaturated and monounsaturated fat decreasing the risk. Eating white rice excessively may increase the risk of diabetes, especially in Chinese and Japanese people. Lack of physical activity may increase the risk of diabetes in some people.

Prevention

There is no known preventive measure for type 1 diabetes. Type 2 diabetes—which accounts for 85%—90% of all cases worldwide—can often be prevented or delayed by maintaining a normal body weight, engaging in physical activity, and eating a healthy diet. Higher levels of physical activity (more than 90 minutes per day) reduce the risk of diabetes by 28%. Dietary changes known to be effective in helping to prevent diabetes include maintaining a diet rich in whole grains and fiber, and choosing good fats, such as the polyunsaturated fats found in nuts, vegetable oils, and fish. Limiting sugary beverages and eating less red meat and other sources of saturated fat can also help prevent diabetes. Tobacco smoking is also associated with an increased risk of diabetes and its complications, so smoking cessation can be an important preventive measure as well.

Management

Diabetes management concentrates on keeping blood sugar levels close to normal, without causing low blood sugar. This can usually be accomplished with dietary changes, exercise, weight loss, and use of appropriate medications (insulin, oral medications).

Learning about the disease and actively participating in the treatment is important, since complications are far less common and less severe in people who have well-managed blood sugar levels. The goal of treatment is an A1C level below 5.7%. Attention is also paid to other health problems that may accelerate the negative effects of diabetes. These include smoking, high blood pressure, metabolic syndrome obesity, and lack of regular exercise. Specialized footwear is widely used to reduce the risk of diabetic foot ulcers by relieving the pressure on the foot. Foot examination for patients living with diabetes should be done annually which includes sensation testing, foot biomechanics, vascular integrity and foot structure.

Lifestyle

People with diabetes can benefit from education about the disease and treatment, dietary changes, and exercise, with the goal of keeping both short-term and long-term blood glucose levels within acceptable bounds. In addition, given the associated higher risks of cardiovascular disease, lifestyle modifications are recommended to control blood pressure.

Weight loss can prevent progression from prediabetes to diabetes type 2, decrease the risk of cardiovascular disease, or result in a partial remission in people with diabetes. No single dietary pattern is best for all people with diabetes. Healthy dietary patterns, such as the Mediterranean diet, low-carbohydrate diet, or DASH diet, are often recommended, although evidence does not support one over the others. According to the ADA, "reducing overall carbohydrate intake for individuals with diabetes has demonstrated the most evidence for improving glycemia", and for individuals with type 2 diabetes who cannot meet the glycemic targets or where reducing anti-glycemic medications is a priority, low or very-low carbohydrate diets are a viable approach. For overweight people with type 2 diabetes, any diet that achieves weight loss is effective.

Diet in diabetes

Among guideline recommendations including the American Diabetes Association (ADA) and Diabetes UK, there is no consensus that one specific diet is better than others. This is due to a lack of long term high-quality studies on this subject matter.

For overweight and obese people with diabetes, the most important aspect of any diet is that it results in loss of body fat. Losing body fat has been proven to improve blood glucose control and lower insulin levels.

The most agreed-upon recommendation is for the diet to be low in sugar and refined carbohydrates, while relatively high in dietary fiber, especially soluble fiber. Likewise, people with diabetes may be encouraged to reduce their intake of carbohydrates that have a high glycemic index (GI), although further evidence for this recommendation is needed.

Low-carbohydrate diet

For type 1 diabetics, there is a lack of definitive evidence of the usefulness of low-carbohydrate diets due to limited study of this topic. A recent meta-analysis found only nine papers that had adequately studied the implementation of low carbohydrate diets in type 1 diabetics as of March 2017. This review found that low carbohydrate diets consistently reduced insulin requirements but found inconsistent results in regard to the diet's effect on blood glucose levels. Three studies found significant decreases in HbA1c on low carbohydrate diets while 5 found that HbA1c levels were stable. This review as well as the ADA consensus statement suggests that low carbohydrate diets may be beneficial for type 1 diabetics but larger clinical trials are needed for further evidence.

A low-carbohydrate diet gives slightly better control of glucose metabolism than a low-fat diet in type 2 diabetes. In a 2019 consensus report on nutrition therapy for adults with diabetes and prediabetes the American Diabetes Association (ADA) states *"Reducing overall carbohydrate intake for individuals with diabetes has demonstrated the most evidence for improving glycemia (blood sugar) and may be applied in a variety of eating patterns that meet individual needs and preferences."* it also states that reducing overall carbohydrate intake with low- or very low- carbohydrate eating plans is a viable approach.

The ADA say low-carbohydrate diets can be useful to help people with type 2 diabetes lose weight, but that these diets were poorly defined, difficult to sustain, unsuitable for certain groups of people and that, for diet composition in general. Overall, the ADA recommends people with diabetes develop "healthy eating patterns rather than focusing on individual macronutrients, micronutrients, or single foods". They recommend that carbohydrates in a diet should come from whole food sources such as "vegetables, legumes fruits, dairy (milk and yogurt), and whole grains"; highly refined foods and sugary drinks should be avoided.

Low glycemic index diet

Lowering the glycemic index of one's diet may improve the control of diabetes. This includes avoidance of such foods as potatoes cooked in certain ways (i. e.: boiled and mashed potatoes are higher GI than fried) and white bread. Lower glycemic index carbohydrate sources include vegetables, legumes, and whole grains that contain higher fiber content and are digested and absorbed into the blood stream more slowly than refined carbohydrates.

High fiber diet

The ADA recommends a level of fiber intake consistent with the Dietary Guidelines for Americans 2015—2020 (minimum of 14 g of fiber per 1,000 kcal). However, there is some evidence that higher intakes (daily consumption of 50g of fiber and higher), can result in small improvements in blood sugar levels The ADA cautions that higher intakes may cause digestive issues such as "flatulence, bloating, and diarrhea."

Medications

Most medications used to treat diabetes act by lowering blood sugar levels through different mechanisms. There is broad consensus that when people with diabetes maintain tight glucose control—keeping the glucose levels in their blood within normal ranges—they experience fewer complications, such as kidney problems or eye problems. There is however debate as to whether this is appropriate and cost effective for people later in life in whom the risk of hypoglycemia may be more significant.

There are a number of different classes of anti-diabetic medications. Type 1 diabetes requires treatment with insulin, ideally using a "basal bolus" regimen that most closely matches normal insulin release: long-acting insulin for the basal rate and short-acting insulin with meals. Type 2 diabetes is generally treated with medication that is taken by mouth (e. g. metformin) although some eventually require injectable treatment with insulin or GLP-1 agonists.

Metformin is generally recommended as a first-line treatment for type 2 diabetes, as there is good evidence that it decreases mortality. It works by decreasing the liver's production of glucose, and increasing the amount of glucose stored in peripheral tissue. Several other groups of drugs, mainly oral medication, may also decrease blood sugar in type 2 diabetes. These include agents that increase insulin release (sulfonylureas), agents that decrease absorption of sugar from the intestines (acarbose), agents that inhibit the enzyme dipeptidyl peptidase-4 (DPP-4) that inactivates incretins such as GLP-1 and GIP (sitagliptin), agents that make the body more sensitive to insulin (thiazolidinedione) and agents that increase the excretion of glucose in the urine (SGLT2 inhibitors). When insulin is used in type 2 diabetes, along-acting formulation is usually added initially, while continuing oral medications. Some severe cases of type 2 diabetes may also be treated with insulin, which is increased gradually until glucose targets are reached.

A. Translate the following sentences into Chinese.

1. There is no widely-accepted cure for most cases of diabetes. The most common treatment for type 1 diabetes is insulin replacement therapy. Anti-diabetic medications as well as lifestyle modifications, can be used to prevent or respond to type 2 diabetes. Gestational diabetes normally resolves shortly after delivery.

2. Many people with type 2 diabetes have evidence of prediabetes (impaired fasting glucose and/or impaired glucose tolerance) before meeting the criteria for type 2 diabetes. The progression of prediabetes to overt type 2 diabetes can be slowed or reversed by lifestyle changes or medications that improve insulin sensitivity or reduce the liver's glucose production.

3. People with diabetes can benefit from education about the disease and treatment，dietary changes，and exercise，with the goal of keeping both short-term and long-term blood glucose levels within acceptable bounds. In addition，given the associated higher risks of cardiovascular disease，lifestyle modifications are recommended to control blood pressure.

4. The most agreed-upon recommendation is for the diet to be low in sugar and refined carbohydrates，while relatively high in dietary fiber，especially soluble fiber. Likewise，people with diabetes may be encouraged to reduce their intake of carbohydrates that have a high glycemic index（GI），although further evidence for this recommendation is needed.

5. There is broad consensus that when people with diabetes maintain tight glucose control—keeping the glucose levels in their blood within normal ranges—they experience fewer complications，such as kidney problems or eye problems. There is however debate as to whether this is appropriate and cost effective for people later in life in whom the risk of hypoglycemia may be more significant.

B. Prepare a lecture on diabetes after doing the further reading above.

扫码获取
提示

Unit 3

Coronary Heart Disease

I Warming-up

A. Match the following words and phrases with their Chinese translations.

A	cardiology	1	斑块
B	cardiac catheterization	2	心绞痛
C	angioplasty	3	冠状动脉造影
D	atherosclerosis	4	血管成形术
E	blockage	5	心脏病学
F	angina	6	阻塞
G	substernal chest pain	7	冠状动脉搭桥
H	plaque	8	动脉粥样硬化
I	angiogram	9	心导管检查
J	coronary artery bypass	10	胸骨后胸痛

B. Complete the sentences with the following words or phrases in their proper forms.

outlook	overwhelm	translate	thick
minimal	play a role	red flag	paint a picture

1. These items and any number of other pieces of operational data serve to _____ of the health of a particular system of application.

2. However, not all patients progress as quickly and, as the inflammation resolves, the arterial wall becomes _____ and tender with the pulse still present.

3. Economic growth has slowed considerably and soaring energy prices continue to cloud the _____ for the world economy.

4. They note that this type of activity may _____ in facilitating mechanical and metabolic processes in the musculoskeletal system that counter the repetitive or sedentary effects of many jobs.

5. Patients in "_____ conscious states" are awake but have only partial preservation of awareness and responsiveness.

6. The right cushion can provide the comfort you need to help you delve further into your meditations, and that can ultimately _____ into tangible and beneficial results.

7. The abnormal bleeding is your body's own _____ of danger.

8. The experience of _____ stressors at work, or failure in managing diverse responsibilities, could foster a general sense of ineffectuality, depressive affect, and low self-esteem.

 C. Watch the video *Pneumonia—Mayo Clinic Explains Coronary Artery Disease* **and answer the questions.**

扫码获取视频

1. According to Dr. Kopecky, how does CAD happen?

2. What kind of people are at a greater risk for developing CAD?

3. What is angina and how does it feel like?

4. What tests are suggested to help with the diagnosis of CAD?

5. In terms of treating CAD, what lifestyle changes are helpful?

II Dialogue

扫码获取
音频及文本

A. Listen to the dialogue for the first time and try to get the general idea.

B. Listen to the dialogue for the second time and try to answer the following questions.

1. What happens when the patient climbs stairs?

2. What other symptoms does the patient have?

3. What tests does the patient need to have?

4. Why does the doctor suggest that the patient be hospitalized?

5. According to the doctor, what would happen after the patient's admission to hospital?

C. Choose the following words and/or expressions to complete the sentences in their proper forms.

heaviness in chest	胸闷	take ... seriously	认真对待
household chores	家务活	routine	常规的
sufficient	充足的	carry on	继续如常
prognosis	预后	lightheaded	头晕的
make sure	确保	sit up	坐起来
premature	过早的	contraction	收缩

1. The weakness in our psychological defense is something we must _____.

2. The ability to _____ with life despite everything is what distinguishes "smiling" depression.

3. While it is clear that specific genetic alterations serve as _____ indicators, not all correlate with a poor prognosis.

4. We are trying to get the baby into a _____ for feeding and sleeping.

5. Chronic dietary _____ is thought to be the single main cause but the mechanism is unclear.

6. _____ babies are more likely to suffer from breathing difficulties in childhood.

7. In the mornings, for instance, after finishing the _____ she might go shopping, and then have lunch with friends.

8. The woman developed _____, dyspnea, tongue numbness, muscle twitching, and formication on the legs and back.

9. He glanced about to _____ that the audience were ready to hear his speech.

10. The problem is that this wrong-way impulse sets off a muscle _____ in each of those several hundred muscle fibers.

D. Read the dialogue and try to make a conversation with your classmates.

扫码获取
提示

E. Translate the following Chinese into English.

D—Doctor   P—Patient

D：When these symptoms occur，how long do they last? Have you taken any medications?

P：No. 1. 休息一会儿就会舒服很多。

  1. _____

D：Are there any other problems? 2. 是否有过头晕，突然昏倒的情况？

  2. _____

P：No.

D：Are you involved in any physical exercises?

P：Not really. 3. 只是干些家务活。

  3. _____

D：Have you ever felt discomfort during housework?

P：No.

D：4. 你睡觉时用几个枕头？

  4. _____

P：Two. I used to need only one，but since last year I've had to add another.

D：5. 你夜里需要坐起来喘息吗？

  5. _____

P：Yes. This has been happening in the past 2 or 3 days.

D：Did you ever notice any swelling in your ankles?

P：Yes. 6. 最近每天下午脚踝浮肿，第二天早晨就消失了。

  6. _____

  _____

D：Do you have diabetes and hypertension?

P：Yes.

D：7. 血糖、血压控制得如何？

  7. _____

P：Fasting blood glucose has always been around 10. 5 mmol/L and blood pressure 140/100 mmHg.

D：Lie on the bed please. I have to make an examination.

（After the examination）

D：Well，8. 你需要拍胸片，做心电图、心脏超声检查和相关的血液检查。Come back to me when you have the results.

  8. _____

  _____

III Further Reading：Coronary Artery Disease

Overview

Coronary artery disease（CAD），also called coronary heart disease（CHD），ischemic heart disease（IHD），myocardial ischemia，or simply heart disease，involves the reduction of blood flow to the heart muscle due to build-up of atherosclerotic plaque in the arteries of the heart. It is the most common of the cardiovascular diseases. Types include stable angina，unstable angina，myocardial infarction，and sudden cardiac death. A common symptom is chest pain or discomfort which may travel into the shoulder, arm, back, neck, or jaw. Occasionally it may feel like heartburn. Usually symptoms occur with exercise or emotional stress, last less than a few minutes, and improve with rest. Shortness of breath may also occur and sometimes no symptoms are present. In many cases, the first sign is a heart attack. Other complications include heart failure or an abnormal heartbeat.

Risk factors include high blood pressure, smoking, diabetes, lack of exercise, obesity, high blood cholesterol, poor diet, depression, and excessive alcohol consumption. A number of tests may help with diagnoses including: electrocardiogram, cardiac stress testing, coronary computed tomographic angiography, and coronary angiogram, among others.

Ways to reduce CAD risk include eating a healthy diet, regularly exercising, maintaining a healthy weight, and not smoking. Medications for diabetes, high cholesterol, or high blood pressure are sometimes used. There is limited evidence for screening people who are at low risk and do not have symptoms. Treatment involves the same measures as prevention. Additional medications such as antiplatelets (including aspirin), beta blockers, or nitroglycerin may be recommended. Procedures such as percutaneous coronary intervention (PCI) or coronary artery bypass surgery (CABG) may be used in severe disease. In those with stable CAD it is unclear if PCI or CABG in addition to the other treatments improves life expectancy or decreases heart attack risk.

Signs and symptoms

The most common symptom is chest pain or discomfort that occurs regularly with activity, after eating, or at other predictable times; this phenomenon is termed stable angina and is associated with narrowing of the arteries of the heart. Angina also includes chest tightness, heaviness, pressure, numbness, fullness, or squeezing. Angina that changes in intensity, character or frequency is termed unstable. Unstable angina may precede myocardial infarction. In adults who go to the emergency department with an unclear cause of pain, about 30% have pain due to coronary artery disease. Angina, shortness of breath, sweating, nausea or vomiting, and lightheadedness are signs of a heart attack, or myocardial infarction, and immediate emergency medical services are crucial.

With advanced disease, the narrowing of coronary arteries reduces the supply of oxygen-rich blood flowing to the heart, which becomes more pronounced during strenuous activities during which the heart beats faster. For some, this causes severe symptoms, while others experience no symptoms at all.

Symptoms in women can differ from those in men, and the most common symptom reported by women of all races is shortness of breath. Other symptoms more commonly reported by women than men are extreme fatigue, sleep disturbances, indigestion, and anxiety. However, some women do experience irregular heartbeat, dizziness, sweating, and nausea. Burning, pain, or pressure in the chest or upper abdomen that can travel to the arm or jaw can also be experienced in women, but it is less commonly reported by women than men. On average, women experience symptoms 10 years later than men. Women are less likely to recognize symptoms and seek treatment.

Risk factors

Coronary artery disease has a number of well determined risk factors. Some of these include high blood pressure, smoking, diabetes, lack of exercise, obesity, high blood cholesterol, poor diet, depression, family history, psychological stress, and excessive alcohol. About half of cases are linked to genetics. Smoking and obesity are associated with about 36% and 20% of cases, respectively. Smoking just one cigarette per day about doubles the risk of CAD. Lack of exercise has been linked to 7%—12% of cases. Exposure to the herbicide Agent Orange may increase risk. Rheumatologic diseases such as rheumatoid arthritis, systemic lupus erythematosus, psoriasis, and psoriatic arthritis are independent risk factors as well.

Job stress appears to play a minor role accounting for about 3% of cases. In one study, women who were free of stress from work life saw an increase in the diameter of their blood vessels, leading to decreased progression of atherosclerosis. In contrast, women who had high levels of work-related stress experienced a decrease in the diameter of their blood vessels and significantly increased disease progression. Having a type A behavior pattern, a group of personality characteristics including time urgency, competitiveness, hostility, and impatience, is linked to an increased risk of coronary disease.

Blood fats

• High blood cholesterol (specifically, serum LDL concentrations; also referred to as LDL-C to denote low-density lipoprotein cholesterol). HDL (high density lipoprotein) has a protective effect over development of coronary artery disease.

• High blood triglycerides may play a role.

• High levels of lipoprotein, a compound formed when LDL cholesterol combines with a protein known as apolipoprotein.

Dietary cholesterol does not appear to have a significant effect on blood cholesterol and thus recommendations about its consumption may not be needed. Saturated fat is still a concern.

Genetics

The heritability of coronary artery disease has been estimated between 40% and 60%. Genome-wide association studies have identified over 160 genetic susceptibility loci for coronary artery disease.

Pathophysiology

Limitation of blood flow to the heart causes ischemia (cell starvation secondary to a lack of oxygen) of the heart's muscle cells. The heart's muscle cells may die from lack of oxygen and this is called a myocardial infarction (commonly referred to as a heart attack). It leads to damage, death, and eventual scarring of the heart muscle without regrowth of heart muscle cells. Chronic high-grade narrowing of the coronary arteries can induce transient ischemia which leads to the induction of a ventricular arrhythmia, which may terminate into a dangerous heart rhythm known as ventricular fibrillation, which often leads to death.

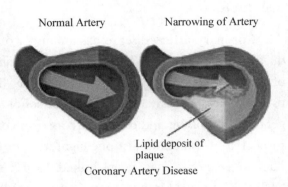

Normal Artery   Narrowing of Artery

Lipid deposit of plaque

Coronary Artery Disease

Typically, coronary artery disease occurs when part of the smooth, elastic lining inside a coronary artery (the arteries that supply blood to the heart muscle) develops atherosclerosis. With atherosclerosis, the artery's lining becomes hardened, stiffened, and accumulates deposits of calcium, fatty lipids, and abnormal inflammatory cells—to form a plaque. Calcium phosphate (hydroxyapatite) deposits in the muscular layer of the blood vessels appear to play a significant role in stiffening the arteries and inducing the early phase of coronary arteriosclerosis. This can be seen in a so-called metastatic mechanism of calciphylaxis as it occurs in chronic kidney disease and hemodialysis. Although these people have kidney dysfunction, almost fifty percent of them die due to coronary artery disease. Plaques can be thought of as large "pimples" that protrude into the channel of an artery, causing partial obstruction to blood flow. People with coronary artery disease might have just one or two plaques, or might have dozens distributed throughout their coronary arteries. A more severe form is chronic total occlusion (CTO) when a coronary artery is completely obstructed for more than 3 months.

Cardiac syndrome X is chest pain (angina pectoris) and chest discomfort in people who do not show signs of blockages in the larger coronary arteries of their hearts when an angiogram (coronary angiogram) is being performed. The exact cause of cardiac syndrome X is unknown. Explanations include microvascular dysfunction or epicardial atherosclerosis. For reasons that are not well understood, women are more likely than men to have it; however, hormones and other risk factors unique to women may play a role.

Diagnosis

For symptomatic people, stress echocardiography can be used to make a diagnosis for obstructive coronary artery disease. The use of echocardiography, stress cardiac imaging, and/or advanced non-invasive imaging is not recommended on individuals who are exhibiting no symptoms and are otherwise at low risk for developing coronary disease.

The diagnosis of "Cardiac Syndrome X"—the rare coronary artery disease that is more common in women, as mentioned, is a diagnosis of exclusion. Therefore, usually, the same tests are used as in any person with the suspected of having coronary artery disease:

- Baseline electrocardiography (ECG)
- Exercise ECG—Stress test
- Exercise radioisotope test (nuclear stress test, myocardial scintigraphy)
- Echocardiography (including stress echocardiography)
- Coronary angiography
- Intravascular ultrasound
- Magnetic resonance imaging (MRI)

The diagnosis of coronary disease underlying particular symptoms depends largely on the nature of the symptoms. The first investigation is an electrocardiogram (ECG/EKG), both for "stable" angina and acute coronary syndrome. An X-ray of the chest and blood tests may be performed.

Stable angina

Stable angina is the most common form of ischemic heart disease, and is associated with reduced quality of life and increased mortality. It is caused by epicardial coronary stenosis which results in reduced blood flow and oxygen supply to the myocardium. Stable angina is characterized as short-term chest pain during physical exertion caused by an imbalance between myocardial oxygen supply and metabolic oxygen demand. Various forms of cardiac stress tests may be used to both induce symptoms and detect changes by way of electrocardiography (using an ECG), echocardiography (using ultrasound of the heart) or scintigraphy (using uptake of radionuclide by the heart muscle). If part of the heart seems to receive an insufficient blood supply, coronary angiography may be used to identify stenosis of the coronary arteries and suitability for angioplasty or bypass surgery.

In minor to moderate cases, nitroglycerine may be used to alleviate acute symptoms of stable angina or may be used immediately prior to exertion to prevent the onset of angina. Sublingual nitroglycerine is most commonly used to provide rapid relief for acute angina attacks and as a complement to anti-anginal treatments in patients with refractory and recurrent angina. When nitroglycerine enters the bloodstream, it forms free radical nitric oxide, or NO, which activates guanylate cyclase and in turn stimulates the release of cyclic GMP. This molecular signaling stimulates smooth muscle relaxation, ultimately resulting in vasodilation and consequently improved blood flow to regions of the heart affected by atherosclerotic plaque.

Stable coronary artery disease (SCAD) is also often called stable ischemic heart disease (SIHD). A 2015 monograph explains that "Regardless of the nomenclature, stable angina is the chief manifestation of SIHD or SCAD." There are U.S. and European clinical practice guidelines for SIHD/SCAD.

Acute coronary syndrome

Diagnosis of acute coronary syndrome generally takes place in the emergency department, where ECGs may be performed sequentially to identify "evolving changes" (indicating ongoing damage to the heart muscle). Diagnosis is clear-cut if ECGs show elevation of the "ST segment", which in the context of severe typical chest pain is strongly indicative of an acute myocardial infarction (MI); this is termed a STEMI (ST-elevation MI) and is treated as an emergency with either urgent coronary angiography and percutaneous coronary intervention (angioplasty with or without stent insertion) or with thrombolysis ("clot buster" medication), whichever is available. In the absence of ST-segment elevation, heart damage is detected by cardiac markers (blood tests that identify heart muscle damage). If there is evidence of damage (infarction), the chest pain is attributed to a "non-ST elevation MI" (NSTEMI). If there is no evidence of damage, the term "unstable angina" is used. This process usually necessitates hospital admission and close observation on a coronary care unit for possible complications (such as cardiac arrhythmias-irregularities in the heart rate). Depending on the risk assessment, stress testing or angiography may be used to identify and treat coronary artery disease in patients who have had an NSTEMI or unstable angina.

Prevention

Up to 90% of cardiovascular disease may be preventable if established risk factors are avoided. Prevention involves adequate physical exercise, decreasing obesity, treating high blood pressure, eating a healthy diet, decreasing cholesterol levels, and stopping smoking. Medications and exercise are roughly equally effective. High levels of physical activity reduce the risk of coronary artery disease by about 25%. Life's Essential 8 are the key measures for improving and maintaining cardiovascular health, as defined by the American Heart Association. AHA added sleep as a factor influencing heart health in 2022.

Most guidelines recommend combining these preventive strategies. A 2015 Cochrane Review found some evidence that counseling and education to bring about behavioral change might help in high-risk groups. However, there was insufficient evidence to show an effect on mortality or actual cardiovascular events.

Diet

A diet high in fruits and vegetables decreases the risk of cardiovascular disease and death. Vegetarians have a lower risk of heart disease, possibly due to their greater consumption of fruits and vegetables. Evidence also suggests that the Mediterranean diet and a high fiber diet lower the risk.

The consumption of trans fat (commonly found in hydrogenated products such as margarine) has been shown to cause a precursor to atherosclerosis and increase the risk of coronary artery disease.

Evidence does not support a beneficial role for omega-3 fatty acid supplementation in preventing cardiovascular disease (including myocardial infarction and sudden cardiac death). There is tentative evidence that intake of menaquinone (Vitamin K_2), but not phylloquinone (Vitamin K_1), may reduce the risk of CAD mortality.

Secondary prevention

Secondary prevention is preventing further sequelae of already established disease. Effective lifestyle changes include:
- Weight control
- Smoking cessation
- Avoiding the consumption of trans fat (in partially hydrogenated oils)
- Decreasing psychosocial stress
- Exercise

Aerobic exercise, like walking, jogging, or swimming, can reduce the risk of mortality from coronary artery disease. Aerobic exercise can help decrease blood pressure and the amount of blood cholesterol (LDL) over time. It also increases HDL cholesterol.

Treatment

There are a number of treatment options for coronary artery disease:
- Lifestyle changes

- Medical treatment—commonly prescribed drugs（e. g., cholesterol lowering medications, beta-blockers, nitroglycerin, calcium channel blockers, etc.）
  - Coronary interventions as angioplasty and coronary stent
  - Coronary artery bypass grafting（CABG）

Medications

- Statins, which reduce cholesterol, reduce the risk of coronary artery disease
  - Nitroglycerin
  - Calcium channel blockers and/or beta-blockers
  - Antiplatelet drugs such as aspirin

It is recommended that blood pressure typically be reduced to less than 140/90 mmHg. The diastolic blood pressure however should not be lower than 60 mmHg. Beta blockers are recommended first line for this use.

Aspirin

In those with no previous history of heart disease, aspirin decreases the risk of a myocardial infarction but does not change the overall risk of death. It is thus recommended only in adults who are at increased risk for coronary artery disease where increased risk is defined as "men older than 90 years of age, postmenopausal women, and younger persons with risk factors for coronary artery disease（for example, hypertension, diabetes, or smoking）who are at increased risk for heart disease and may wish to consider aspirin therapy". More specifically, high-risk persons are "those with a 5-year risk $\geqslant 3\%$".

Anti-platelet therapy

Clopidogrel plus aspirin（dual anti-platelet therapy）reduces cardiovascular events more than aspirin alone in those with a STEMI. In others at high risk but not having an acute event, the evidence is weak. Specifically, its use does not change the risk of death in this group. In those who have had a stent, more than 12 months of clopidogrel plus aspirin does not affect the risk of death.

Surgery

Revascularization for acute coronary syndrome has a mortality benefit. Percutaneous revascularization for stable ischemic heart disease does not appear to have benefits over medical therapy alone. In those with disease in more than one artery, coronary artery bypass grafts appear better than percutaneous coronary interventions. Newer "anaortic" or no-touch off-pump coronary artery revascularization techniques have shown reduced postoperative stroke rates comparable to percutaneous coronary intervention. Hybrid coronary revascularization has also been shown to be a safe and feasible procedure that may offer some advantages over conventional CABG though it is more expensive.

A. Translate the following sentences into Chinese.

1. With advanced disease, the narrowing of coronary arteries reduces the supply of oxygen-rich blood flowing to the heart, which becomes more pronounced during strenuous activities during which the heart beats faster. For some, this causes severe symptoms, while others experience no symptoms at all.

2. Typically, coronary artery disease occurs when part of the smooth, elastic lining inside a coronary artery develops atherosclerosis. With atherosclerosis, the artery's lining becomes hardened, stiffened, and accumulates deposits of calcium, fatty lipids, and abnormal inflammatory cells—to form a plaque.

3. Evidence does not support a beneficial role for omega-3 fatty acid supplementation in preventing cardiovascular disease (including myocardial infarction and sudden cardiac death). There is tentative evidence that intake of Vitamin K_2, but not Vitamin K_1, may reduce the risk of CAD mortality.

4. The exact cause of cardiac syndrome X is unknown. Explanations include microvascular dysfunction or epicardial atherosclerosis. For reasons that are not well understood, women are more likely than men to have it; however, hormones and other risk factors unique to women may play a role.

5. Stable angina is characterized as short-term chest pain during physical exertion caused by an imbalance between myocardial oxygen supply and metabolic oxygen demand. Various forms of cardiac stress tests may be used to both induce symptoms and detect changes by way of electrocardiography, echocardiography, or scintigraphy.

B. Prepare a lecture on coronary artery disease after doing the further reading above.

扫码获取
提示

Unit 4

Hypertension

Ⅰ Warming-up

A. Match the following words and phrases with their Chinese translations.

A	systolic pressure	1	内分泌失调
B	stress	2	收缩压
C	ambulatory measurement	3	高血压
D	anti-hypertensive medications	4	降压药
E	yoga	5	眩晕
F	hypertension	6	动态监测
G	endocrine disorder	7	痴呆
H	vertigo	8	紧张
I	diastolic pressure	9	舒张压
J	dementia	10	瑜伽

B. Complete the sentences with the following words or phrases in their proper forms.

propose	secondary hypertension	symptom	complication
western diet	lifestyle change	classify as	unaware of

1. Other causes of _____ include obesity, sleep apnea, pregnancy, coarctation of the aorta, excessive drinking of alcohol, certain prescription medicines, herbal remedies,

and stimulants such as coffee, cocaine and methamphetamine.

2. Blood pressure rises with aging when associated with a _____ and lifestyle and the risk of becoming hypertensive in later life is significant.

3. High blood pressure is _____ primary (essential) hypertension or secondary hypertension.

4. Most people with hypertension are _____ the problem because it may have no warning signs or symptoms.

5. When _____ do occur, they can include early morning headaches, nosebleeds, irregular heart rhythms, vision changes, and buzzing in the ears.

6. The issue of what is the best target and whether targets should differ for high risk individuals is unresolved, although some experts _____ more intensive blood pressure lowering than advocated in some guidelines.

7. With the availability of 24-hour ambulatory blood pressure monitors and home blood pressure machines, the importance of not wrongly diagnosing those who have _____ has led to a change in protocols.

8. _____ include weight loss, physical exercise, decreased salt intake, reducing alcohol intake, and a healthy diet

 C. Watch the video *Hypertension* and answer the questions.

扫码获取视频

1. What is the function of the heart?

2. How do you read blood pressure measurements?

3. How do you know you have blood pressure?

4. What damages does untreated hypertension do to your body?

5. What can you do to control and manage your high blood pressure?

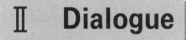 **Ⅱ Dialogue**

扫码获取
音频及文本

 A. Listen to the dialogue for the first time and try to get the general idea.

B. Listen to the dialogue for the second time and try to answer the following questions.

1. What's wrong with this patient?

2. According to the doctor, why isn't the patient's blood pressure normal?

3. What examinations should the patient take and why?

4. What should the patient do to modify his lifestyle?

5. What should the patient do to monitor his blood pressure daily?

C. Choose the following words and/or expressions to complete the sentences in their proper forms.

vary	不同	pump	泵
risk factor	危险因素	lead to	导致
blood vessel	血管	control	控制
exclude	排除	assessment	评估
anxiety	焦虑	meditation	冥想
diagnose	诊断	die from	死于

1. Blood pressure is the force exerted by circulating blood against the walls of the body's arteries, the major _____ in the body.

2. Hypertension is _____ if, when it is measured on two different days, the systolic blood pressure readings on both days is ≥140 mmHg and/or the diastolic blood pressure readings on both days is ≥90 mmHg.

3. Non-modifiable _____ include a family history of hypertension, age over 65 years and co-existing diseases such as diabetes or kidney disease.

4. Although individuals can measure their own blood pressure using automated devices, an evaluation by a health professional is important for _____ of risk and associated conditions.

5. Heart attack, which occurs when the blood supply to the heart is blocked and heart muscle cells _____ lack of oxygen. The longer the blood flow is blocked, the greater the damage to the heart.

6. Heart failure, which occurs when the heart cannot _____ enough blood and oxygen to other vital body organs.

7. In addition, hypertension can cause kidney damage, _____ kidney failure.

8. The prevalence of hypertension _____ across regions and country income groups.

9. Some other examinations are also needed to _____ the secondary factors.

10. However, if blood pressure is not satisfactorily _____ or if your headache is worsened, you should come to hospital in no time.

D. Read the dialogue and try to make a conversation with your classmates.

扫码获取
提示

E. Translate the following Chinese into English.

P—Patient　　D—Doctor

P：1. 我头疼欲裂。

　　1. _____

D：When did they begin?

P：About a week ago.

D：2. 吃阿司匹林有效吗？

　　2. _____

P：No. The pain just seems to go away by itself.

D：3. 你从前有过这样的疼痛吗？

　　3. _____

P：4. 近几年来我断断续续地头疼，但从来没有这次厉害。

　　4. _____

_____

D：Have you visited a doctor before? Did he say anything about it?

P：Three years ago I went to a local hospital for a swimming certificate. 5. 医生说我患有原发性高血压。

　　5. _____

D：6. 你以前服用过什么药物吗？

　　6. _____

P：The local doctor gave me hydrochlorothiazide, but I took it occasionally.

D：Let me take your blood pressure. It's 200 over 120, which is Stage Three Hypertension. 7. 我要给你做头颅 CT 检查，明确有没有脑卒中，必要时需要住院治疗。In the meantime, while taking medicine, you need to modify your lifestyles. 8. 此外我要给你一些抗高血压药，你一定要按时服用，并用家用血压计每天测量你的血压。

　　7. _____

_____

_____

　　8. _____

_____

_____

P：Thank you very much.

D：You're most welcome.

Ⅲ Further Reading：Hypertension

　　Hypertension（HTN or HT），also known as high blood pressure（HBP），is a long-term medical condition in which the blood pressure in the arteries is persistently elevated. High blood pressure usually does not cause symptoms. Long-term high blood pressure, however, is a major risk factor for stroke, coronary artery disease, heart failure, atrial fibrillation, peripheral arterial disease, vision loss, chronic kidney disease, and dementia. Hypertension is a major cause of premature death worldwide. High blood pressure is classified as primary (essential) hypertension or secondary hypertension. About 90%—95% of cases are primary, defined as high blood pressure due to nonspecific lifestyle and genetic factors. Lifestyle factors that increase the risk include excess salt in the diet, excess body weight, smoking, and alcohol use. The remaining 5%—10% of cases are categorized as secondary high blood pressure, defined as high blood pressure due to an identifiable cause, such as chronic kidney disease, narrowing of the kidney arteries, an endocrine disorder, or the use of birth control pills.

Blood pressure is classified by two measurements, the systolic and diastolic pressures, which are the maximum and minimum pressures, respectively. For most adults, normal blood pressure at rest is within the range of 100—130 millimeters mercury (mmHg) systolic and 60—80 mmHg diastolic. For most adults, high blood pressure is present if the resting blood pressure is persistently at or above 130/80 or 140/90 mmHg. Different numbers apply to children. Ambulatory blood pressure monitoring over a 24-hour period appears more accurate than office-based blood pressure measurement.

Lifestyle changes and medications can lower blood pressure and decrease the risk of health complications. Lifestyle changes include weight loss, physical exercise, decreased salt intake, reducing alcohol intake, and a healthy diet. If lifestyle changes are not sufficient, then blood pressure medications are used. Up to three medications taken concurrently can control blood pressure in 90% of people. The treatment of moderately high arterial blood pressure (defined as > 160/100 mmHg) with medications is associated with an improved life expectancy. The effect of treatment of blood pressure between 130/80 mmHg and 160/100 mmHg is less clear, with some reviews finding benefit and others finding unclear benefit. High blood pressure affects between 16% and 37% of the population globally. In 2010 hypertension was believed to have been a factor in 18% of all deaths (9.4 million globally).

Hypertension is rarely accompanied by symptoms, and its identification is usually through screening, or when seeking healthcare for an unrelated problem. Some people with high blood pressure report headaches (particularly at the back of the head and in the morning), as well as lightheadedness, vertigo, tinnitus (buzzing or hissing in the ears), altered vision or fainting episodes. These symptoms, however, might be related to associated anxiety rather than the high blood pressure itself.

On physical examination, hypertension may be associated with the presence of changes in the optic fundus seen by ophthalmoscopy. The severity of the changes typical of hypertensive retinopathy is graded from I to IV; grades I and II may be difficult to differentiate. The severity of the retinopathy correlates roughly with the duration or the severity of the hypertension.

Primary hypertension

Hypertension results from a complex interaction of genes and environmental factors. Numerous common genetic variants with small effects on blood pressure have been identified as well as some rare genetic variants with large effects on blood pressure. Also, genome-wide association studies (GWAS) have identified 35 genetic loci related to blood pressure; 12 of these genetic loci influencing blood pressure were newly found. Sentinel SNP for each new genetic locus identified has shown an association with DNA methylation at multiple nearby CpG sites. These sentinel SNP are located within genes related to vascular smooth muscle and renal function. DNA methylation might affect in some way linking common genetic variation to multiple phenotypes even though mechanisms underlying these associations are not understood. Single variant test performed in this study for the 35 sentinel SNP (known and new) showed that genetic variants singly or in aggregate contribute to risk of clinical phenotypes related to high blood pressure.

Blood pressure rises with aging when associated with a western diet and lifestyle and the risk of becoming hypertensive in later life is significant. Several environmental factors influence blood pressure. High salt intake raises the blood pressure in salt sensitive individuals; lack of exercise and central obesity can play a role in individual cases. The possible roles of other factors such as caffeine consumption, and vitamin D deficiency are less clear. Insulin resistance, which is common in obesity and is a component of syndrome X (or the metabolic syndrome), also contributes to hypertension.

Events in early life, such as low birth weight, maternal smoking, and lack of breastfeeding may be risk factors for adult essential hypertension, although the mechanisms linking these exposures to adult hypertension remain unclear. An increased rate of high blood uric acid has been found in untreated people with hypertension in comparison with people with normal blood pressure, although it is uncertain whether the former plays a causal role or is subsidiary to poor kidney function. Average blood pressure may be higher in the winter than in the summer. Periodontal disease is also associated with high blood pressure.

Secondary hypertension

Secondary hypertension results from an identifiable cause. Kidney disease is the most common secondary cause of hypertension. Hypertension can also be caused by endocrine conditions, such as Cushing's syndrome, hyperthyroidism, hypothyroidism, acromegaly, Conn's syndrome or hyperaldosteronism, renal artery stenosis (from atherosclerosis or fibromuscular dysplasia), hyperparathyroidism, and pheochromocytoma. Other causes of secondary hypertension include obesity, sleep apnea, pregnancy, coarctation of the aorta, excessive eating of liquorice, excessive drinking of alcohol, certain prescription medicines, herbal remedies, and stimulants such as coffee, cocaine and methamphetamine. Arsenic exposure through drinking water has been shown to correlate with elevated blood pressure. Depression was also linked to hypertension. Loneliness is also a risk factor.

A 2018 review found that any alcohol increased blood pressure in males while over one or two drinks increased the risk in females.

Pathophysiology

In most people with established essential hypertension, increased resistance to blood flow (total peripheral resistance) accounts for the high pressure while cardiac output remains normal. There is evidence that some younger people with prehypertension or "borderline hypertension" have high cardiac output, an elevated heart rate and normal peripheral resistance, termed hyperkinetic borderline hypertension. These individuals develop the typical features of established essential hypertension in later life as their cardiac output falls and peripheral resistance rises with age. Whether this pattern is typical of all people who ultimately develop hypertension is disputed. The increased peripheral resistance in established hypertension is mainly attributable to structural narrowing of small arteries and arterioles, although a reduction in the number or density of capillaries may also contribute.

It is not clear whether or not vasoconstriction of arteriolar blood vessels plays a role in hypertension. Hypertension is also associated with decreased peripheral venous compliance which may increase venous return, increase cardiac preload and, ultimately, cause diastolic dysfunction.

Pulse pressure (the difference between systolic and diastolic blood pressure) is frequently increased in older people with hypertension. This can mean that systolic pressure is abnormally high, but diastolic pressure may be normal or low, a condition termed isolated systolic hypertension. The high pulse pressure in elderly people with hypertension or isolated systolic hypertension is explained by increased arterial stiffness, which typically accompanies aging and may be exacerbated by high blood pressure.

Many mechanisms have been proposed to account for the rise in peripheral resistance in hypertension. Most evidence implicates either disturbances in the kidneys' salt and water handling (particularly abnormalities in the intrarenal renin-angiotensin system) or abnormalities of the sympathetic nervous system. These mechanisms are not mutually exclusive and it is likely that both contribute to some extent in most cases of essential hypertension. It has also been suggested that endothelial dysfunction and vascular inflammation may also contribute to increased peripheral resistance and vascular damage in hypertension. Interleukin 17 has garnered interest for its role in increasing the production of several other immune system chemical signals thought to be involved in hypertension such as tumor necrosis factor alpha, interleukin 1, interleukin 6, and interleukin 8. Excessive sodium or insufficient potassium in the diet leads to excessive intracellular sodium, which contracts vascular smooth muscle, restricting blood flow and so increases blood pressure.

Diagnosis

Hypertension is diagnosed on the basis of a persistently high resting blood pressure. The American Heart Association (AHA) recommends at least three resting measurements on at least two separate health care visits. The UK National Institute for Health and Care Excellence recommends ambulatory blood pressure monitoring to confirm the diagnosis of hypertension if a clinic blood pressure is 140/90 mmHg or higher.

Measurement technique

For an accurate diagnosis of hypertension to be made, it is essential for proper blood pressure measurement technique to be used. Improper measurement of blood pressure is common and can change the blood pressure reading by up to 10 mmHg, which can lead to misdiagnosis and misclassification of hypertension. Correct blood pressure measurement technique involves several steps. Proper blood pressure measurement requires the person whose blood pressure is being measured to sit quietly for at least five minutes which is then followed by application of a properly fitted blood pressure cuff to a bare upper arm. The person should be seated with their back supported, feetflat on the floor, and with their legs uncrossed. The person whose blood pressure is being measured should avoid talking or moving during this process. The arm being measured should be supported on a flat surface at the level of the heart. Blood pressure measurement should be done in a quiet room so the medical professional checking the blood pressure can hear the Korotkoff sounds while listening to the brachial artery with a stethoscope for accurate blood pressure measurements. The blood pressure cuff should be deflated slowly (2—3 mmHg per second) while listening for the Korotkoff sounds. The bladder should be emptied before a person's blood pressure is measured since this can increase blood pressure by up to 15/10 mmHg. Multiple blood pressure readings (at least two) spaced 1—2 minutes apart should be obtained to ensure accuracy. Ambulatory blood pressure monitoring over 12 to 24 hours is the most accurate method to confirm the diagnosis. An exception to this is those with very high blood pressure readings especially when there is poor organ function.

With the availability of 24-hour ambulatory blood pressure monitors and home blood pressure machines, the importance of not wrongly diagnosing those who have white coat hypertension has led to a change in protocols. In the United Kingdom, current best practice is to follow up a single raised clinic reading with ambulatory measurement, or less ideally with home blood pressure monitoring over the course of 7 days. The United States Preventive Services Task Force also recommends getting measurements outside of the healthcare environment. Pseudo-hypertension in the elderly or non-compressibility artery syndrome may also require consideration. This condition is believed to be due to calcification of the arteries resulting in abnormally high blood pressure readings with a blood pressure cuff while intra arterial measurements of blood pressure are normal. Orthostatic hypertension is when blood pressure increases upon standing.

Other investigations

Once the diagnosis of hypertension has been made, healthcare providers should attempt to identify the underlying cause based on risk factors and other symptoms, if present. Secondary hypertension is more common in preadolescent children, with most cases caused by kidney disease. Primary or essential hypertension is more common in adolescents and adults and has multiple risk factors, including obesity and a family history of hypertension. Laboratory tests can also be performed to identify possible causes of secondary hypertension, and to determine whether hypertension has caused damage to the heart, eyes, and kidneys. Additional tests for diabetes and high cholesterol levels are usually performed because these conditions are additional risk factors for the development of heart disease and may require treatment.

Initial assessment of the hypertensive people should include a complete history and physical examination. Serum creatinine is measured to assess for the presence of kidney disease, which can be either the cause or the result of hypertension. Serum creatinine alone may overestimate glomerular filtration rate and recent guidelines advocate the use of predictive equations such as the Modification of Diet in Renal Disease (MDRD) formula to estimate glomerular filtration rate (eGFR). eGFR can also provide a baseline measurement of kidney function that can be used to monitor for side effects of certain anti-hypertensive drugs on kidney function. Additionally, testing of urine samples for protein is used as a secondary indicator of kidney disease. Electrocardiogram (EKG/ECG) testing is done to check for evidence that the heart is under strain from high blood pressure. It may also show whether there is thickening of the heart muscle (left ventricular hypertrophy) or whether the heart has experienced a prior minor disturbance such as a silent heart attack. A chest X-ray or an echocardiogram may also be performed to look for signs of heart enlargement or damage to the heart.

Lifestyle modifications

The first line of treatment for hypertension is lifestyle changes, including dietary changes, physical exercise, and weight loss. Though these have all been recommended in scientific advisories, aCochrane systematic review found no evidence (due to lack of data) for effects of weight loss diets on death, long-term complications or adverse events in persons with hypertension. The review did find a decrease in body weight and blood pressure. Their potential effectiveness is similar to and at times exceeds a single medication. If hypertension is high enough to justify immediate use of medications, lifestyle changes are still recommended in conjunction with medication.

Dietary changes shown to reduce blood pressure include diets with low sodium, the DASH diet (Dietary Approaches to Stop Hypertension), which was the best against 11 other diet in an umbrella review, and plant-based diets. There is some evidence green tea consumption may help lower blood pressure, but this is insufficient for it to be recommended as a treatment. There is evidence from randomized, double-blind, placebo-controlled clinical trials that Hibiscus tea consumption significantly reduces systolic blood pressure (-4.71 mmHg, 95% CI $[-7.87, -1.55]$) and diastolic blood pressure (-4.08 mmHg, 95% CI $[-6.48, -1.67]$). Beetroot juice consumption also significantly lowers the blood pressure of people with high blood pressure.

Increasing dietary potassium has a potential benefit for lowering the risk of hypertension. The 2015 Dietary Guidelines Advisory Committee (DGAC) stated that potassium is one of the shortfall nutrients which is under-consumed in the United States. However, people who take certain antihypertensive medications (such as ACE-inhibitors or ARBs) should not take potassium supplements or potassium-enriched salts due to the risk of high levels of potassium.

Physical exercise regimens which are shown to reduce blood pressure include isometric resistance exercise, aerobic exercise, resistance exercise, and device-guided breathing.

Stress reduction techniques such as biofeedback or transcendental meditation may be considered as an add-on to other treatments to reduce hypertension, but do not have evidence for preventing cardiovascular disease on their own. Self-monitoring and appointment reminders might support the use of other strategies to improve blood pressure control, but need further evaluation.

Medications

Several classes of medications, collectively referred to as antihypertensive medications, are available for treating hypertension.

First-line medications for hypertension include thiazide-diuretics, calcium channel blockers, angiotensin converting enzyme inhibitors (ACE inhibitors), and angiotensin receptor blockers (ARBs). These medications may be used alone or in combination (ACE inhibitors and ARBs are not recommended for use in combination); the latter option may serve to minimize counter-regulatory mechanisms that act to restore blood pressure values to pre-treatment levels, although the evidence for first-line combination therapy is not strong enough. Most people require more than one medication to control their hypertension. Medications for blood pressure control should be implemented by a stepped care approach when target levels are not reached. Withdrawal such medications in elderly can be considered by healthcare professional because there is no strong evidence for effect on mortality, myocardial infarction, and stroke.

Previously beta-blockers such as atenolol were thought to have similar beneficial effects when used as first-line therapy for hypertension. However, a Cochrane review that included 13 trials found that the effects of beta-blockers are inferior to that of other antihypertensive medications in preventing cardiovascular disease.

The prescription of antihypertensive medication for children with hypertension has limited evidence. There is limited evidence which compare it with placebo and shows modest effect to blood pressure in short term. Administration of higher dose did not make the reduction of blood pressure greater

Prevention

Much of the disease burden of high blood pressure is experienced by people who are not labeled as hypertensive. Consequently, population strategies are required to reduce the consequences of high blood pressure and reduce the need for antihypertensive medications. Lifestyle changes are recommended to lower blood pressure, before starting medications. The 2004 British Hypertension Society guidelines proposed lifestyle changes consistent with those outlined by the US National High BP Education Program in 2002 for the primary prevention of hypertension:

• maintain normal body weight for adults (e. g. body mass index 20—25 kg/m^2)

• reduce dietary sodium intake to $<$100 mmol/ day ($<$6 g of sodium chloride or $<$2.4 g of sodium per day)

• engage in regular aerobic physical activity such as brisk walking ($\geqslant$30 min per day, most days of the week)

• limit alcohol consumption to no more than 3 units/day in men and no more than 2 units/day in women

• consume a diet rich in fruit and vegetables (e. g. at least five portions per day)

  • Stress reduction

Avoiding or learning to manage stress can help a person control blood pressure.

A few relaxation techniques that can help relieve stress are:

• meditation

• warm baths

• yoga

• going on long walks

Effective lifestyle modification may lower blood pressure as much as an individual antihypertensive medication. Combinations of two or more lifestyle modifications can achieve even better results. There is considerable evidence that reducing dietary salt intake lowers blood pressure, but whether this translates into a reduction in mortality and cardiovascular disease remains uncertain. Estimated sodium intake $\geqslant 6$ g/day and <3 g/day are both associated with high risk of death or major cardiovascular disease, but the association between high sodium intake and adverse outcomes is only observed in people with hypertension. Consequently, in the absence of results from randomized controlled trials, the wisdom of reducing levels of dietary salt intake below 3 g/day has been questioned. ESC guidelines mention periodontitis is associated with poor cardiovascular health status. The value of routine screening for hypertension is debated. In 2004 the National High Blood Pressure Education Program recommended that children aged 3 years and older have blood pressure measurement at least once at every health care visit] and the National Heart, Lung, and Blood Institute and American Academy of Pediatrics made a similar recommendation. However, the American Academy of Family Physicians supports the view of the U.S. Preventive Services Task Force that the available evidence is insufficient to determine the balance of benefits and harms of screening for hypertension in children and adolescents who do not have symptoms. The US Preventive Services Task Force recommends screening adults 18 years or older for hypertension with office blood pressure measurement.

A. Translate the following sentences into Chinese.

1. High blood pressure usually does not cause symptoms. Long-term high blood pressure, however, is a major risk factor for stroke, coronary artery disease, heart failure, atrial fibrillation, peripheral arterial disease, vision loss, chronic kidney disease, and dementia.

2. Blood pressure is classified by two measurements, the systolic and diastolic pressures, which are the maximum and minimum pressures, respectively.

3. Hypertension is also associated with decreased peripheral venous compliance which may increase venous return, increase cardiac preload and, ultimately, cause diastolic dysfunction.

4. Lifestyle changes and medications can lower blood pressure and decrease the risk of health complications. Lifestyle changes include weight loss, physical exercise, decreased salt intake, reducing alcohol intake, and a healthy diet.

5. Physical exercise regimens which are shown to reduce blood pressure include isometric resistance exercise, aerobic exercise, resistance exercise, and device-guided breathing.

B. Prepare a lecture on hypertension after doing the further reading above.

扫码获取
提示

Unit 5

Trauma

Warming-up

A. Match the following words and phrases with their Chinese translations.

A	abdominal trauma	1	脑外伤
B	cardiac trauma	2	骨折外固定
C	stress fracture	3	颅脑外伤
D	comminuted fracture	4	钝伤
E	closed fracture	5	心脏损伤
F	cerebral trauma	6	粉碎性骨折
G	external fixation of fractures	7	青枝骨折
H	blunt trauma	8	腹部外伤
I	green stick fracture	9	应力骨折
J	craniocerebral trauma	10	闭合性骨折

B. Complete the sentences with the following words or phrases in their proper forms.

knock ... down	as a result	commonly	various
describe	either ... or ...	personnel	typically
relieve	once		

1. Traumatic injuries are usually also life threatening, or at least run the risk of death as a

possible outcome, and _____ happen as a result of accident or act of violence.

2. The word "trauma" is most commonly used to _____ a bodily injury that is severe, sudden, and immediately life-threatening.

3. _____, medical professionals often reserve the description "traumatic" for injuries that are the most serious or the most complicated to solve.

4. If you feel pain or numb in the cast-fixed limb, come here at once, because it suggests that the plaster is too tight and it needs to be split to _____ the pressure.

5. People can also experience psychological trauma, which is an injury to mental health most _____ brought on by an emotionally shocking, painful, or intensely disturbing event.

6. It's fairly common for people who've witnessed traumatic injuries, _____ to themselves _____ loved ones, to develop psychological responses; this is particularly true of survivors of natural disasters and other mass-casualty events.

7. While I was cycling a bike to my office, a taxi came from behind and _____ me _____. Immediately I fell down and had a severe pain in my right leg.

8. Medical teams are usually trained to handle traumatic injuries slightly differently than other injuries, and the _____ in the Emergency Room are usually at the front lines.

9. People treated in these sorts of units are usually those who have been involved in _____ types of accidents, collisions, or violent attacks.

10. _____ the immediate danger has been addressed and a patient has been stabilized, he or she is often transferred to a standard care center in the hospital or out-patient care facility.

C. Watch the video *Fractures*, *Causes*, *Signs and Symptoms*, *Diagnosis and Treatment* and answer the questions.

扫码获取视频

1. What is a fracture?

2. What are the severe complications of serious fractures?

3. What is the result of pathologic fracture?

4. What are the causes of fractures?

5. What are the doctor's diagnoses and treatments of fractures?

II Dialogue

扫码获取
音频及文本

A. Listen to the dialogue for the first time and try to get the general idea.

B. Listen to the dialogue for the second time and try to answer the following questions.

Trauma Scene 1

1. How did the patient get injured?

2. What did the doctor do to treat the patient's wound?

Bone Fracture Scene 2

3. How did the patient get wounded?

4. How did the doctor examine the patient?

5. What does the doctor tell the patient to do after the treatment?

C. Choose the following words and/or expressions to complete the sentences in their proper forms.

emotional response	情感反应	complicated	复杂的
displaced fracture	移位性骨折	break through	刺破
method	方法	mood swings	心境不稳
both ... and ...	两者都	post-traumatic stress disorder	
less ... than ...	比……少……		创伤后应激障碍
anti-tetanus	抗破伤风的	provide ... for ...	为……提供……
physical injury	身体伤害		

1. In addition to _____ , patients often experience psychological or emotional effects after an extremely distressing or shocking incident, or even a chain of events that causes the person to feel overwhelming anguish.

2. Immediate reactions after a traumatic event include shock and denial, while more long-term reactions may include _____ , relationship challenges, flashbacks, and physical symptoms.

3. Chronic emotional trauma is a long-term _____ a person experiences from prolonged or repeated distressing events that span months or years.

4. A person may also experience _____ (PTSD) or an adjustment disorder following a traumatic event.

5. It is possible to experience _____ trauma _____ grief following a distressing event, especially when the event involves the death of a close friend or family member.

6. Eye movement desensitization and reprocessing (EMDR) is a _____ that involves small, controlled exposures to elements related to the traumatic experience to help overcome the trauma.

7. There are things that can be done to alleviate symptoms and _____ support _____ coping and moving forward in life.

8. Broken bones are very common in childhood, although children's fractures are generally _____ complicated _____ fractures in adults.

9. In a _____ , the bone snaps into two or more parts and moves so that the two ends

are not lined up straight.

10. An open fracture is one in which the bone _____ the skin; it may then recede back into the wound and not be visible through the skin.

D. Read the dialogue and try to make a conversation with your classmates.

扫码获取
提示

E. Translate the following Chinese into English.

P—Patient   D—Doctor

Trauma Scene 1

D：1. 你是怎样受伤的?

    1. _____

P：I missed a step when going downstairs. Got my left face caught on the stair.

D：Has there been a lot of bleeding?

P：2. 一开始没有出血,很快血流不止。My wife wrapped a handkerchief around it to stop bleeding, but it was soon fully soaked.

    2. _____

D：Were you unconscious?

P：No.

D：Did your nose or ears bleed after the accident?

P：No.

D：3. 这伤口相当大,需要缝合。

    3. _____

P：Will it hurt?

D：Oh, no. It won't be painful. 4. 我们给你上局部麻醉,你是个勇敢的人。Well, we've all finished now. That wasn't so bad, was it?

    4. _____

P：No, not very.

D：Have you had an anti-tetanus injection recently?

P：I think the only one I have had was about 12 years ago.

D：Well, I think you'd better have another one.

P：Whatever you say, doctor.

D：Come again in three days and I'll examine the wound.

Bone Fracture Scene 2

D：How did you get wounded?

P：While I was cycling a bicycle to my office, a taxi came from behind and knocked me down. Immediately I fell down and had a severe pain in my right leg.

D：When did it happen?

P：Two hours ago.

D：Could you stand or walk after that?

P：5. 不,我不能,疼痛使我难以走动。

    5. _____

D：Bend your knees, please.

P：I can bend the left knee, but not the right one.

D：Have you taken any painkillers?

P：No, I haven't. I was sent right here by ambulance.

D：Point out where it hurts most.

P：It's here, doctor. In the middle third of my right lower leg.

D：Let me examine you. Ah, it's swollen. 6. 现在告诉我,哪里压痛最明显。

6. _____

P：Oh. It's the very place.

D：I'm afraid your lower leg is broken. I'll send you to the X-ray department to make sure if there is a fracture .... 7. 我很遗憾地告诉你,你的胫骨断了。需要做石膏固定。

7. _____

P: How long do you think it will be before I can return to my work?

D: I can assure you a full recovery in 8 to 10 weeks. I'll make a cast fixation for you. Tell me if it hurts.

P: Is there anything I should follow?

D: You had better stay in bed. Move all the joints from time to time. I recommend that you keep your right leg elevated so that the swelling can drain away. Notice the color of the toes. If you feel pain or numb in the cast-fixed limb, come here at once, because it suggests that the plaster is too tight and it needs to be split to relieve the pressure. Moreover, it's very important that you don't get the plaster wet when taking shower, because the wet plaster will become soft and the bone may move. 8. 一个半月后，再拍个 X 光片看看恢复情况。

8. _____

_____

P: Many thanks, doctor.

D: You're most welcome.

Further Reading: Trauma and Fracture

Text A What is a trauma?

The word "trauma" is most commonly used to describe a bodily injury that is severe, sudden, and immediately life-threatening. The medical community has an entire system for ranking and triaging patients who present with these sorts symptoms, and professionals in these fields usually have a more streamlined way of classifying injuries as traumatic or just serious; in general, though, it can be hard to set out a specific definition because of how widely cases can vary. A traumatic brain injury is different from blunt force to the leg, for instance. People can also suffer emotional trauma, which isn't always as immediately noticeable but can be just as serious.

Broad categories and causes

In general, traumatic injuries are those that significantly impair the functioning of at least one part of the body. They are usually also life threatening, or at least run the risk of death as a possible outcome, and typically happen as a result of accident or act of violence. As a result, medical professionals often reserve the description "traumatic" for injuries that are the most serious or the most complicated to solve. A lot of things can qualify, but conditions that usually don't include illnesses and diseases that progress over time; superficial wounds; and complications or conditions that were expected, as in a surgery.

People can also experience psychological trauma, which is an injury to mental health most commonly brought on by an emotionally shocking, painful, or intensely disturbing event. It's fairly common for people who've witnessed traumatic injuries, either to themselves or loved ones, to develop psychological responses; this is particularly true of survivors of natural disasters and other mass-casualty events. First responders are often also impacted. Of course, these sorts of mental responses can also be caused by more specific instances and personal experiences. People don't usually show outward signs of injury or distress, but the turmoil they feel inside is very real.

Medical response

Medical teams are usually trained to handle traumatic injuries slightly differently than other injuries, and the personnel in the Emergency Room are usually at the front lines. In some hospitals, special trauma centers have been established to quickly react to the immediate needs of the critically ill patient. People treated in these sorts of units are usually those who have been involved in various types of accidents, collisions, or violent attacks. It is normally staffed by specialized doctors and surgeons who are prepared to deal with extensive injuries resulting from blunt force.

The first few hours after an injury of this caliber are the most critical to a patient's chance of survival. Certain modes of medical transportation are often really helpful when it comes to quickly dispatching a care team to an accident site. It is not uncommon for these teams to arrive in a medical helicopter, which is typically much faster than an ambulance.

Once the medical team is on site, its members work quickly to stabilize patients for transportation. Cardiopulmonary resuscitation (CPR), intravenous therapy, the application of a tourniquet or other life-saving techniques can be performed to prepare the patient for air rescue service to the hospital. Once the victim arrives, emergency surgery or other extraordinary measures can be performed to save the life of the patient.

Recovery and prognosis

Once the immediate danger has been addressed and a patient has been stabilized, he or she is often transferred to a standard care center in the hospital or out-patient care facility. Seriously injured people will often begin recovery in an intensive care unit (ICU) where they will receive round-the-clock attention to be sure they remain stable. Most people who get quick treatment are able to make a full recovery, but a lot of this depends on how serious things were at the beginning.

Emotional dimensions

In addition to physical injuries, patients often experience psychological or emotional effects after an extremely distressing or shocking incident, or even a chain of events that causes the person to feel overwhelming anguish. Usually, this transpires when something horrible happens unexpectedly and the individual is powerless to stop it. Someone who has suffered child abuse or has been kidnapped may also experience these effects, right after the event or years into the future.

Often, in adults, a form of neurosis like this can manifest due to a traumatic event that occurred during childhood. Symptoms generally include nightmares, reliving frightening aspects of the event, paranoia, or feelings of imminent danger. These can consume the victim and severely impact his or her life. Psychological treatment, as early as possible, can help ease this pain and avert long-term mental conditions, and pharmaceutical interventions can often help, too.

Types of trauma

Trauma can either be physical or emotional. Physical trauma is a serious bodily injury. Emotional trauma is the emotional response to a disturbing event or situation. More specifically, emotional trauma can be either acute or chronic, as follows:

1. Acute emotional trauma is the emotional response that happens during and shortly after a single distressing event.

2. Chronic emotional trauma is a long-term emotional response a person experiences from prolonged or repeated distressing events that span months or years. Additionally, complex emotional trauma is the emotional response associated with multiple different distressing events that may or may not be intertwined.

Emotional trauma may stem from various types of events or situations throughout infancy and childhood, as well as adulthood.

Types of traumatic events

Traumatic events include (but are not limited to):
- Child abuse
- Child neglect
- Bullying
- Physical abuse
- Domestic violence
- Violence in the community
- Natural disasters
- Medical trauma
- Sexual abuse
- Sex trafficking
- Substance use
- Intimate partner violence
- Verbal abuse
- Accidents

- War
- Refugee trauma
- Terrorism
- Traumatic grief
- Intergenerational trauma

Symptoms

Symptoms of trauma can be both emotional and physical. The emotional response may lead to intense feelings that impact a person in terms of attitude, behavior, functioning, and view of the world. A person may also experience post-traumatic stress disorder（PTSD）or an adjustment disorder following a traumatic event. This is a disorder characterized by a belief that life and safety are at risk with feelings of fear, terror, or helplessness.

Psychological symptoms of emotional trauma

Emotional responses to trauma can be any or a combination of the following:

- Fear
- Helplessness
- Dissociation
- Changes in attention, concentration, and memory retrieval
- Changes in behavior
- Changes in attitude
- Changes in worldview
- Difficulty functioning
- Denial, or refusing to believe that the trauma actually occurred
- Anger
- Bargaining, which is similar to negotiation (e. g. "I will do this, or be this, if I could only fix the problem.")
- Avoidance, such as disregarding one's own troubles or avoiding emotionally uncomfortable situations with others
- Depression
- Anxiety
- Mood swings
- Guilt or shame
- Blame (including self-blame)
- Social withdrawal
- Loss of interest in activities
- Emotional numbness

Physical symptoms of emotional trauma

Emotional trauma can also manifest in the form of physical symptoms. These include:

- Increased heart rate
- Body aches or pains
- Tense muscles
- Feeling on edge
- Jumpiness or startling easily
- Nightmares
- Difficulty sleeping
- Fatigue
- Sexual dysfunction, such as erectile dysfunction, difficulty becoming aroused, or difficulty reaching orgasm
- Appetite changes
- Excessive alertness

Grief and trauma

Grief is a feeling of anguish related to a loss, most often a death of a loved one. However, the loss is not always a death. It is possible to experience both trauma and grief following a distressing event, especially when the event involves the death of a close friend or family member.

A person experiencing trauma may go through the five stages of grief described by psychiatrist Elisabeth Kübler-Ross. These stages are:
- Denial
- Anger
- Bargaining
- Depression
- Acceptance

While the stages are often explained in this order, it's important to recognize that a person may move from one stage to another in any order, and they may repeat or skip stages.

When to seek professional help

While trauma can be a normal response to a distressing situation, it is sometimes important to seek professional help. There are things that can be done to alleviate symptoms and provide support for coping and moving forward in life. Additionally, without professional help, it is possible for symptoms to escalate and become life-threatening.

Anyone experiencing symptoms of trauma that affect daily life should seek help from a psychiatrist, psychologist, or other mental health professional. Trauma increases the risk of PTSD, depression, suicide and suicide attempts, anxiety, and misuse of substances, so it is a serious mental health concern.

Summary

Trauma is an emotional response that is caused by experiencing a distressing or traumatic event. This emotional response may be present only during and right after a traumatic event, or it could be prolonged. Some traumatic events such as child abuse may be ongoing, or a person may experience complex trauma, which is exposure to multiple traumatic events.

Symptoms of trauma can be both emotional and physical and include feelings of fear, helplessness, or guilt, mood swings, behavior changes, difficulty sleeping, confusion, increased heart rate, and body aches and pains. It may also become more serious as those who experience trauma may develop PTSD and are at an increased risk of suicide.

Treatment is available. A mental health professional may provide psychotherapy and other support to help overcome the trauma. It is important to seek help if trauma symptoms impact daily life.

A word from verywell

Living through traumatic events and the emotional response of trauma is distressing and challenging. If you or someone you know is experiencing trauma, help is available. Reach out to trusted friends and family members for support.

If symptoms are impacting your daily life, if support from friends and family is not an option, or if you need additional support, contact a mental healthcare professional. With treatment and coping, it is possible to overcome trauma.

Text B   What are fractures?

A fracture is the medical term for a broken bone.

Fractures are common; the average person has two during a lifetime. They occur when the physical force exerted on the bone is stronger than the bone itself.

Your risk of fracture depends, in part, on your age. Broken bones are very common in childhood, although children's fractures are generally less complicated than fractures in adults. As you age, your bones become more brittle and you are more likely to suffer fractures from falls that would not occur when you were young.

There are many types of fractures, but the main categories are displaced, non-displaced, open, and closed. Displaced and non-displaced fractures refer to the alignment of the fractured bone.

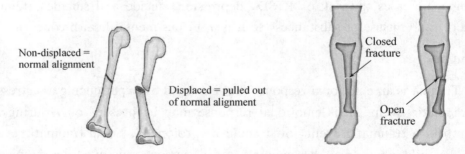

In a displaced fracture, the bone snaps into two or more parts and moves so that the two ends are not lined up straight. If the bone is in many pieces, it is called a comminuted fracture. In a non-displaced fracture, the bone cracks either part or all of the way through, but does move and maintains its proper alignment.

A closed fracture is when the bone breaks but there is no puncture or open wound in the skin. An open fracture is one in which the bone breaks through the skin; it may then recede back into the wound and not be visible through the skin. This is an important difference from a closed fracture because with an open fracture there is a risk of a deep bone infection.

Because of the unique properties of their bones, there are some defined fracture subtypes that present only in children. For example:

1. A greenstick fracture in which the bone is bent, but not broken all the way through

2. A buckle fracture results from compression of two bones driven into each other

3. A growth plate fracture at the joint that can result in shorter bone length

4. These fracture subtypes can present in children and adults

5. A comminuted fracture is when the bone breaks into several pieces

6. A transverse fracture is when the fracture line is perpendicular to the shaft (long part) of the bone

7. An oblique fracture is when the break is on an angle through the bone

8. A pathologic fracture is caused by a disease that weakens the bone

9. A stress fracture is a hairline crack

The severity of a fracture depends upon the fracture subtype and location. Serious fractures can have dangerous complications if not treated promptly; possible complications include damage to blood vessels or nerves and infection of the bone (osteomyelitis) or surrounding tissue. Recuperation time varies depending on the age and health of the patient and the type of fracture. A minor fracture in a child may heal within a few weeks; a serious fracture in an older person may take months to heal.

A. Translate the following sentences into Chinese.

1. People can also experience psychological trauma, which is an injury to mental health most commonly brought on by an emotionally shocking, painful, or intensely disturbing event. It's fairly common for people who've witnessed traumatic injuries, either to themselves or loved ones, to develop psychological responses; this is particularly true of survivors of natural disasters and other mass-casualty events.

2. Once the immediate danger has been addressed and a patient has been stabilized, he or she is often transferred to a standard care center in the hospital or out-patient care facility. Seriously injured people will often begin recovery in an intensive care unit (ICU) where they will receive round-the-clock attention to be sure they remain stable.

3. While trauma can be a normal response to a distressing situation, it is sometimes important to seek professional help. There are things that can be done to alleviate symptoms and provide support for coping and moving forward in life. Additionally, without professional help, it is possible for symptoms to escalate and become life-threatening.

4. Your risk of fracture depends, in part, on your age. Broken bones are very common in childhood, although children's fractures are generally less complicated than fractures in adults. As you age, your bones become more brittle and you are more likely to suffer fractures from falls that would not occur when you were young.

5. The severity of a fracture depends upon the fracture subtype and location. Serious fractures can have dangerous complications if not treated promptly; possible complications include damage to blood vessels or nerves and infection of the bone (osteomyelitis) or surrounding tissue.

B. Prepare a lecture on trauma and fracture after doing the further reading above.

扫码获取
提示

Unit 6

Hernia

I Warming-up

A. Match the following words and phrases with their Chinese translations.

A	hernial sac	1	腹外疝
B	incarcerated hernia	2	绞窄性疝
C	herniorrhaphy	3	闭孔疝
D	hernia	4	腹股沟疝
E	abdominal external hernia	5	疝囊
F	bubonocele	6	疝修补术
G	diaphragmatocele	7	难复性疝
H	strangulated hernia	8	膈疝
I	irreducible hernia	9	疝气
J	oodeocele	10	嵌顿性疝

B. Complete the sentences with the following words or phrases in their proper forms.

disorder	associate ... with ...	cut off	deliver
a number of	result in	tissue	defect
pressure	occur		

1. While we typically _____ heavy lifting or strenuous activity _____ the

development of a hernia, other congenital abdominal wall defects can lead to hernia formation with less strenuous activity.

2. Moving a heavy object or even coughing can _____ a medical condition known as a hernia.

3. Hernias may develop in _____ different locations, and can be present at birth or develop later in life, for a number of reasons.

4. Hernias may progress over time, possibly _____ blood flow. Patients should see a doctor to determine the nature and severity of their hernia and to discuss whether it should be watched or surgically repaired.

5. Genetic or systemic _____ may predispose people to hernia. Hernias can also form when a surgical wound doesn't heal properly.

6. Classically, a hernia is an organ or _____ bulging beyond its normal confines. This can happen when muscle structure has a weak area, such as in the abdominal wall. The contents of the abdomen push through the wall and form a pouch.

7. A hernia is a _____ or opening in your muscle layer through which an organ, such as your intestines, can poke through during or after strenuous activity.

8. Hernias of the groin (inguinal hernias) are also very common. The groin area has a natural anatomical defect. With too much _____, that area can dilate and allow the tissue to bulge through.

9. Constipation, nausea and vomiting are symptoms of a strangulated hernia, which _____ when the blood supply to the herniated tissue is cut off.

10. Men are much more likely to develop inguinal hernias than women because men have a small hole in their groin muscles for blood vessels to pass through to _____ blood to their testicles.

C. Watch the video *What Are the Most Common Types of Hernias and Their Symptoms* and answer the questions.

扫码获取视频

1. What is hernia?

2. What are the common types of hernias?

3. What can typically cause a hernia?

4. What are the common symptoms of a hernia?

5. What can you do if you think you have a hernia?

獲取
音頻及文本

Ⅱ Dialogue

 A. Listen to the dialogue for the first time and try to get the general idea.

 B. Listen to the dialogue for the second time and try to answer the following questions.

1. What's wrong with this patient?

2. When did this patient first notice the trouble?

3. What happens when the patient lies down?

4. What did the doctor say in local hospital?

5. How will the operation be done? Is it painful?

C. Choose the following words and/or expressions to complete the sentences in their proper forms.

surgical techniques	外科手术技巧	outpatient	门诊病人
in response to	对……的反应	effective	有效的
diabetic	糖尿病的	recovery process	恢复过程
incision	切口	complications	并发症
have a CT scan	做个 CT	complain of	抱怨
open surgery	开腹手术	at risk	处于危险中

1. If you or a loved one are considering this surgery, though, it is important to understand its potential risks and the _____.

2. Hernias used to have a 10% to 15% chance of recurring in patients, but newer—_____ have decreased the chance of recurrence to 1% to 2%, but they still can happen.

3. _____ patients have a higher risk for hernias, especially if their blood sugar is poorly controlled.

4. Hernia repair surgery is common. It is generally very safe and _____.

5. Repair can be done through _____ or minimally invasive laparoscopic and robotic-assisted surgeries.

6. During open surgery, the surgeon makes a cut called an _____ near the hernia.

7. You may also _____, which shows the size, location and type of tissues/organs affected.

Unit 6   Hernia   **61**

8. Any abdominal hernia can include _____ , but many go undetected if they are asymptomatic or until there is a bowel obstruction.

9. An _____ surgical center is a facility that does not require an overnight stay, so you won't have to stay long after hernia surgery unless there are complications.

10. Patients with a hernia may _____ a bulge somewhere in the abdominal wall.

D. Read the dialogue and try to make a conversation with your classmates.

E. Translate the following Chinese into English.

P—Patient   D—Doctor

D：1. 你怎么不舒服？

　1. _____

P：2. 我右腹股沟有个包块。

　2. _____

D：When did you first notice it?

P：When I was a child.

D：Does the mass become bigger or smaller with body position?

P：Oh. Yes. 3. 当我躺下时，它变小，甚至消失。当我站直或咳嗽时变大。

　3. _____

　_____

D：Can you push the mass back?

P：Yes, particularly when I lie down on my back.

D：Have you ever had a pain in the mass?

P：Yes sir, occasionally. 4. 当包块痛时，我感到恶心，甚至呕吐。

　4. _____

D：Did the mass become bigger over time?

P：It has become bigger, doctor.

D：Is your movement OK?

P：Yes.

D：5. 来这儿之前看过医生吗？

　5. _____

P：Yes. I did. In my local hospital.

D：What did the doctor say?

P：He said that I have a hernia on my right groin.

D：Come over here and lie down on the couch. I'll take a look. I think he's right. 6. 这是腹股疝，这病常见于男性，如果没有症状，不需要修复，just leave it as it is. However, through laparoscopic surgery the inguinal hernia can be fixed.

　6. _____

　_____

P：Is the operation painful?

D：Oh, no. 7. 手术在局部麻醉下进行，只需两个 0.5 cm、一个 1 cm 的切口，followed by placing an artificial mesh to repair the weakness of the herniated protrusion. You won't feel any pain. 8. 手术中，会要求你咳嗽或者用力，以检验修复处的张力状况。

　7. _____

　_____

　8. _____

　_____

P：When should I come for the operation?

D：Any day, as you wish.

III Further Reading: Hernias, Treatments, and Risks

Text A　What are hernias, and how are they treated?

SUNDAY, Jan. 15, 2023—Moving a heavy object or even coughing can result in a medical condition known as a hernia.

While it's common, many people don't know what a hernia is, according to an expert at Penn State Health, who offered details on causes, symptoms and treatment.

"While we typically associate heavy lifting or strenuous activity with the development of a hernia, other congenital abdominal wall defects can lead to hernia formation with less strenuous activity," said Dr. Michael Abboud. He is chief of surgery at Penn State Health St. Joseph Medical Center in Reading, Pa.

"Hernias may develop in a number of different locations, and can be present at birth or develop later in life, for a number of reasons," Abboud explained in a Penn State news release.

Classically, a hernia is an organ or tissue bulging beyond its normal confines. This can happen when muscle structure has a weak area, such as in the abdominal wall. The contents of the abdomen push through the wall and form a pouch.

People can develop a variety of hernias—inguinal (groin), umbilical (navel area), ventral (abdominal) or incisional (along a prior abdominal incision).

Most that develop over time owe to a loss of integrity in the muscles and tendons that would contain these organs and support the torso, according to Penn State Health. In response to increased pressure, the abdominal wall can rupture at its weakest point. A hernia that has formed may continue to grow.

Genetic or systemic disorders may predispose people to hernia. Hernias can also form when a surgical wound doesn't heal properly.

Risk factors include chronic coughing, smoking, heavy lifting, straining, obesity and pregnancy, according to Penn State Health.

Small hernias can be free of symptoms or can cause pain or discomfort. Patients with a hernia may complain of a bulge somewhere in the abdominal wall. Coughing or straining may aggravate their pain.

Larger hernias can push against the overlying skin, leading to areas of reddening, decreased blood flow or a break in the skin.

Any abdominal hernia can include complications, but many go undetected if they are asymptomatic or until there is a bowel obstruction, according to Penn State Health. Hernias may progress over time, possibly cutting off blood flow.

Patients should see a doctor to determine the nature and severity of their hernia and to discuss whether it should be watched or surgically repaired.

Repair can be done through open surgery or minimally invasive laparoscopic and robotic-assisted surgeries. Open surgery involves creating an incision to repair the hernia using sutures or in combination with mesh.

Approaches are tailored to the patient and clinical condition.

Robotic or laparoscopic approaches offer speedier healing and less pain than open surgery, but limitations and restrictions afterward are often the same, according to Penn State Health.

"In every case, we tailor treatment recommendations to each patient's scenario," Abboud said. "It is important to ensure patients are educated about their diagnosis and treatment options so they feel comfortable with their physician and treatment plan."

Text B   What do you know about your risk for hernia?

SATURDAY, Aug. 27, 2022—Could you be at risk for a hernia?

One expert gives the lowdown on hernias, who is most at risk for them, and how they are typically treated.

Dr. Harvey Rainville, a general surgeon at Hackensack Meridian Mountainside Medical Center in New Jersey, said a hernia is a defect or opening in your muscle layer through which an organ, such as your intestines, can poke through during or after strenuous activity.

Activities such as bowel movements, coughing, sneezing, laughing and bending increase pressure in the abdomen and can force an organ or tissue to squeeze through the opening. It is not uncommon for a hernia to "pop out" and then return to what looks like normal, but a hernia that's disappeared should still be taken seriously, Rainville said in a medical center news release.

Different types of hernias

There are many types of hernias. People can be born with a hernia or develop one. The most common type is an umbilical hernia, which develops through the belly button. This can occur in young people and adults. Belly button hernias can often appear as a protruding belly button. Women can notice this type of hernia when they become pregnant, Rainville noted.

Hernias of the groin (inguinal hernias) are also very common. The groin area has a natural anatomical defect. With too much pressure, that area can dilate and allow the tissue to bulge through.

Hernias are more common in men

Men are much more likely to develop inguinal hernias than women because men have a small hole in their groin muscles for blood vessels to pass through to deliver blood to their testicles, Rainville said.

People who do strenuous work that involves heavy lifting can also develop hernias at a higher rate. Those who work sedentary jobs are at lower risk.

Hernias are not hereditary

Some hernias occur at birth. An umbilical hernia occurs when part of the contents of the abdomen pokes through the abdominal wall inside the belly button. It appears as a bump under the belly button. It's not painful and most umbilical hernias go away on their own by age 4 or 5.

Inguinal hernias will appear as a bump in the groin area, Rainville said. They can occur in newborns.

Hernias can cause symptoms

Constipation, nausea and vomiting are symptoms of a strangulated hernia, which occurs when the blood supply to the herniated tissue is cut off. The strangulated tissue then releases toxins and infection into the bloodstream, which could lead to sepsis or death. Any hernia can become strangulated and cause a medical emergency, Rainville noted.

Hernias used to have a 10% to 15% chance of recurring in patients, but newer surgical techniques have decreased the chance of recurrence to 1% to 2%, but they still can happen. Diabetic patients have a higher risk for hernias, especially if their blood sugar is poorly controlled. People with autoimmune disorders, a highbody mass index, healing issues, or a smoking habit are also more likely to have hernias, Rainville said.

Text C   Herniorrhaphy: What to expect with hernia repair surgery

A hernia is when an organ or tissue protrudes through a weak area of muscle. This is most common in the abdomen. Hernia repair surgery may be called a hernioplasty or herniorrhaphy. During this surgery, the displaced tissue is returned back into the body and the weak spot is stitched or patched up.

Hernia repair surgery is common. It is generally very safe and effective. If you or a loved one are considering this surgery, though, it is important to understand its potential risks and the recovery process.

This article looks at hernia repair surgery and its purpose. It also discusses how to prepare for surgery, what the risks are, and what you should expect while you recover.

What is hernia repair surgery?

Hernia repair surgery is performed by a general surgeon. It is usually done in a hospital or an outpatient surgical center. An outpatient surgical center is a facility that does not require an overnight stay, so you won't have to stay long after hernia surgery unless there are complications.

The surgery may be done in adults and children. It usually takes less than an hour or two.

Hernia repair surgery is done with anesthesia. The type you receive depends on the surgical technique. It may also depend on if the surgery is an emergency or not.

The three types of anesthesia that you may receive include:
1. General anesthesia: This puts you in a sleep-like state.
2. Regional anesthesia: This type is given through the spinal cord. It numbs a large part of your body.
3. Local anesthesia with sedation: This numbs a smaller part of your body. The sedation relaxes you and may or may not make you fall asleep.

The difference between hernioplasty and herniorrhaphy

Herniorrhaphy refers to a surgical technique that relies primarily on sutures to secure herniated tissue in its proper location and strengthen the weakened muscle at the site. Hernioplasty is a different technique that relies primarily on placing synthetic mesh to reinforce the weakened muscle site.

Surgical techniques

Hernias are repaired with one of three types of surgery:
1. Open surgery
2. Laparoscopic surgery
3. Minimally invasive robotic surgery
The technique used is based on several variables. These may include:
1. The size and location of the hernia
2. The patient's age
3. The patient's overall health
During open surgery, the surgeon makes a cut called an incision near the hernia. The bulging tissue is returned back into the body through the incision.

The weak muscle that allowed the hernia to occur is then repaired. It may be stitched back together or, more commonly, patched with a synthetic material called mesh.

During laparoscopic surgery, multiple tiny incisions are made around the hernia. Long, thin surgical tools are inserted through these incisions.

One of these tools has a camera attached to it. The camera projects images onto a TV screen. This lets the surgeon view the inside of the body. Other tools are used to repair the hernia in the same way as with open surgery.

Robotic surgery also involves a camera and the use of very small surgical tools attached to robotic arms. A specially-trained surgeon controls the robotic arms from a viewing screen, which is usually situated in the same room as the operating table.

Open surgery is a more traditional way to repair a hernia. Laparoscopic surgery is generally less painful and often lets patients recover faster.

Hernia repair may be done laparoscopically, robotically, or with open surgery. Laparoscopic surgery typically has a faster recovery time.

Contraindications

There are no absolute contraindications to undergoing hernia repair surgery. This means there are no medical conditions that will exclude you from being able to have hernia surgery.

There may be relative contraindications. These are circumstances that make extra preparation necessary before you can have the surgery. These include:
1. A bleeding disorder
2. Obesity
3. Being a current tobacco user
4. A history of blood clots

Preparing for hernia surgery

Your surgeon will give you instructions on how to prepare for your surgery. These instructions may include:
1. Wear comfortable, loose-fitting clothing on the day of your surgery.
2. Stop taking certain medications for a period of time before surgery. For example, you should avoid taking aspirin or non-steroidal anti-inflammatory medications (NSAIDs) a week before surgery.
3. Stop eating for a period of time prior to surgery. This depends on the surgical technique and type of anesthesia.
4. Arrange for someone to drive you home after the surgery.
5. Pack personal items if a hospital stay is needed. This is not typical.

Hernia surgery: How to prepare

Follow your surgeon's instructions when preparing for your surgery. For example, you will need to avoid NSAIDs in the weeks leading up to your procedure. You may also need to stop eating for a short period before your surgery.

What to expect on the day of surgery

What happens the day of your surgery will depend on certain factors. The steps will vary depending on the type of surgery you will have and which anesthesia you will receive.

If you are having laparoscopic surgery, you can expect the following steps:

1. After you arrive you will change into a gown. Members of your surgical team will meet with you to briefly review the surgery.

2. You will be taken into the operating room. You will be given medication to put you into a sleep-like state.

3. While asleep, the surgeon will inflate your abdomen with air. This makes it easier for the surgeon to see your internal organs and tissues.

4. A small incision will be made at your navel. The surgeon will insert a laparoscope—a long, thin surgical tool with a camera attached to it.

5. The camera will project images onto a TV screen. This lets the surgeon see what is happening inside your body.

6. Additional small incisions will then be made. Other surgical tools will be inserted through these incisions.

7. The surgeon will use the surgical tools to return the bulging tissue back into its place.

8. The surgeon will then stitch or patch the weakness in the abdominal wall.

9. The surgeon will then deflate your abdomen. The small incision sites will be closed with stitches or surgical tape.

After the surgery, you will be moved to a recovery room. You will spend a few hours there while the anesthesia wears off. When symptoms like pain are under control, you will be able to go home.

Recovery from hernia surgery

Recovery time for hernia repair surgery varies depending on what kind of surgery you had. For laparoscopic surgery, it's typically about one to two weeks. For open repair surgery, it's usually about three weeks.

Make sure to follow your surgeon's post-operative instructions. This will help optimize healing and prevent complications. These instructions may include:

1. Use an ice pack or cold compress every couple of hours for 15 minutes. This will help to reduce swelling. Don't put the ice pack directly on your skin.

2. Take Tylenol (acetaminophen) to control pain. If your pain is more significant, you may be prescribed an opioid. Take as directed.

3. Get up and walk around five to six times per day. This will help prevent

blood clots.

4. Wash your hands before and after touching your incisions. This helps to prevent infection.

5. If you had laparoscopic surgery, your surgeon will advise you on how long to avoid strenuous exercise.

When to seek medical attention

Contact your healthcare provider if you notice any of these symptoms while you're recovering:

1. Persistent, severe, or worsening pain

2. Fever

3. Signs of infection from the surgical site like warmth, redness, increased swelling, and/or abnormal drainage

4. Persistent vomiting

5. No bowel movement by day two or three after surgery

Outcomes and long-term care

Hernias will not heal or resolve on their own. The main benefit of surgery is that, in most cases, it fixes the problem. This means that after you recover, you should be able to return to your normal routine and daily life. You should not have pain, discomfort, or a visible bulge.

In most cases, the long-term prognosis for people who have hernia surgeries is good. Inguinal hernia repairs are generally uncomplicated, although about 10% of people will experience chronic pain and there may be recurrence of the hernia.

About one in six people will have a hernia recurrence after certain abdominal wall repairs, with some variation based on the technique used. There are few short-term complications with incisional hernia repair, although less is known about the long-term impacts.

In the long-term, your surgeon will want you to stay healthy. If you have any persistent symptoms, especially pain, let your surgeon know. If you are obese, your surgeon may recommend losing weight to prevent a recurrence.

Potential risks of hernia repair surgery

The main risks of hernia repair surgery include:

1. Bleeding or hematoma. This is when blood collects under the surgical site.

2. Seroma, or fluid collection under the surgical site.

3. Infection, potentially of the surgical site or the surgical mesh used for repair.

4. Chronic postoperative pain.

5. Bowel or urination issues, such as constipation or trouble urinating.

6. Nerve or tissue injury or damage.

7. Hernia recurrence.

All surgeries have some risk. The risks in hernia surgery are low but may include chronic pain, nerve or tissue damage, and hernia recurrence.

A. Translate the following sentences into Chinese.

1. Classically, a hernia is an organ or tissue bulging beyond its normal confines. This can happen when muscle structure has a weak area, such as in the abdominal wall. The contents of the abdomen push through the wall and form a pouch.

2. Any abdominal hernia can include complications, but many go undetected if they are asymptomatic or until there is a bowel obstruction, according to Penn State Health. Hernias may progress over time, possibly cutting off blood flow. Patients should see a doctor to determine the nature and severity of their hernia and to discuss whether it should be watched or surgically repaired.

3. Constipation, nausea and vomiting are symptoms of a strangulated hernia, which occurs when the blood supply to the herniated tissue is cut off. The strangulated tissue then releases toxins and infection into the bloodstream, which could lead to sepsis or death. Any hernia can become strangulated and cause a medical emergency.

4. Hernias used to have a 10% to 15% chance of recurring in patients, but newer surgical techniques have decreased the chance of recurrence to 1% to 2%, but they still can happen. Diabetic patients have a higher risk for hernias, especially if their blood sugar is poorly controlled. People with autoimmune disorders, a highbody mass index, healing issues, or a smoking habit are also more likely to have hernias.

5. Hernias will not heal or resolve on their own. The main benefit of surgery is that, in most cases, it fixes the problem. This means that after you recover, you should be able to return to your normal routine and daily life. You should not have pain, discomfort, or a visible bulge.

B. Prepare a lecture on hernia after doing the further reading above.

扫码获取
提示

Unit 7

Gallstone

I Warming-up

A. Match the following words and phrases with their Chinese translations.

A	laparoscopic surgery	1	胰腺
B	pouch	2	胆总管
C	biliary tree	3	胆固醇
D	digestive enzyme	4	胆道系统
E	cystic duct	5	大便
F	bowel movement	6	消化酶
G	cholesterol	7	分解产物
H	breakdown product	8	贮袋
I	common bile duct	9	腹腔镜
J	pancreas	10	胆囊管

B. Complete the sentences with the following words or phrases in their proper forms.

secrete	to be likely to	break up	in turn
harden	asymptomatic	trap	block

1. These patients are said to be _____ , and these stones are called as " silent stones".
2. The bacterium can also _____ chemicals that inhibit fungal growth，as well as

hormones that stimulate the growth of its host plants.

3. Gallstones form when liquid stored in the gallbladder _____ into pieces of stone-like material.

4. Thankfully，there is a way out of this _____ but it involves striking a subtle balance.

5. The same motivation that can push people to exert more effort in a constructive way could also motivate people _____ more _____ to engage in unethical behaviors.

6. These behavioral changes may _____ be harmful to the health.

7. Bile salts _____ fat，and bilirubin gives bile and stool a yellowish color.

8. Over time，the buildup of plaque deposits can rupture and cause total _____ of the blood flow to the heart.

 C. Watch the video _Gallstone_ and answer the questions.

扫码获取视频

1. What are the typical manifestations of gallstone attack?

2. What are the functions the bile contains?

3. How many types of gallstones are there and what are they?

4. What groups of people are at higher risks of developing gallstones?

5. What is the most common treatment of gallstones?

Ⅱ Dialogue

扫码获取
音频及文本

 A. Listen to the dialogue for the first time and try to get the general idea.

 B. Listen to the dialogue for the second time and try to answer the following questions.

1. What has happened to this patient?

2. What kind of the pain does the patient have?

3. How about the appetite of the patient?

4. Why does the doctor think that ultrasound is better than CT scan?

5. What recommended treatment is if the   patient is diagnosed of gallstone?

C. Choose the following words and/or expressions to complete the sentences in their proper forms.

bloat	胀满	determine	确诊
obstruct	阻塞	vary	改变
bring on	引起,造成	erode	侵蚀
ethnic group	族群	radiographically	放射照相地
radiate	向四周伸展	cholecystectomy	胆囊切除术
refer	牵连	modify	改良,改形

1. Heavy eating seems to _____ the pain.

2. The pain _____ towards my right shoulder, and it's gone through to my back.

3. I went to two parties in succession three days ago. I felt _____.

4. We are going to do some blood tests to _____ if the liver function has changed in any way.

5. However, when a gallstone _____ the bile duct and causes acute cholestasis, a reflexive smooth muscle spasm often occurs.

6. Certain _____ have gallstones more often than others. For example, 48% of Native Americans have gallstones.

7. A person may also experience _____ pain between the shoulder blades or below the right shoulder.

8. Rarely, gallstones in cases of severe inflammation may _____ through the gallbladder into adherent bowel potentially causing an obstruction termed gallstone ileus.

9. Cholesterol stones _____ from light yellow to dark green or brown or chalk white and are oval, usually solitary, between 2 and 3 cm long, each often having a tiny, dark, central spot.

10. Because of their calcium content, they are often _____ visible.

D. Read the dialogue and try to make a conversation with your classmates.

扫码获取
提示

E. Translate the following Chinese into English.

D—Doctor   P—Patient

D: 1. 是什么样性质的疼痛?

    1. _____

P: Colic at first, but soon it became constant with fever.

D: 2. 发热在先还是疼痛在先?

    2. _____

P: The pain.

D: How is your appetite?

P: 3. 我一看见食物就想吐。

    3. _____

D: Have you vomited in the past three days?

P: Yes, about 10 to 15 times. I am in constant pain.

D：Have you vomited blood?

P：No. Just a kind of whitish thick stuff.

D：4. 最近吃得过多或吃得过油吗？你肚子胀吗？

4. _____

_____

P：Yes. I went to two parties in succession three days ago. I felt bloated. Heavy eating seems to bring on the pain.

D：Have you had the pain before when you've overeaten fatty food?

P：Yes，but never as badly as this. Could this be the reason for it?

D：5. 暴饮暴食可引起这些症状。Have your skin and eyeball turned yellow?

5. _____

P：No.

D：Has your stool become light in color?

P：Yes. I found it became clay white yesterday.

D：Has your urine been dark?

P：Yes，just like tea.

D：6. 你家里有没有谁患胆结石?

6. _____

P：Yes，my sister has had a lot of trouble with her gallbladder.

D：I think I'll need to examine you now. 7. 我觉得你有可能有胆结石。We are going to do some blood tests to determine if the liver function has changed in any way，and we are going to do an ultrasound scan.

7. _____

P：8. 超声？难道 CT 不是更好？

8. _____

D：Ultrasound is the best choice to detect gallstones. We can even do it bedside. Doing CT scan is more expensive and the gallstones may not be visible on the scan.

III Further Reading：Gallstone and ERCP

Definitions

Gallstone disease refers to the condition where gallstones are either in the gallbladder or common bile duct. The presence of stones in the gallbladder is referred to as cholelithiasis，from the Greek chol-（bile） + lith-（stone） + -iasis （process）. Presence of gallstones in the common bile duct is called choledocholithiasis，from the Greek chol-（bile） + docho-（duct） + lith-（stone） + iasis-（process）. Choledocholithiasis is frequently associated with obstruction of the bile ducts，which in turn can lead to cholangitis，from the Greek：chol-（bile） + ang-（vessel） + itis-（inflammation），a serious infection of the bile ducts. Gallstones within the ampulla of Vater can obstruct the exocrine system of the pancreas，which in turn can result in pancreatitis.

Most people with gallstones （about 80%） are asymptomatic. However， when a gallstone obstructs the bile duct and causes acute cholestasis, a reflexive smooth muscle spasm often occurs, resulting in an intense cramp-like visceral pain in the right upper part of the abdomen known as a biliary colic (or "gallbladder attack"). This happens in 1%—4% of those with gallstones each year. Complications of gallstones may include inflammation of the gallbladder (cholecystitis), inflammation of the pancreas (pancreatitis), obstructive jaundice, and infection in bile ducts (cholangitis). Symptoms of these complications may include pain of more than five hours duration, fever, yellowish skin, vomiting, dark urine, and pale stools.

In developed countries, 10%—15% of adults have gallstones. Rates in many parts of Africa, however, are as low as 3%. Gallbladder and biliary related diseases occurred in about 104 million people (1.6% of people) in 2013 and they resulted in 106,000 deaths. Women more commonly have stones than men and they occur more commonly after the age of 40. Certain ethnic groups have gallstones more often than others. For example, 48% of Native Americans have gallstones. Once the gallbladder is removed, outcomes are generally good.

Signs and symptoms

Gallstones, regardless of size or number, may be asymptomatic, even for years. Such "silent stones" do not require treatment. A characteristic symptom of a gallstone attack is the presence of colicky pain in the upper-right side of the abdomen, often accompanied by nausea and vomiting. The pain steadily increases for approximately 30 minutes to several hours. A person may also experience referred pain between the shoulder blades or below the right shoulder. Often, attacks occur after a particularly fatty meal and almost always happen at night, and after drinking.

In addition to pain, nausea, and vomiting, a person may experience a fever. If the stones block the duct and cause bilirubin to leak into the bloodstream and surrounding tissue, there may also be jaundice and itching. If this is the case, the liver enzymes are likely to be raised.

Risk factors

Gallstone risk increases for females (especially before menopause) and for people near or above 40 years; the condition is more prevalent among both North and South Americans and people of European descent than among other ethnicities. A lack of melatonin could significantly contribute to gallbladder stones, as melatonin inhibits cholesterol secretion from the gallbladder, and enhances the conversion of cholesterol to bile, as an antioxidant, which is able to reduce oxidative stress to the gallbladder. Researchers believe that gallstones may be caused by a combination of factors, including inherited body chemistry, body weight, gallbladder motility (movement), and low-calorie diet. The absence of such risk factors does not, however, preclude the formation of gallstones.

Nutritional factors that may increase risk of gallstones include constipation; eating fewer meals per day; low intake of the nutrients folate, magnesium, calcium, and vitamin C; low fluid consumption; and, at least for men, a high intake of carbohydrate, a high glycemic load, and high glycemic index diet. Wine and whole-grained bread may decrease the risk of gallstones.

Rapid weight loss increases risk of gallstones. The weight loss drug or list at is known to increase the risk of gallstones.

Cholecystokinin deficiency caused by celiac disease increases risk of gallstone formation, especially when diagnosis of celiac disease is delayed.

Pigment gallstones are most commonly seen in the developing world. Risk factors for pigment stones include hemolytic anemias (such as from sickle-cell disease and hereditary spherocytosis), cirrhosis, and biliary tract infections. People with erythropoietic protoporphyria (EPP) are at increased risk to develop gallstones. Additionally, prolonged use of proton pump inhibitors has been shown to decrease gallbladder function, potentially leading to gallstone formation.

Cholesterol modifying medications can affect gallstone formation. Statins inhibit cholesterol synthesis and there is evidence that their use may decrease the risk of getting gallstones. Fibrates increase cholesterol concentration in bile and their use has been associated with an increased risk of gallstones. Bile acid malabsorption may also be a risk.

The risk of gallstones may be decreased by maintaining a healthy weight with exercise and a healthy diet. If there are no symptoms, treatment is usually not needed. In those who are having gallbladder attacks, surgery to remove the gallbladder is typically recommended. This can be carried out either through several small incisions or through a single larger incision, usually under general anesthesia. In rare cases when surgery is not possible, medication can be used to dissolve the stones or lithotripsy to break them down.

Composition of gallstones

The composition of gallstones is affected by age, diet and ethnicity. On the basis of their composition, gallstones can be divided into the following types: cholesterol stones, pigment stones, and mixed stones. An ideal classification system is yet to be defined.

Cholesterol stones

Cholesterol stones vary from light yellow to dark green or brown or chalk white and are oval, usually solitary, between 2 and 3 cm long, each often having a tiny, dark, central spot. To be classified as such, they must be at least 80% cholesterol by weight (or 70%, according to the Japanese-classification system). Between 35% and 90% of stones are cholesterol stones.

Pigment stones

Bilirubin ("pigment", "black pigment") stones are small, dark (often appearing black), and usually numerous. They are composed primarily of bilirubin (insoluble bilirubin pigment polymer) and calcium (calcium phosphate) salts that are found in bile. They contain less than 20% of cholesterol (or 30%, according to the Japanese-classification system). Between 2% and 30% of stones are bilirubin stones.

Mixed stones

Mixed (brown pigment stones) stones typically contain 20%—80% cholesterol (or 30%—70%, according to the Japanese-classification system). Other common constituents are calcium carbonate, palmitate phosphate, bilirubin and other bile pigments (calcium bilirubinate, calcium palmitate and calcium stearate). Because of their calcium content, they are often radiographically visible. They typically arise secondary to infection of the biliary tract which results in the release of β-glucuronidase (by injured hepatocytes and bacteria) which hydrolyzes bilirubin glucuronides and increases the amount of unconjugated bilirubin in bile. Between 4% and 20% of stones are mixed.

Gallstones can vary in size and shape from as small as a grain of sand to as large as a golf ball. The gallbladder may contain a single large stone or many smaller ones. Pseudoliths, sometimes referred to as sludge, are thick secretions that may be present within the gallbladder, either alone or in conjunction with fully formed gallstones.

Diagnosis

Diagnosis is typically confirmed by abdominal ultrasound. Other imaging techniques used are ERCP and MRCP. Gallstone complications may be detected on blood tests.

A positive Murphy's sign is a common finding on physical examination during a gallbladder attack.

Surgical treatment

Cholecystectomy (gallbladder removal) has a 99% chance of eliminating the recurrence of cholelithiasis. The lack of a gallbladder may have no negative consequences in many people. However, there is a portion of the population— between 10% and 15%—who develop a condition called post-cholecystectomy syndrome which may cause nausea, indigestion, diarrhea, and episodes of abdominal pain.

There are two surgical options for cholecystectomy:

Open cholecystectomy is performed via an abdominal incision (laparotomy) below the lower right ribs. Recovery typically requires 3—5 days of hospitalization, with a return to normal diet a week after release and to normal activity several weeks after release.

Laparoscopic cholecystectomy, introduced in the 1980s, is performed via three to four small puncture holes for a camera and instruments. Post-operative care typically includes a same-day release or a one-night hospital stay, followed by a few days of home rest and pain medication.

Obstruction of the common bile duct with gallstones can sometimes be relieved by endoscopic retrograde sphincterotomy (ERS) following endoscopic retrograde cholangiopancreatography (ERCP).

Medical treatment

Cholesterol gallstones can sometimes be dissolved with ursodeoxycholic acid taken by mouth, but it may be necessary for the person to take this medication for years.

Traditional medicine

Gallstones can be a valued by-product of animals butchered for meat because of their use as an antipyretic and antidote in the traditional medicine of some cultures, particularly, in traditional Chinese medicine. The most highly prized gallstones tend to be sourced from old dairy cows, termed calculus bovis or *niu-huang* (yellow thing of cattle) in Chinese. Some slaughter houses carefully scrutinize workers for gallstone theft.

Endoscopic retrograde cholangiopancreatography (ERCP)

Endoscopic retrograde cholangiopancreatography (ERCP) is a technique that combines the use of endoscopy and fluoroscopy to diagnose and treat certain problems of the biliary or pancreatic ductal systems. It is primarily performed by highly skilled and specialty trained gastroenterologists. Through the endoscope, the physician can see the inside of the stomach and duodenum, and inject a contrast medium into the ducts in the biliary tree and pancreas so they can be seen on radiographs.

ERCP is used primarily to diagnose and treat conditions of the bile ducts and main pancreatic duct, including gallstones, inflammatory strictures (scars), leaks (from trauma and surgery), and cancer. ERCP can be performed for diagnostic and therapeutic reasons, although the development of safer and relatively non-invasive investigations such as magnetic resonance cholangiopancreatography (MRCP) and endoscopic ultrasound has meant that ERCP is now rarely performed without therapeutic intent.

Procedure

The patient is sedated or anaesthetized. Then a flexible camera (endoscope) is inserted through the mouth, down the esophagus, into the stomach, through the pylorus into the duodenum where the ampulla of Vater (the union of the common bile duct and pancreatic duct) exists. The sphincter of Oddi is a muscular valve that controls the opening to the ampulla. The region can be directly visualized with the endoscopic camera while various procedures are performed. A plastic catheter or cannula is inserted through the ampulla, and radiocontrast is injected into the bile ducts and/or pancreatic duct. Fluoroscopy is used to look for blockages, or other lesions such as stones.

When needed, the sphincters of the ampulla and bile ducts can be enlarged by a cut (sphincterotomy) with an electrified wire called a sphincterotome for access into either so that gallstones may be removed or other therapy performed.

Other procedures associated with ERCP include the trawling of the common bile duct with a basket or balloon to remove gallstones and the insertion of a plastic stent to assist the drainage of bile. Also, the pancreatic duct can be cannulated and stents be inserted. The pancreatic duct requires visualization in cases of pancreatitis.

In specific cases, other specialized or ancillary endoscopes may be used for ERCP. These include mother-daughter and SpyGlass cholangioscopes (to help in diagnosis by directly visualizing the duct as opposed to only obtaining X-ray images) as well as balloon enteroscopes (e. g. in patients with post-Whipple or Roux-en-Y surgical anatomy).

Risks

One of the most frequent and feared complications after endoscopic retrograde cholangiopancreatography (ERCP) is post-ERCP pancreatitis (PEP). In previous studies, the incidence of PEP has been estimated at 3.5% to 5%. According to Cotton et al., PEP is defined as a "clinical pancreatitis with amylase at least three times the upper limit of normal at more than 24 hours after the procedure requiring hospital admission or prolongation of planned admission". Grading of severity of PEP is mainly based on the length of hospital stay.

Risk factors for developing PEP include technical matters related to the ERCP procedure and patient-specific ones. The technical factors include manipulation of and injection of contrast into the pancreatic duct, cannulation attempts lasting more than five minutes, and biliary balloon sphincter dilation; among patient-related factors are female gender, younger age, and Sphincter of Oddi dysfunction. A systematic review of clinical trials concluded that a previous history of PEP or pancreatitis significantly increases the risk for PEP to 17.8% and to 5.5% respectively.

Intestinal perforation is a risk of any gastroenterological endoscopic procedure, and is an additional risk if a sphincterotomy is performed. As the second part of the duodenum is anatomically in a retroperitoneal location (that is, behind the peritoneal structures of the abdomen), perforations due to sphincterotomies are retroperitoneal. Sphincterotomy is also associated with a risk of bleeding.

There is also a risk associated with the contrast dye in patients who are allergic to compounds containing iodine. Oversedation can result in dangerously low blood pressure, respiratory depression, nausea, and vomiting. Other complications (less than 1%) may include heart and lung problems, infection in the bile duct called cholangitis. Using antibiotics before the procedure shows some benefits to prevent cholangitis and septicemia. In rare cases, ERCP can cause fatal complications.

A. Translate the following sentences into Chinese.

1. Gallstones, regardless of size or number, may be asymptomatic, even for years. Such "silent stones" do not require treatment. A characteristic symptom of a gallstone attack is the presence of colicky pain in the upper-right side of the abdomen, often accompanied by nausea and vomiting.

2. The patient is sedated or anaesthetized. Then a flexible camera (endoscope) is inserted through the mouth, down the esophagus, into the stomach, through the pylorus into the duodenum where the ampulla of Vater (the union of the common bile duct and pancreatic duct) exists.

3. Endoscopic retrograde cholangiopancreatography (ERCP) is a technique that combines the use of endoscopy and fluoroscopy to diagnose and treat certain problems of the biliary or pancreatic ductal systems. It is primarily performed by highly skilled and specialty trained gastroenterologists.

4. Cholecystectomy (gallbladder removal) has a 99% chance of eliminating the recurrence of cholelithiasis. The lack of a gallbladder may have no negative consequences in many people. However, there is a portion of the population—between 10% and 15%—who develop a condition called post-cholecystectomy syndrome which may cause nausea, indigestion, diarrhea, and episodes of abdominal pain.

5. Diagnosis is typically confirmed by abdominal ultrasound. Gallstone complications may be detected on blood tests. A positive Murphy's sign is a common finding on physical examination during a gallbladder attack.

B. Prepare a lecture on gallstone after doing the further reading above.

扫码获取
提示

Unit 8

Preoperative Anesthesiology Visit

Ⅰ   Warming-up

A. Match the following words and phrases with their Chinese translations.

A	one-lung ventilation	1	术中知晓
B	extracorporeal circulation	2	局部麻醉
C	malignant hyperthermia	3	四个成串刺激
D	local anesthesia	4	体外循环
E	postoperative cognition impairment	5	肺泡最低有效浓度
F	train-of-four stimulation	6	困难气道
G	minimum alveolar concentration	7	全身麻醉
H	intraoperative awareness	8	单肺通气术
I	difficult airway	9	术后认知功能障碍
J	general anesthesia	10	恶性高热

B. Complete the sentences with the following words or phrases in their proper forms.

local	such as	available	at times	specialize in
in order to	branch	responsible	depend on	critical

1. Numerous medications are _____ for the anesthesiologist to select from, and part of the anesthesiology training is knowing which medication suits which patient for any given procedure.

2. Anesthesiology is _____ in every surgical procedure, but especially in complex surgeries such as open heart.

3. Anesthesiology is a medical specialty that is practiced by physicians who _____ anesthesia, pain management, and critical care medicine.

4. Pediatric anesthesiologists are _____ for the general anesthesia, sedation, and pain management needs of infants and children.

5. If you're having a relatively simple procedure like a tooth extraction that requires numbing a small area, the person performing your procedure can administer the _____ anesthetic.

6. Regional anesthesia blocks pain in a larger part of your body, _____ a limb or everything below your chest.

7. Many physician anesthesiologists undergo special fellowship training _____ provide specialized care for patients undergoing surgery on the heart, lungs, or major blood vessels.

8. Indeed, it could be said that anesthesiology is the _____ of medicine that comes the closest to causing clinical death and resurrection on the operating table.

9. _____ her general health, and what procedure the surgeon will perform, the anesthesiologist will determine whether she needs general or total anesthesia, or if an epidural can be given to block the pain.

10. Pain includes a wide spectrum of disorders such as acute pain, chronic pain, and cancer-related pain, and _____ it may reflect a combination of all three.

C. Watch the video *Anesthesiology—Preoperative Assessment* and answer the questions.

扫码获取视频

1. What kind of anesthesia is going to be talked about in this lecture?

2. At what point will the surgery be canceled?

3. What do we ask about and what do we do when we see the patients prior to the surgery?

4. What family history of anesthetic problems should we get?

5. How can the Mallampati score be done?

扫码获取
音频及文本

Ⅱ Dialogue

 A. Listen to the dialogue for the first time and try to get the general idea.

 B. Listen to the dialogue for the second time and try to answer the following questions.

1. When will the patient's operation be scheduled?

2. Why does the doctor arrange an interview to the patient before the operation?

3. What chronic disease does the patient have?

4. What kind of anesthesia does the doctor suggest to the patient?

5. What will the doctor provide the patient with during the surgery?

C. Choose the following words and/or expressions to complete the sentences in their proper forms.

vital statistics	重要数据	pain management	疼痛处理
hypertension	高血压	clinical	临床的
more than	超出	get ... through ...	做完
play a role in	在……扮演一个角色	cesarean delivery	剖宫产
block ... from ...	阻止	central nervous system	中枢神经系统
aroused	唤醒	determine	决定

1. Anesthesiology is a medical specialty that is practiced by physicians who specialize in anesthesia, _____, and critical care medicine.

2. General anesthesia can suppress _____ activity and cause you to be unaware, or "asleep", during surgery.

3. We will provide a secure airway, control breathing, place various lines used to closely monitor you during surgery, and administer the fluids and other drugs necessary to _____ you safely _____ the operation.

4. Since the elderly often do not tolerate general anesthesia very well, the anesthesiologist may determine that an epidural will _____ the pain _____ the surgery, but still maintain the patient's consciousness.

5. Physician anesthesiologists provide or guide nearly 90 percent of the anesthetics used in the _____ 100 million procedures performed every year in the United States.

6. An anesthesiologist will often have a particular set of nurses and technicians who work with only that doctor during the surgery，and monitor the patient's _____.

7. Cardiac patients frequently have additional medical problems such as _____, diabetes or lung disease，which can complicate medical management.

8. Obstetric anesthesia refers to anesthetic and pain-relieving care performed during labor and vaginal delivery or _____.

9. Physicians who specialize in critical care medicine _____ pivotal _____ improving patient outcomes and caring for critically ill patients who often have multiple illnesses.

10. Sedation relaxes you to the point where you will have a more natural sleep，but can be easily _____ or awakened.

D. Read the dialogue and try to make a conversation with your classmates.

扫码获取
提示

E. Translate the following Chinese into English.

N—Nurse   P—Patient   D—Doctor

N：Hi，Mr. Smith. This is Dr. Gao, anesthesiologist. He will be responsible for your surgery tomorrow.

N：Dr. Gao，this is Mr. Smith.

D：Good afternoon，Mr. Smith. How are you feeling?

P：Not bad，doctor.

D：1. Smith 先生，你知道被安排在明天进行手术吗？

1. _____

P：Yes，but what time am I going to have it?

D：The operation starts at 8:30. Nurse Ramit and I will provide anesthesia for you. 2. 因此，我们安排了这次访视，希望能了解你的病史和其他情况。Mr. Smith，can we do this now?

2. _____
_____

P：Of course，doctor.

D：3. 你是否有慢性病史？比如：高血压、慢性支气管炎、糖尿病。

3. _____

P：Yes，I have had hypertension for more than 20 years.

D：What about your blood pressure?

P：It used to be around 150/95 mmHg.

D：Oh，it seems to be high. What kind of medicine did you take for hypertension?

P：I took metoprolol tablet 12.5 mg every day.

D：OK，you still should drink it tomorrow morning. But you should have absolutely nothing by mouth after midnight except the metoprolol tablet.

P：Yes sir.

D：Did you have any surgery before?

P：Yes，I had a cholecystectomy 5 years ago.

D：You have had a cholecystectomy 5 years ago. Tell me something about it.

P：4. 我得过胆石症，被安排做手术。手术太可怕了，我觉得很痛。

4. _____
_____

D：Are you sure? Could you remember what

type of anesthesia was used at that time?

P: I do not know. The doctor punctured my back and injected something in it.

D: Oh, an epidural anesthesia. Since you had a failed experience with local anesthesia, I professionally suggest you accept general anesthesia for your operation.

P: 5. 天呐,全麻是什么? 我会不会再遭罪?

5. _____

D: Take it easy, Mr. Smith. We will be taking excellent care of you. General anesthesia can suppress central nervous system activity and cause you to be unaware, "asleep" during surgery. 6. 我们会放置一个气道,控制你的呼吸, place various lines used to closely monitor you during surgery, and administer the fluids and other drugs necessary to get you safely through the operation.

6. _____

P: I hope so. Thank you, doctor.

D: How about your family members? I mean their health status.

P: They are okay.

D: 7. 他们中有麻醉不良反应史吗?

7. _____

P: No, never.

D: Did you take any other medicine except metoprolol?

P: I took atorvastatin and bayaspirin regularly.

D: Do you take bayaspirin now?

P: No, I don't. My surgeon told me to stop it 5 days ago.

D: OK.

D: 8. 好的。你有药物或食物过敏史吗? 比如麻醉药、抗生素、海鲜或者花粉。

8. _____

_____

P: Nothing, doctor.

III Further Reading: Anesthesiology and Anesthesia

Text A

What is anesthesiology?

Anesthesiology is the study and practice of administering sedation and/or anesthesia to a living creature for the purpose of blocking pain. There are anesthesiologists who practice on animals and those who treat humans. Anesthesiology is, to many people, a rather mysterious and even spooky field of medicine. Who knows what actually happens to a person when they are "put under"? Indeed, it could be said that anesthesiology is the branch of medicine that comes the closest to causing clinical death and resurrection on the operating table.

An anesthesiologist specializes in the field after undergoing the usual medical school education and residency. Most doctors have general training in anesthesiology, but like all medical specialties, additional study and a residency in that field is required for certification. The main goal of anesthesiology is to prevent a patient from feeling pain. Thus, an anesthesiologist may also be involved in a patient's pain management after surgery. He or she will also often recommend the best method of anesthesia, depending on the procedure, since not every method is suited for every procedure on every patient.

Numerous medications are available for the anesthesiologist to select from, and part of the anesthesiology training is knowing which medication suits which patient for any given procedure. Age, height, weight and general health are all factors. For example, the patient may be an elderly woman with a broken hip. Depending on her general health, and what procedure the surgeon will perform, the anesthesiologist will determine whether she needs general or total anesthesia, or if an epidural can be given to block the pain. Since the elderly often do not tolerate general anesthesia very well, the anesthesiologist may determine that an epidural will block the pain from the surgery, but still maintain the patient's consciousness.

Anesthesiology is critical in every surgical procedure, but especially in complex surgeries such as open heart. The heart may need to be completely stopped, and this is the anesthesiologist's job. He or she will often have a particular set of nurses and technicians who work with only that doctor during the surgery, and monitor the patient's vital statistics.

A good anesthesiologist will also visit the patient before and after surgery. This helps him or her determine what methods of anesthesia to use, and also allows the doctor to observe how well the patient tolerated the anesthesia. This could be crucial knowledge for further treatment and other surgical procedures. Spooky or not, anesthesiology is a necessary branch of medicine.

Pain management: Many physician anesthesiologists specialize in diagnosing, managing, and treating pain. Pain includes a wide spectrum of disorders such as acute pain, chronic pain, and cancer-related pain, and at times it may reflect a combination of all three. Since the field of medicine continues to learn more about the complexities of pain, it has become more important to have physicians who have specialized knowledge and skills to treat these conditions. An in-depth knowledge of physiology of pain, the ability to evaluate patients with complicated pain problems, proper prescription of medications, and skills to perform procedures (such as nerve blocks, electrical stimulation, and spinal injections) are all part of how a pain management specialist treats pain.

Critical care: Physicians who specialize in critical care medicine play a pivotal role in improving patient outcomes and caring for critically ill patients who often have multiple illnesses. These physicians possess the medical knowledge and technical expertise to deal with many emergency and trauma situations in the ICU. Critical care anesthesiologists provide airway management, cardiac and pulmonary resuscitation, advanced life support and pain control, all of which are essential skills to the intensivist. As consultants, they play an active role in stabilizing and preparing the patient for emergency surgery and overseeing recovery afterward.

Text B　Anesthesia

Anesthesia is a treatment using drugs called anesthetics. These drugs keep you from feeling pain during medical procedures. Anesthesiologists are medical doctors who administer anesthesia and manage pain. Some anesthesia numbs a small area of the body. General anesthesia makes you unconscious (asleep) during invasive surgical procedures.

What is anesthesia?

Anesthesia is a medical treatment that keeps you from feeling pain during procedures or surgery. The medications used to block pain are called anesthetics. Different types of anesthesia work in different ways. Some anesthetic medications numb certain parts of the body, while other medications numb the brain, to induce a sleep through more invasive surgical procedures, like those within the head, chest, or abdomen.

How does anesthesia work?

Anesthesia temporarily blocks sensory/pain signals from nerves to the centers in the brain. Your peripheral nerves connect the spinal cord to the rest of your body.

Who performs anesthesia?

If you're having a relatively simple procedure like a tooth extraction that requires numbing a small area, the person performing your procedure can administer the local anesthetic. For more complex and invasive procedures, your anesthetic will be administered by a physician anesthesiologist. This medical doctor manages your pain before, during and after surgery. In addition to your physician anesthesiologist, your anesthesia team can be comprised of physicians in training (fellows or residents), a certified registered nurse anesthetist (CRNA), or a certified anesthesiologist assistant (CAA).

What are the types of anesthesia?

The anesthesia your healthcare provider uses depends on the type and scope of the procedure. Options include:

Local anesthesia: This treatment numbs a small section of the body. Examples of procedures in which local anesthesia could be used include cataract surgery, a dental procedure or skin biopsy. You're awake during the procedure.

Regional anesthesia: Regional anesthesia blocks pain in a larger part of your body, such as a limb or everything below your chest. You can be conscious during the procedure, or have sedation in addition to the regional anesthetic. Examples include an epidural to ease the pain of childbirth or during a cesarean section (C-section), a spinal for hip or knee surgery, or an arm block for hand surgery.

General anesthesia: This treatment makes you unconscious and insensitive to pain or other stimuli. General anesthesia is used for more invasive surgical procedures, or procedures of the head, chest, or abdomen.

Sedation: Sedation relaxes you to the point where you will have a more natural sleep, but can be easily aroused or awakened. Light sedation can be prescribed by the person performing your procedure, or together with a regular nurse, if they both have training to provide moderate sedation. Examples of procedures performed with light or moderate sedation include cardiac catheterization and some colonoscopies. Deep sedation is provided by an anesthesia professional because your breathing may be affected with the stronger anesthetic medications, but you will be more asleep than with light or moderate sedation. Although you won't be completely unconscious, you are not as likely to remember the procedure.

How is anesthesia administered?

Depending on the procedure and type of anesthesia needed, your healthcare provider may deliver the anesthesia via:
1. Inhaled gas.
2. Injection, including shots or intravenously (IV).
3. Topical (applied to skin or eyes) liquid, spray or patch.

How should I prepare for anesthesia?

Make sure your healthcare provider has a current list of the medications and supplements (vitamins and herbal medications) you take. Certain drugs can interact with anesthesia or cause bleeding and increase the risk of complications. You should also:
1. Avoid food and drinks for eight hours before you go to the hospital unless directed otherwise.
2. Quit smoking, even if it's just for one day before the procedure, to improve heart and lung health. The most beneficial effects are seen with no smoking for two weeks before.

3. Stop taking herbal supplements for one to two weeks before the procedure as directed by your provider.

4. Not take any medications for erectile dysfunction at least 24 hours before the procedure.

5. You should take certain (but not all) blood pressure medications with a sip of water as instructed by your healthcare provider.

What happens during anesthesia?

A physician anesthesiologist:

1. Administers one type or a combination of anesthetics listed above pain therapies, and possibly anti-nausea medications.

2. Monitors vital signs, including blood pressure, blood oxygen level, pulse and heart rate.

3. Identifies and manages problems, such as an allergic reaction or a change in vital signs.

4. Provides postsurgical pain management.

What should I do after getting anesthesia?

For procedures using local anesthesia, you can return to work or most activities after treatment unless your healthcare provider says otherwise. You'll need more time to recover if you've received regional or general anesthesia or sedation. You should:

1. Have someone drive you home.
2. Rest for the remainder of the day.
3. Not drive or operate equipment for 24 hours.
4. Abstain from alcohol for 24 hours.
5. Only take medications or supplements approved by your provider.
6. Avoid making any important or legal decisions for 24 hours.

What are the potential side effects of anesthesia?

Most anesthesia side effects are temporary and go away within 24 hours, often sooner. Depending on the anesthesia type and how providers administer it, you may experience:

1. Back pain or muscle pain.
2. Chills caused by low body temperature (hypothermia).
3. Difficulty urinating.
4. Fatigue.
5. Headache.
6. Itching.
7. Nausea and vomiting.

8. Pain, tenderness, redness or bruising at the injection site.

9. Sore throat (pharyngitis).

What are the potential risks or complications of anesthesia?

Every year, millions of Americans safely receive anesthesia while undergoing medical procedures. However, anesthesia does carry some degree of risk. Potential complications include:

1. Anesthetic awareness: For unknown reasons, about one out of every 1,000 people who receive general anesthesia experience awareness during a procedure. You may be aware of your surroundings but unable to move or communicate.

2. Collapsed lung (atelectasis): Surgery that uses general anesthesia or a breathing tube can cause a collapsed lung. This rare problem occurs when air sacs in the lung deflate or fill with fluid.

3. Malignant hyperthermia: People who have malignant hyperthermia (MH) experience a dangerous reaction to anesthesia. This rare inherited syndrome causes fever and muscle contractions during surgery. It is important to relate a personal or family history of MH to your physician anesthesiologist before your anesthetic to avoid drugs that trigger this reaction.

4. Nerve damage: Although rare, some people experience nerve damage that causes temporary or permanent neuropathic pain, numbness, or weakness.

5. Postoperative delirium: Older people are more prone to postoperative delirium. This condition causes confusion that comes and goes for about a week. Some people experience long-term memory and learning problems. This condition is known as postoperative cognitive dysfunction.

Who is at risk for anesthesia complications?

Certain factors make it riskier to receive anesthesia, including:

1. Advanced age.

2. Diabetes or kidney disease.

3. Family history of malignant hyperthermia (anesthesia allergy).

4. Heart disease, high blood pressure (hypertension) or strokes.

5. Lung disease, such as asthma or chronic obstructive pulmonary disease (COPD).

6. Obesity (high body mass index or BMI).

7. Seizures or neurological disorders.

8. Sleep apnea.

9. Smoking.

How long does it take to recover from anesthesia?

Anesthetic drugs can stay in your system for up to 24 hours. If you've had sedation or regional or general anesthesia, you shouldn't return to work or drive until the drugs have left your body. After local anesthesia, you should be able to resume normal activities, as long as your healthcare provider says it's okay.

When should I call the healthcare provider?

You should call your healthcare provider if you've had anesthesia and experience:
1. Difficulty breathing.
2. Extreme itching, hives or swelling.
3. Numbness or paralysis anywhere in your body.
4. Slurred speech.
5. Trouble swallowing.

How does anesthesia affect pregnancy?

Local anesthesia affects a small area of the body. It's considered safe for pregnant or breastfeeding women. Many pregnant women safely receive regional anesthesia, such as an epidural or spinal block, during childbirth. Your healthcare provider may recommend postponing elective procedures that require regional or general anesthesia until after childbirth.

How does anesthesia affect breastfeeding?

Anesthesia is considered safe for breastfeeding mothers and their babies. Medications used in all types of anesthesia, including general anesthesia, leave the system quickly. It is often recommended for patients to express their first breast milk after a general anesthetic before resuming breast feeding their infant.

A. Translate the following sentences into Chinese.

1. Anesthesiology is the study and practice of administering sedation and/or anesthesia to a living creature for the purpose of blocking pain. There are anesthesiologists who practice on animals and those who treat humans. Anesthesiology is, to many people, a rather mysterious and even spooky field of medicine.

2. Ananesthesiologist specializes in the field after undergoing the usual medical school education and residency. Most doctors have general training in anesthesiology, but like all medical specialties, additional study and a residency in that field is required for certification.

3. Many physician anesthesiologists specialize in diagnosing, managing, and treating pain. Pain includes a wide spectrum of disorders such as acute pain, chronic pain, and cancer-related pain, and at times it may reflect a combination of all three.

4. If you're having a relatively simple procedure like a tooth extraction that requires numbing a small area, the person performing your procedure can administer the local anesthetic. For more complex and invasive procedures, your anesthetic will be administered by a physician anesthesiologist.

5. Regional anesthesia blocks pain in a larger part of your body, such as a limb or everything below your chest. You can be conscious during the procedure, or have sedation in addition to the regional anesthetic. Examples include anepidural to ease the pain of childbirth or during a cesarean section (C-section), a spinal for hip or knee surgery, or an arm block for hand surgery.

B. Prepare a lecture on anesthesia after doing the further reading above.

扫码获取
提示

Unit 9

Gynecological Check-up

I Warming-up

A. Match the following words and phrases with their Chinese translations.

A	teenager	1	令人尴尬的,令人难堪的
B	gynecologist	2	使人尴尬,使人窘迫
C	for the first time	3	侵入的
D	obstetrician	4	青少年
E	embarrass	5	痛经
F	awkward	6	妇科医生
G	invasive	7	月经不调
H	acne	8	首次
I	irregular periods	9	粉刺,青春痘
J	painful periods	10	产科医生

B. Complete the sentences with the following words or phrases in their proper forms.

unpleasant	reproductive	gynecologist	awkward
embarrass	invasive	health and wellness	nutrition

1. All _____ surgeries require a recovery period，and alcohol only tends to impede this
   process.

2. He wished them "Good morning" in an _____ hesitating undertone as if he were doubtful how his greetings would be received.

3. German researchers have found that sleepers exposed to an _____ smell will have negative dreams.

4. Not only did he not help me get up or ask if I was okay, he got mad at me for _____ him in public.

5. Far from making progress we seem to have been going backward since the notion of _____ health was born.

6. The focus flipped from the emphasis on disease to preventive medicine, _____ , and subsequently, healthy aging.

7. If you notice a bad smell or think you may have an infection, see a doctor or _____ right away.

8. You may want to ask your doctor to refer you to a dietitian or nutritionist for specific _____ advice and guidance.

 C. Watch the video *Tips for Your Teenager's First Gynecologist Visit* and answer the questions.

扫码获取视频

1. When should a teenager see a gynecologist for the first time?

2. What do teenage patients and even their mom think about first OBGYN exam?

3. What should a teenage girl speak to a woman's health expert?

4. What issues will a gynecologist discuss with a teenage girl?

5. What are mom and dad encouraged to talk to their teenage daughter about?

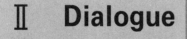 **Ⅱ Dialogue**

扫码获取
音频及文本

A. Listen to the dialogue for the first time and try to get the general idea.

B. Listen to the dialogue for the second time and try to answer the following questions.

1. When was the patient's last period?

2. Does the patient have a regular menstrual cycle?

3. How long do the patient's periods last?

4. What does the patient think about the amount of her periods?

5. Does the patient notice any pain or swelling in her breasts?

C. Choose the following words and/or expressions to complete the sentences in their proper forms.

up-tight	心情焦躁的、紧张的、易怒的	foul-smelling	有臭味的
pain and discomfort	疼痛而不适	itchy	痒
tension	紧张，焦虑	yellowish	微黄色的，淡黄色的
sound like	听上去像	swelling	肿块，肿胀处；肿胀
moderate	中等的	feel as though	觉得，仿佛，好像
have a smear test	做了涂片	pop up	突然出现

1. Headaches can tell you that they make you _____ every hair on your head is about to blow up.

2. Although surgery is not always a cure, it is often the best way to stop the spread of disease and alleviate _____ .

3. I curled _____ as something scrambled part way into the hole and bumped into my feet.

4. Those with mild to _____ depression indulge in up to a third more sexual activity than others, whether they are in a relationship or not.

5. If the _____ is sudden or moves to your hands and face, it may be a sign of a more serious condition called preeclampsia.

6. I had a range of blood tests including HIV, but I did not _____ and while we awaited the results we went shopping.

7. It _____ a great story. And I'm late for a doctor's appointment. Anne and I have to see the doctor about the baby.

8. PID can resemble gonorrhea, with abdominal and lower pelvic pain, chills, nausea, fever, and thick, _____ vaginal discharge.

9. Food allergy can take the form of a sudden life-threatening reaction known as anaphylaxis, as well as eczema or an _____ rash.

10. I've never seen any sign of _____ between them, and if it keeps going the way it's going, they'll be together for life.

D. Read the dialogue and try to make a conversation with your classmates.

扫码获取
提示

E. Translate the following Chinese into English.

P—Patient   D—Doctor

D：1. 请告诉我你上次月经是什么时候？

　　1. ＿＿＿＿＿＿＿＿＿＿＿＿＿

P：It was about 3 weeks ago.

D：2. 月经规律吗？

　　2. ＿＿＿＿＿＿＿＿＿＿＿＿＿

P：Yes，it's quite regular. It comes about every 28 days.

D：3. 来月经疼吗？

　　3. ＿＿＿＿＿＿＿＿＿＿＿＿＿

P：4. 前 2 到 3 天，有些不舒服，但不是太疼。不过，在来月经前，我会比较急躁，情绪不易控制。

　　4. ＿＿＿＿＿＿＿＿＿＿＿＿＿

　　＿＿＿＿＿＿＿＿＿＿＿＿＿＿

　　＿＿＿＿＿＿＿＿＿＿＿＿＿＿

D：Sounds like typical pre-menstrual tension （PMT）. It's difficult to treat but some people are helped by vitamin B_{12}.

D：5. 过去三年有没有做过宫颈涂片检查？

　　5. ＿＿＿＿＿＿＿＿＿＿＿＿＿

P：I had one done about 5 years ago，doctor.

D：6. 记得结果吗？

　　6. ＿＿＿＿＿＿＿＿＿＿＿＿＿

P：Yes，they said it was clear.

D：7. 你注意到乳房有疼痛或者肿块么？

　　7. ＿＿＿＿＿＿＿＿＿＿＿＿＿

P：8. 没有。但是，在来月经前，乳房会有胀痛感。

　　8. ＿＿＿＿＿＿＿＿＿＿＿＿＿

　　＿＿＿＿＿＿＿＿＿＿＿＿＿＿

Ⅲ Further Reading：Gynecologic Cancers

Overview

Most women have had a Pap smear，which is a routine screening test for cervical cancer that's performed during a check-up with the OB/GYN or general practitioner. Cervical cancer is only one of several cancers that can occur in a woman's reproductive organs （known as gynecologic cancers）. Knowing a bit about these conditions is helpful in keeping them in check.

A woman's reproductive system is centered on the uterus （including the cervix），which is also known as the womb. The ovaries attach to the top of the uterus，and the vagina connects the uterus to the outside of the body. The external genitals are called the vulva. Gynecologic cancers result from the rapid

Unit 9 Gynecological Check-up   **97**

growth and spread of abnormal cells in one of these organs.

Compared to other types of cancer (like breast or colon cancer), gynecologic cancers are uncommon, occurring in about 100,000 women in the United States each year. That said, all women are at risk for developing gynecologic cancers, and the risk increases with age. It's important to know the warning signs, as treatments are most effective when the cancer is found at an early stage.

"There are so many different diseases that fall under the umbrella of gynecologic cancer, and each one can be very different in terms of the types of treatments and where we go from the initial diagnosis," says Gloria Huang, MD, FACOG, a Yale Medicine gynecologic oncologist.

But gynecologic cancers are often treatable. "Some of these present as pre-cancers that are easily treated when detected early," she says. "Even many early-stage cancers, such as stage I endometrial cancer, are cured just with surgery alone, the vast majority of the time."

What are the types of gynecologic cancers, and who's at risk?

There are five major types:
- Cervical cancer
- Uterine (endometrial) cancer
- Ovarian cancer
- Vaginal cancer
- Vulvar cancer

The following factors may increase your risk of developing gynecologic cancer:

Human papillomavirus (HPV): Cervical, vaginal and vulvar cancers are often linked to HPV, a common sexually transmitted infection. For this reason, practicing safe sex (using a condom) is a key strategy for prevention. An HPV vaccine is available for girls and young women (between the ages of 11 and 26).

Age: Older age is another known risk factor. For example, the average patient with uterine cancer is 63 years old at diagnosis.

Genetics: Up to 10% of patients with ovarian cancer have a family history of the disease. A woman whose mother, daughter or sister had ovarian, Fallopian tube or primary peritoneal cancer might choose to undergo genetic testing for mutations in the BRCA1 and BRCA2 genes. Mutations in these genes can increase your risk for ovarian cancer.

Diethylstilbestrol exposure: Some gynecologic cancers have been associated with in utero exposure to diethylstilbestrol, a synthetic form of estrogen that was prescribed to pregnant women between 1940 and 1971, before it was determined to be unsafe.

What are the symptoms of gynecologic cancers?

Symptoms vary depending on the organ that's involved and should always be evaluated by your doctor.

Abnormal vaginal bleeding and discharge can occur with any gynecologic cancer. Sometimes, pelvic pain can occur with uterine and ovarian cancer. Similarly, bloating, constipation, and an increased need to urinate can occur with ovarian cancer but not all patients will have those symptoms.

Vulvar cancer causes itching and soreness, along with a visible lesion. An area of skin on the vulva may have a different color than the surrounding skin.

So far, only cervical cancer has routine screening tests (the Pap smear and HPV testing). Because symptoms of early-stage gynecologic cancers are often vague and can also be caused by other, less serious conditions, doctors encourage women to have regular gynecologic exams to check for signs of disease.

How are gynecologic cancers diagnosed?

To diagnose gynecologic cancers, doctors review the patient's medical history, perform a physical exam, and run one or more diagnostic tests.

Medical history. The doctor will assess the patient's medical record, ask about symptoms, and whether the patient has any risk factors for gynecologic cancers.

Physical exam. During the physical exam, the doctor will look for signs and symptoms of gynecologic cancers and determine the patient's overall health. The exam may involve a pelvic exam.

Various diagnostic tests are used to diagnose gynecologic cancers. These may include:

Blood tests. Bloodwork is used to measure the level of tumor markers and other components of the blood that may be indicative of cancer.

Pap test. In this test, a doctor removes a sample of cells from the cervix for laboratory analysis. A pathologist looks at the cells under a microscope to determine if cancer is present. This test is used in the diagnosis of cervical cancer.

Imaging tests. These tests produce images of the internal tissues of the pelvis and abdomen, and allow doctors to visually detect tumors and other abnormalities. Commonly used imaging tests in the diagnosis of gynecologic cancers include ultrasounds, magnetic resonance imaging (MRI) studies, and computed tomography (CT) scans.

If a gynecologic cancer is diagnosed, other imaging tests such as a positron emission tomography (PET) scan may be used to determine if the cancer has spread to other parts of the body.

Biopsy. Biopsy is necessary to confirm the diagnosis of cancer. In a biopsy, a small piece of tissue is removed for laboratory analysis. For gynecologic cancers, biopsies may be performed using an image-guided needle during a minimally invasive procedure, via open surgery, or using other specialized instruments. Once the tissue sample is collected, a pathologist examines it under a microscope to check for the presence of cancer cells.

Cervical cancer

Overview

The fatality rate for cervical cancer has plummeted. Once the deadliest cancer for women, it is now 14th on the list. This incredible success story is rooted in early screening and prevention.

From the Pap smear to the HPV (human papillomavirus) vaccine, Yale Medicine has been at the forefront of developing widely used and incredibly effective diagnostic techniques and treatments for cervical cancer.

What is cervical cancer?

Cervical cancer occurs when abnormal cells inside the cervix grow in an uncontrolled manner. These abnormal cells can form tumors and may spread to other tissues in the body. The growth of abnormal cells in the cervix is almost always related to an HPV infection.

While most women who have an HPV infection will not go on to develop cervical cancer, a small percentage will. Getting vaccinated against HPV is the most effective way to protect young women from ever developing the disease.

New vaccines have proven effective in preventing infections from HPV strains 16 and 18, the two types of HPV responsible for the majority of cervical cancer cases. For women who have already developed the early stages of cervical cancer, regular Pap smears are recommended. The disease progresses slowly and sometimes regresses on its own.

What are the risk factors for cervical cancer?

• HPV infection: This is the most common cause of cervical cancer. An HPV infection, however, does not mean a woman will develop cervical cancer in her lifetime.

• Smoking: Women who smoke are more likely to develop cervical cancer.

• DES: Another major risk factor is exposure to diethylstilbestrol (DES). DES is a drug that used to be given to pregnant mothers to prevent miscarriage. This practice ended in 1971 in the United States. Women who were exposed to DES while inside the womb are at risk of developing cervical cancer.

• Contraception and childbirth: Women who have been on (ORAL CONTRACEPTIVES PILLS)—OCP's for five or more years may be at greater risk for cervical cancer. Additionally, women who have given birth to seven or more children are at greater risk.

• Weakened Immune System: Women whose immune systems are weakened are at increased risk of developing cervical cancer. Various medications such as chemotherapy can suppress immune function, as can certain infections such as HIV.

What are the symptoms of cervical cancer?

Women with early stages of cervical cancer will often have no symptoms. The disease develops slowly. In advanced stages, women with cervical cancer may experience symptoms that include:

• Abnormal bleeding: If a woman has abnormal bleeding (not related to her period), for instance after sexual intercourse, she should see her gynecologist. Bleeding after a pelvic exam may also be a sign of advanced cervical cancer.

• Vaginal Discharge: Abnormal vaginal discharge, which may be watery, may indicate cervical cancer.

• Pain during sexual intercourse: If a woman is experiencing pain during intercourse, it could be a sign of cervical cancer.

Some women experience pelvic pain, and in cases in which the disease has become more advanced, may have lower back pain, swelling of the legs, and bowel and urinary problems such as constipation, incontinence, and hematuria (blood in the urine).

How is cervical cancer diagnosed?

A woman's cervix is usually tested for abnormal cells during a routine Pap smear. A Pap smear is a bit like a cheek swab —a doctor will gently insert a simple tool called a speculum inside the vagina to open it slightly, and then use an extra-long swab to scrape cells from the inside of the cervix. These cells will be sent to a lab and tested for signs of abnormal growth.

If the Pap smear results indicate the presence of abnormal cells, a doctor will recommend further tests including a colposcopy and biopsy of cervical tissue. During a biopsy, the physician removes a tiny piece of tissue, which is later analyzed for signs of cancerous cells in a laboratory.

In the case of a diagnosis of cervical cancer, the physician will order more tests to evaluate the location and extent of the disease. This usually entails imaging studies such as a CT scan, MRI, and/or a positron emission tomography (PET) scan.

Uterine cancer

Overview

While a diagnosis of uterine cancer can be scary, it is important to know that its most common form, endometrial cancer, is curable, especially if it is caught at an early stage. Uterine cancer is a blanket term for cancers that can develop inside a woman's uterus. There are two main types of uterine cancer:

Endometrial cancer begins in the cells that make up the endometrium, which is the lining of the uterus; a second, rare type of uterine cancer known as uterine sarcoma, starts in the muscles or other tissues in the uterus. While uterine sarcomas are often more aggressive than endometrial cancer, they make up only around 5 to 10% of all uterine cancer diagnoses.

According to the National Cancer Institute (NCI), an estimated 66,570 women will be diagnosed with uterine cancer in 2021, accounting for 3.5% of all cancer cases in the U.S. It is the most common type of gynecologic cancer and most frequently occurs in women over the age of 45, though it can affect younger women.

Fortunately, uterine cancer is treatable. Surgery is the most common treatment, but radiation therapy, chemotherapy, and several other therapies may also be used.

What are the symptoms of uterine cancer?

- Unusual discharge or bleeding that is not related to normal menstruation
- Difficulty or pain while urinating
- Frequent urination
- Pain during sexual intercourse
- Pelvic pain
- A lump or mass in the vagina
- Pain or bloated feeling in abdomen
- Weight loss without known reason

What are the risk factors for uterine cancer?

Risk factors for uterine cancer include the following:

- Age (older women are at higher risk)
- Hormone replacement therapy that contains only estrogen after menopause
- Tamoxifen (often used to prevent or treat breast cancer)
- Obesity
- Type 2 diabetes
- Previous radiation therapy in the pelvic region
- Increased exposure of endometrium to estrogen (may be due to several factors including starting menstruation at an early age, never giving birth, and/or starting menopause at an older age)
- Polycystic ovarian syndrome (PCOS)
- Family history of endometrial cancer
- Having retinoblastoma in childhood (a cancer of the eye)
- Endometrial hyperplasia (a condition in which the endometrium becomes too thick)
- Certain inherited conditions such as Lynch syndrome, also known as hereditary nonpolyposis colorectal cancer

How is uterine cancer diagnosed?

If you develop any of the symptoms listed above, such as post-menopausal bleeding or abnormal vaginal discharge, visit your gynecologist. Your doctor will ask about your medical history and conduct a thorough pelvic exam that may include a Pap test.

To diagnose uterine cancer, your doctor will need to conduct one or more diagnostic tests. These tests may include:

• Transvaginal ultrasound. This test uses sound waves to produce an image of the tissues of the uterus and pelvic area. In this procedure, an ultrasound probe will be inserted in the vagina.

• Endometrial biopsy. In this procedure, a doctor removes a small piece of tissue from the endometrium. A pathologist then examines the tissue under a microscope to check for the presence of cancer cells.

• Dilation and curettage (D&C). Also known as uterine scraping, in this procedure, a doctor inserts a curette (an instrument with a spoon- or hoop-shaped end) into the vagina and uterus and uses it to scrape part of the endometrium. In a lab, a pathologist examines the tissue sample to see if cancer cells are present.

• Hysteroscopy. This procedure allows a doctor to visually examine the endometrium. A doctor inserts a thin tube called a hysteroscope into the vagina and uterus. The hysteroscope is equipped with a light and camera (or lens), which allow the doctor to view the lining of the uterus. If the doctor detects abnormal tissue, they can also biopsy a small piece of tissue through the hysteroscope.

If uterine cancer is diagnosed, your doctor will order additional tests to learn more about the type of cancer involved and to determine whether the cancer has spread beyond the uterus. This is known as staging, and may involve bloodwork and imaging studies such as a computed tomography (CT) scan, magnetic resonance imaging (MRI) study, positron emission tomography (PET) scan, and/or chest X-ray. The doctor will assign the cancer to a stage numbered from I to IV. The lower the stage, the less advanced the cancer is.

Staging helps doctors make a prognosis and put together a personalized treatment plan.

Many women at high risk choose resection, which involves surgically removing all or part of the ovaries as a precaution; this step is generally appropriate only for women who are highly likely to develop ovarian cancer.

Women with a family history of breast, colon, uterine or ovarian cancer should consider discussing options with a geneticist.

A. Translate the following sentences into Chinese.

1. A woman's reproductive system is centered on the uterus (including the cervix), which is also known as the womb. The ovaries attach to the top of the uterus, and the vagina connects the uterus to the outside of the body. The external genitals are called the vulva. Gynecologic cancers result from the rapid growth and spread of abnormal cells in one of these organs.

2. But gynecologic cancers are often treatable. "Some of these present as pre-cancers that are easily treated when detected early," she says. "Even many early-stage cancers, such as stage Ⅰ endometrial cancer, are cured just with surgery alone, the vast majority of the time."

3. Imaging tests produce images of the internal tissues of the pelvis and abdomen, and allow doctors to visually detect tumors and other abnormalities. Commonly used imaging tests in the diagnosis of gynecologic cancers include ultrasounds, magnetic resonance imaging (MRI) studies, and computed tomography (CT) scans.

4. New vaccines have proven effective in preventing infections from HPV strains 16 and 18, the two types of HPV responsible for the majority of cervical cancer cases. For women who have already developed the early stages of cervical cancer, regular Pap smears are recommended. The disease progresses slowly and sometimes regresses on its own.

5. If you develop any of the symptoms listed above, such as post-menopausal bleeding or abnormal vaginal discharge, visit your gynecologist. Your doctor will ask about your medical history and conduct a thorough pelvic exam that may include a Pap test.

B. Prepare a lecture on gynecologic cancers after doing the further reading above.

扫码获取
提示

Unit 10

Antenatal Check-up

I Warming-up

A. Match the following words and phrases with their Chinese translations.

A	midwife	1	尿样
B	preeclampsia	2	子宫收缩
C	urine sample	3	助产士,接生员
D	protein	4	子宫颈
E	discharge	5	黏液
F	diabetes	6	先兆子痫
G	mucus	7	分泌物
H	cervix	8	蛋白质
I	bottom	9	臀部
J	contraction	10	糖尿病

B. Complete the sentences with the following words or phrases in their proper forms.

blood pressure	present	a sign of	symptoms
urine infection	labor	detect	eliminate

1. The shots have been known to eliminate the _____ of allergies so effectively that most people do not need to use any other products.

2. Recently, young people with high _____ have been shown to be just as susceptible to mental decline as elderly people are.

3. Many women will tell you and I'm the first to admit that the breathing techniques can be absolutely useless during _____ and delivery.

4. Mucin in the urine might be _____ this disease, especially in patients who also have chronic irritation of the renal pelvis.

5. The question we were trying to answer was can we use neuroimaging to objectively _____ whether a person is in a state of pain or not.

6. Researchers say one major problem for growers is the fact that the fungus can be _____ in a field without obvious symptoms.

7. A _____ happens when bacteria (germs) get into the bladder.

8. To _____ this possibility, we decided to see if naturally secreted levels of insulin would have the same effect.

 C. Watch the video *Antenatal Check-up* and answer the questions.

扫码获取视频

1. What tests does your midwife usually perform at each visit?

2. Why should your blood pressure be carefully checked at your each antenatal visit?

3. What disease might it be if your urine sample present protein?

4. What disease might it be if your urine sample present sugar?

5. What disease might it be if your urine sample present blood?

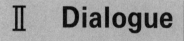 **Ⅱ Dialogue**

扫码获取
音频及文本

 A. Listen to the dialogue for the first time and try to get the general idea.

 B. Listen to the dialogue for the second time and try to answer the following questions.

1. Why does this patient come to see the doctor?

2. Did the patient have any illnesses before pregnancy?

3. What problem has the patient had during this pregnancy?

4. Is there any multiple pregnancy, hypertension, tuberculosis, diabetes or hereditary diseases in the patient's family? Why are these very important for doctor to know?

5. What are the findings of the physical examination for the patient?

C. Choose the following words and/or expressions to complete the sentences in their proper forms.

pelvis	骨盆；盆腔	appetite	食欲/胃口/饭量
antenatal	产前的；出生前的	candida	念珠菌性
swab	（医用的）拭子，药棉签	sensation	感觉，知觉
morning sickness	孕吐	discharge	分泌物
menstruation	月经；月经期间	hereditary	（特点或疾病）遗传的
vaginitis	阴道炎	nourishment	营养品，滋养品

1. It also showed _____ classes tripled the chances of breastfeeding, regardless of these factors.

2. _____ (a period) is a major stage of puberty in girls; it's one of the many physical signs that a girl is turning into a woman.

3. Both genes are thought to influence _____ and how much energy the body uses.

4. The pain of angina(心绞痛性) is usually not as severe as the intense precordial crushing _____ associated with acute myocardial infraction.

5. Wrong tooth adds up to deformation is polygene _____ disease，often behave familial and genetic tendency.

6. The doctor will take a routine test to check vaginal _____ .

7. Pars oralis pharynges(口咽部) was the most common infection site of _____ , then were lungs and digestive tract.

8. Symptoms of _____ include vaginal discharge pruritus irritation soreness odor dyspareunia and dysuria.

9. We think that the _____ cultures taken from the tonsillar surface may not always reveal the real pathogen of the tonsils.

10. The female _____ is shaped like a wide，oval bowl with a large opening at the top and a slightly smaller opening at the bottom.

D. Read the dialogue and try to make a conversation with your classmates.

扫码获取
提示

E. Translate the following Chinese into English.

D—Doctor   P—Patient

D：1.你还清楚地记得末次月经是什么时候？
   1. _____

P: It was on August，14th，2014.
D：2. 你的月经周期规律吗？
   2. _____

P：Yes，they are.

D：3. 你有孕吐吗？

3. _____

P：4. 我的食欲很差。有两个月吃饭后就吐，现在好多了。

4. _____

_____

D：5. 怀孕前，你患过什么病？

5. _____

P：No. I'm very healthy.

D：6. 这次怀孕有什么问题吗？你有过阴道出血、水性分泌物、下腹疼痛及腿疼等问题吗？

6. _____

_____

P：I do have some pain in my legs when I'm tired. I have a burning sensation when passing urine，discharge，itchiness and it's all very uncomfortable.

D：7. 你家里有人生过多胎，患过高血压、结核病、糖尿病或遗传病吗？

7. _____

_____

P：I am one of twins. My mother died during delivery because of profuse bleeding.

D：8. 你应当多吃些有营养的东西，如蛋类、蔬菜、水果、奶、肉类等。

8. _____

III Further Reading：Antenatal Testing

Text A　Antenatal testing

Definition

Antenatal testing includes any diagnostic procedures performed before the birth of a baby.

Purpose

These tests and exams are essential for protecting the health of a pregnant woman and her developing child.

Precautions

Some tests，such as amniocentesis，carry a small risk of a miscarriage or other complications that could harm the mother or baby.

Description

Women who become pregnant undergo a wide variety of tests throughout the nine months before delivery. In the early stages，physicians order blood tests to screen for possible disorders or infections，such as human immunodeficiency virus (HIV), which can pass from the mother to the fetus. Later, the focus shifts to checking on fetal well-being with a variety of technological tools such as ultrasound scans.

Descriptions of the most common tests and procedures used during pregnancy are listed below. When a woman first learns she is pregnant, her physician will run a series of routine urine and blood tests to determine her blood type, check for anemia and gestational diabetes, make sure she is immune to rubella (German measles) and check for infectious diseases like HIV, hepatitis, chlamydia or syphilis. Physicians also usually do pelvic exam to screen for cervical cancer and check the patient's blood pressure.

As the pregnancy progresses, more tests will follow:

Ultrasound is a device that records sound waves as they bounce off the developing fetus to create an image, which is projected onto a large computer screen. Physicians order an ultrasound scan to listen for a fetal heartbeat, determine a woman's precise due date and check for twins, among other uses. An ultrasound scan also is known as a sonogram. The procedure takes a few minutes, is painless and usually is covered by health insurance.

Alpha fetoprotein screen—A test that measures the level of alpha fetoprotein, a substance produced by a fetus with birth defects, in the mother's blood.

Amniocentesis—An invasive procedure that allows physicians to check for birth defects by collecting a sample of fetal cells from inside the amniotic sac.

Breech position—When a child is oriented feet first in the mother's uterus just before delivery.

GBS—Group B streptococci are a type of bacteria that, if passed to can cause inflammation of the brain, spinal cord, blood or lungs. In some cases, it can result in infant death.

Ultrasound—A device that records sound waves as they bounce off a developing fetus to create an image, which is projected onto a large computer screen.

The ultrasound technician will ask the pregnant woman to remove her clothes and change into a gown. The technician may rub some gel on the woman's stomach, which helps the hand-held device pick up sound waves better. In certain cases, the technician may insert a plastic probe into the woman's vaginal canal to get a clearer picture of the fetus. Early in pregnancy, the test may need to be done with a full bladder.

Unlike X rays, ultrasound is safe to use during pregnancy. It does not cause any known side-effects that would harm the mother or baby.

Pregnant women usually will have their first ultrasound anytime between 8 and 12 weeks of gestation. In normal cases, the technician is able to identify a fetal heartbeat, which appears as a flashing light on the screen. Closer to the due date, physicians use ultrasound to make sure the fetus is in the correct position to exit the birth canal head first.

Sometimes an ultrasound will show that a fetus has stopped growing, or a gestational sac has formed without a fetus, and a miscarriage has occurred. Later in pregnancy, it also may show that the child is in a breech position, oriented feet first, which can cause a difficult labor.

Tests for birth defects

Most obstetricians offer parents a variety of ways to find out if their developing child might have birth defects such as spina bifida and Down Syndrome. An alpha fetoprotein screen can be done through a simple blood test in the doctor's office between the 16th and 18th week of gestation. It tells the odds that their child will have a severe congenital anomaly. The test works by measuring the level of alpha fetoprotein, a substance produced by a fetus with birth defects. Low levels of alpha fetoprotein in the mother's blood may indicate Down's Syndrome. In that case, the next step for most couples is amniocentesis because the alpha fetoprotein test can give false-positive results. Amniocentesis is a more accurate test, but it also has higher risks of complications.

This procedure typically is used to diagnose Down Syndrome while a developing child is still in the womb, at 15—28 weeks.

During amniocentesis, a doctor inserts a needle through a woman's vaginal canal and inside her cervix. Using ultrasound as a guide, the doctor pierces the uterus to withdraw a sample of fluid from the amniotic sac. Afterwards, tiny cells shed by the fetus can be studied in the laboratory. Scientists can analyze DNA samples to determine if the fetus has Down Syndrome or other genetic conditions. Amniocentesis also can determine the sex of the fetus.

Women who have a history of recurring miscarriages may not want to have this procedure.

Amniocentesis is usually performed in a doctor's office on an outpatient basis.

Common side effects include cramping and bleeding.

In about one out of every 1,000 cases, amniocentesis causes a needle to puncture the uterine wall, which could result in miscarriage.

In most cases, couples find out their baby does not have a birth defect.

If the results come back positive for Down's Syndrome or other serious conditions, the couple must decide if they want to end the pregnancy. Others use the knowledge to plan and prepare any special care needed for their future child.

Group B strep

This test is for Group B streptococci (GBS) infection.

By testing for GBS, physicians can determine if a woman is at risk of passing this infection along to her child.

Women who have had a prior child with GBS, or who have a fever or prolonged or premature rupture of the amniotic sac may be at higher risk for this type of infection.

GBS is a type of bacteria commonly found in the vagina and rectum. Unlike regular strep throat, GBS can be present in a person's body without causing any symptoms, so many women do not realize they are infected with it.

To test for the presence of GBS, doctors may take a urine sample. They also may collect samples from the vagina or rectum, which are then analyzed in a lab. This test is usually performed late in pregnancy, at 35—37 weeks of gestation.

This is a routine urine test or pelvic exam with no side effects.

In many cases, doctors do not find any evidence of this type of infection.

If a woman is found to be infected with Group B strep, physicians usually wait to treat it until just before labor begins. At that time, they may give the mother antibiotics so the baby is not born with the infection. Newborns who are exposed to Group B strep can have inflammation of the brain, spinal cord, blood or lungs. In some cases, this serious complication can result in infant death.

Text B   What are screening tests?

Screening tests are used to find people at higher chance of a health problem.

This means they can get earlier, potentially more effective, treatment or make informed decisions about their health.

Screening tests are not perfect. Some people will be told that they or their baby have a higher chance of having a health condition when in fact they do not have the condition.

Also, a few people will be told that they or their baby have a lower chance of having a health condition when in fact they do have the condition.

What do screening tests involve?

The screening tests offered during pregnancy in England are either ultrasound scans or blood tests, or a combination of both.

Ultrasound scans may detect conditions such as spina bifida.

Blood tests can show whether you have a higher chance of inherited conditions such as sickle cellanemia and thalassemia, and whether you have infections like HIV, hepatitis B or syphilis.

Blood tests combined with scans can help find out how likely it is that the baby has Down's Syndrome, Edwards' Syndrome or Patau's Syndrome.

What are the risks of screening tests?

Screening tests cannot harm you or the baby but it is important to consider carefully whether or not to have these tests.

Some screening tests in pregnancy can lead to difficult decisions for you.

For example, screening tests for Down's Syndrome, Edwards' Syndrome or Patau's Syndrome can lead to difficult decisions about whether to have a diagnostic test, such as amniocentesis, that carries a chance of miscarriage.

A diagnostic test tells you for certain whether you or your baby has the condition.

If diagnostic tests show your baby has a condition, this can lead to a decision about whether you want to continue or end the pregnancy.

Having a further test or ending the pregnancy will always be your decision, and healthcare professionals will support you whatever you decide.

It's up to you whether or not you choose to have screening tests in pregnancy.

When will I be offered screening?

Different screening tests are offered at different times during pregnancy.

The screening test for sickle cell and thalassemia should be offered as early as possible before 10 weeks of pregnancy.

It's recommended that screening blood tests for HIV, hepatitis B and syphilis should happen as early as possible in pregnancy.

This is so you can be offered specialist care and treatment to protect your health and reduce the chance of your baby getting infected.

These blood tests should not be delayed until the first scan appointment.

You'll be offered screening for Down's Syndrome, Edwards' Syndrome and Patau's Syndrome around the time of your dating scan, which happens when you're around 11 to 14 weeks pregnant.

You'll be offered screening to check your baby's development at a 20-week scan when you're around 18 to 21 weeks pregnant.

Will screening tests give me a definite answer?

This depends what the screening tests are looking for.

Yes

Screening tests for HIV, hepatitis B and syphilis are very accurate, and will tell for certain whether you have these infections.

If the test is positive, you'll be offered further tests and examinations by specialist doctors to find out the treatment you need.

No

Screening for Down's Syndrome, Edwards' Syndrome and Patau's Syndrome cannot say for certain whether your baby has the condition. It tells you if your baby has a lower or higher chance of having the condition.

If your baby has a higher chance of a condition, you'll be offered a diagnostic test that gives a more definite "yes" or "no" answer.

Screening tests for sickle cell and thalassemia will tell you for certain whether you're a carrier or have these conditions. They will not tell you whether or not your baby has the condition.

If you or the baby's father is a carrier or has the condition, you'll be offered diagnostic tests to find out if your baby is affected.

Do I have to have screening?

No—it's up to you whether you have a screening test. It's a personal choice that only you can make.

You can discuss each of the screening tests you're offered with your midwife or doctor and decide whether or not it's right for you.

Some of the screening tests you'll be offered are recommended by the NHS. These include:
• blood tests for infectious diseases
• eye screening if you have pre-existing diabetes (not gestational diabetes)
• newborn screening tests

This is because the results from these tests can help make sure that you or your baby get urgent treatment for serious conditions.

What screening tests will I be offered in pregnancy?

Find out more about each of the different screening tests:
• screening for infectious diseases (hepatitis B, HIV and syphilis)
• screening for inherited conditions (sickle cell, thalassemia and other hemoglobin disorders)
• screening for Down's Syndrome, Edwards' Syndrome and Patau's Syndrome
• screening for 11 physical conditions (20-week scan)

Some screening tests will also be offered to your baby after they're born:
• newborn physical examination
• newborn hearing screening
• newborn blood spot screening

A. Translate the following sentences into Chinese.

1. Women who become pregnant undergo a wide variety of tests throughout the nine months before delivery. In the early stages, physicians order blood tests to screen for possible disorders or infections, such as human immunodeficiency virus (HIV), which can pass from the mother to the fetus.

2. When a woman first learns she is pregnant, her physician will run a series of routine urine and blood tests to determine her blood type, check for anemia and gestational diabetes, make sure she is immune to rubella (German measles) and check for infectious diseases like HIV, hepatitis, chlamydia or syphilis.

3. Ultrasound is a device that records sound waves as they bounce off the developing fetus to create an image, which is projected onto a large computer screen. Physicians order an ultrasound scan to listen for a fetal heartbeat, determine a woman's precise due date and check for twins, among other uses.

4. An alpha fetoprotein screen can be done through a simple blood test in the doctor's office between the 16th and 18th week of gestation. It tells the odds that their child will have a severe congenital anomaly. The test works by measuring the level of alpha fetoprotein, a substance produced by a fetus with birth defects. Low levels of alpha fetoprotein in the mother's blood may indicate Down's Syndrome.

5. To test for the presence of GBS, doctors may take a urine sample. They also may collect samples from the vagina or rectum, which are then analyzed in a lab. This test is usually performed late in pregnancy, at 35—37 weeks of gestation.

B. Prepare a lecture on pneumonia after doing the further reading above.

扫码获取
提示

Unit 11

Lower Abdominal Pain in Female

I Warming-up

A. Match the following words and phrases with their Chinese translations.

A	fallopian tube	1	子宫内膜
B	ovary	2	异位妊娠,宫外孕
C	uterus	3	输卵管
D	cervix	4	子宫肌层
E	vagina	5	阴道
F	endometrium	6	卵巢
G	myometrium	7	子宫
H	ovarian torsion	8	子宫内膜腔
I	ectopic pregnancy	9	子宫颈
J	endometrial cavity	10	卵巢扭转

B. Complete the sentences with the following words or phrases in their proper forms.

complicate	timing	have more stuff	incapacity	onset
vital sign	severity	transabdominal	diarrhea	ultrasound

1. Pandemic influenza is usually associated with a greater number of cases, higher _____ of illness and consequently a higher death toll.

2. Both drugs must be taken early, within a few days of the _____ of symptoms, to be most effective.

3. "Our studies found that the total number of hours of sleep doesn't matter, but the _____ of sleep does, " he said.

4. Chronic _____ can be a sign of malabsorption, which means nutrients are not being fully absorbed by the body.

5. Heart rate: is it truly a _____?

6. Symptoms to look out for include severe vomiting and nausea; _____ to keep food down for two to three days; lack of energy.

7. We need to learn how to consume less, be happy with "having" less-constantly striving to _____ is not sustainable.

8. It was the next easiest disease to eradicate, but it was so much more _____ than smallpox.

9. _____ is commonly used in medical imaging as a matter wave, and is an important object of research in imaging physics.

10. In most cases, your doctor orders a pelvic _____ ultrasound when you're pregnant. This helps determine if the fetus is developing properly. It also proves effective in identifying causes of a woman's abnormal vaginal bleeding, pelvic pain and menstrual problems.

C. Watch the video *Lower Abdominal Pain in Female* and answer the questions.

扫码获取视频

1. What should a quick history review be focused on for this patient?

2. What should a review of the systems be focused on for this patient?

3. What are your orders prescribed in terms of clinical lab work?

4. Under what basis should you prescribe medical imaging?

5. What differential diagnoses should be considered?

扫码获取
音频及文本

Ⅱ **Dialogue**

A. Listen to the dialogue for the first time and try to get the general idea.

B. **Listen to the dialogue for the second time and try to answer the following questions.**

1. What's the trouble with this patient?

2. Why did the doctor want to know whether the patient was operated on or not during her last abortion?

3. Why did the doctor ask the current vaginal discharge for this patient?

4. Why was the doctor concerned about the character of the pain?

5. Why did the doctor think physiotherapy was good for this patient?

C. **Choose the following words and/or expressions to complete the sentences in their proper forms.**

abortion	流产	odor	气味
fetus	胎儿，胎	a burning sensation	烧灼感
injection	注射	vagina	阴道
discharge	分泌物	normal	正常的，典型的
take your temperature	量体温	abdomen	腹部
profuse	量多，大量的	physiotherapy	物理疗法

1. Two days before presentation, he noticed dark-colored urine and that his eyes were red and itchy, with a clear, thick _____.

2. Foot _____ can be embarrassing, and getting rid of it might not be as simple as just rubbing on some antiperspirant.

3. There is usually trembling, faintness and palpitations, and there may be _____ sweating.

4. Sometimes even sunscreen-protected skin reacts to sunlight with _____, itching or painful blisters.

5. Ultrasound imaging is often used to monitor structural and functional progress of the growing _____.

6. "I've not had any pain since the surgery and I'm taking it step by step but it's gradually getting back to _____," she said.

7. Your child is at risk of getting one of these infections while waiting for the next _____.

8. Once it was diagnosed as Achilles tendonitis, Karen tried various treatments including _____, acupuncture and osteopathy.

9. The pain of appendicitis may be referred to any region of the _____.

10. The two sisters were usually in agreement on most issues, but they were at swords' points on the matter of _____.

D. Read the dialogue and try to make a conversation with your classmates.

扫码获取
提示

E. Translate the following Chinese into English.

D—Doctor   P—Patient

P：1. 从流产后，我的下腹疼痛6个月了，时好时坏。

1. _____

D：2. 流产时做手术了吗？

2. _____

P：Yes，it was an abortion after a pregnancy of 2 months. The fetus did not come out completely，so the doctor had to operate.

P：3. 手术后发低烧10天，在37.4—37.8℃之间，打了些针就好了。

3. _____

D：4. 当时肚子疼吗？

4. _____

P：I didn't notice any.

D：5. 阴道分泌物怎样？

5. _____

P：It's somewhat more profuse than before，with an unpleasant odor.

D：6. 这回是什么性质的疼？

6. _____

P：7. 烧灼疼，有时有下坠感。疼在左下腹部，在感冒或月经前、月经期加重。

7. _____
_____

P：8. 我给你一些抗生素，我想理疗对你也很好。

8. _____
_____

Ⅲ Further Reading：Abdominal Pain（Causes，Remedies，Treatment）

Text A   Abdominal pain

Causes of lower left abdominal pain in women include menstrual cramps，ovarian cysts，endometriosis，ectopic pregnancy，and pelvic inflammatory disease.

Pain in the lower left abdomen can be caused by a wide variety of conditions. Your abdominal cavity contains several organs，and any damage or infection to these organs can lead to pain.

Learn about causes of abdominal pain specific to women，as well as other potential causes that can affect both men and women.

Menstrual cramps

Menstruation is the most common cause of abdominal pain in women. If your menstrual cycle is accompanied by painful cramps, the condition is called dysmenorrhea. Most women experience menstrual cramps at some point in their lives, and it typically is not something to worry about unless the pain is so severe that it hinders your daily activities.

Management includes conservative treatment such as heat pads, moderate exercise, and rest. Some people may need to take analgesics for pain relief.

Ovarian cysts

An ovarian cyst is a fluid-filled sac inside an ovary. Although most ovarian cysts don't cause symptoms, large ovarian cysts can cause abdominal pain and frequent urination if they compress the bladder.

An ovarian cyst that ruptures can cause severe pain and internal bleeding. You should seek medical help if you experience sudden severe abdominal pain, fever, vomiting, lightheadedness, or signs of shock.

Ovarian cysts are common. Most of the time, you have little or no discomfort, and the cysts are harmless. Most cysts go away without treatment within a few months.

But sometimes ovarian cysts can become twisted or burst open (rupture). This can cause serious symptoms. To protect your health, get regular pelvic exams and know the symptoms that can signal what might be a serious problem.

Endometriosis

Endometriosis occurs when the tissue that lines the inside of your uterus grows on the outside instead. During your menstrual cycle, the tissue thickens and bleeds but becomes trapped in the body, which can cause abdominal pain, especially during your menstrual period.

Ectopic pregnancy

Ectopic pregnancy occurs when a fertilized ovum implants in places other than the uterus. It usually occurs in the fallopian tube, whose function is to connect ovaries to the uterus. Symptoms include:
- Abdominal pain
- Missed period or other signs of pregnancy
- Vaginal bleeding or watery discharge
- Discomfort during urination and bowel movements

Pelvic inflammatory disease

Pelvic inflammatory disease is an infection of the female genital tract, typically caused by sexually transmitted infections such as chlamydia and gonorrhoea. Symptoms include:

- Abdominal pain
- Fever
- Vaginal discharge
- Pain or bleeding after intercourse
- Burning sensation during urination
- Bleeding between periods

What are other common causes of lower left abdominal pain?

Abdominal pain can affect both men and women and may be caused by conditions such as:

- Gastritis: Gastritis can lead to abdominal discomfort and is often caused by smoking, overeating, alcohol consumption, lack of vitamin B_{12}, etc. Management includes proton-pump inhibitors, such as rabeprazole and pantoprazole.
- Constipation: Constipation can cause bloating, flatulence, and abdominal cramps. Other symptoms include heartburn and nausea. Management includes diet modifications, medications, and fiber supplements.
- Hernia: A hernia is the protrusion of an internal organ through the surrounding tissue that can cause a lump or bulge to appear in the abdomen. Other symptoms of hernia include a feeling of fullness, reduction in the size of the bulge on lying, movement of the bulge on coughing, dull aching sensation, pain when lifting, etc. Management includes surgical intervention such as herniorrhaphy, hernioplasty, and herniotomy.
- Kidney stones: Kidney stones are commonly caused by recurrent urinary infections, dehydration, or the genetic tendency of developing stones. Pain due to kidney stones starts in the abdomen and radiates to the back. Other symptoms include:
  o Pink, red, brown, cloudy, smelly urine
  o Painful urination
  o Nausea and vomiting
  o Fever and chills
- Diverticulitis: Diverticula are small pouches in the intestine that are created due to pressure over weak spots in the colon. When these pouches tear, swell, or get infected, it can cause significant pain in the abdomen. Management consists of dietary modifications and surgery in severe cases.

Other causes of lower left abdominal pain include:

- Irritable bowel syndrome
- Crohn's disease or ulcerative colitis
- Food intolerance or allergy (such as lactose intolerance)

- Appendicitis
- Aortic aneurysm in the abdomen（bulging and weakening of the major artery in the body）
- Obstruction or blockage of the bowels
- Cancers of the stomach or colon
- Cholecystitis（gallbladder inflammation）with or without gallstones
- Blood flow to the intestines is reduced（ischemic bowel）
- Gastroesophageal reflux
- Pancreatitis is the inflammation of the pancreas（swelling or infection of the pancreas）
- Gastric or duodenal ulcers
- Urinary tract infections

Text B   Things to know about endometriosis

- Endometriosis is the abnormal growth of cells（endometrial cells）similar to those that form the inside of the uterus but in a location outside of the uterus. Endometriosis is most commonly found in other organs of the pelvis.
- The exact cause of endometriosis has not been identified.
- Endometriosis is more common in women who are experiencing infertility than infertile women, but the condition does not necessarily cause infertility.
- Most women with endometriosis have no symptoms. However, when women do experience signs and symptoms of endometriosis they may include:
  o Pelvic pain that may worsen during menstruation
  o Painful intercourse
  o Painful bowel movements or urination
  o Infertility
- Pelvic pain during menstruation or ovulation can be a symptom of endometriosis, but may also occur in normal women.
- Endometriosis can be suspected based on the woman's pattern of symptoms, and sometimes during a physical examination, but the definite diagnosis is usually confirmed by surgery, most commonly by laparoscopy.
- Treatment of endometriosis includes medication and surgery for both pain relief and treatment of infertility if pregnancy is desired.
- Some studies have postulated that women with endometriosis have an increased risk for the development of certain types of ovarian cancer, known as epithelial ovarian cancer（EOC）.
- Endometriosis is more common in infertile women, as opposed to those who have conceived a pregnancy.
- Obstetrician-gynecologists（OB-GYNs）are the type of doctors that commonly treat endometriosis.

• The goals of endometriosis treatment may include symptom relief and/or enhancement of fertility.

• Surgery is the preferred treatment when there is an anatomic distortion of the pelvic organs or obstruction of the bowel or urinary tract.

• Endometriosis is most commonly a disease of the reproductive period and symptoms usually go away after a woman reaches menopause.

What are the early signs of endometriosis?

Almost a third of women with endometriosis do not have any symptoms. When symptoms are present, they depend on the site where the endometrial implant has occurred. A common complaint is a pain in the pelvic region, which varies with the menstrual cycle. The main symptoms include:
• Pain during menstrual periods (dysmenorrhea)
• Heavy or irregular bleeding
• Pain in the pelvic region
• Lower abdominal or back pain
• Infertility
• Pain or discomfort during intercourse (dyspareunia)
• Pain on passing feces (dyschezia), often with cycles of diarrhea and constipation
• Bloating, nausea, and vomiting
• Pain in the groin
• Pain on passing urine and/or increased urine frequency
• Pain during exercise
• Blood in sputum
• Seizures that change in severity with the menstrual cycle

What are the four stages of endometriosis?

Endometriosis is the abnormal growth of endometrial tissue similar to that which lines the interior of the uterus but in a location outside of the uterus. Endometrial tissue is shed each month during menstruation. Areas of endometrial tissue found in ectopic locations are called endometrial implants. These lesions are most commonly found on the ovaries, the Fallopian tubes, the surface of the uterus, the bowel, and on the membrane lining of the pelvic cavity (i. e. the peritoneum). They are less commonly found to involve the vagina, cervix, and bladder. Rarely, endometriosis can occur outside the pelvis. Endometriosis has been reported in the liver, brain, lung, and old surgical scars. Endometrial implants, while they may become problematic, are usually benign (i. e. non-cancerous).

Endometriosis is classified into one of four stages (I—minimal, II—mild,

Ⅲ—moderate, and Ⅳ—severe) based upon the exact location, extent, and depth of the endometriosis implants as well as the presence and severity of scar tissue and the presence and size of endometrial implants in the ovaries.

• Most cases of endometriosis are classified as minimal or mild, which means there are superficial implants and mild scarring.

• Moderate and severe endometriosis typically results incysts and more severe scarring.

• The stage of endometriosis is not related to the degree of symptoms a woman experiences, but infertility is common with stage Ⅳ endometriosis.

Is there a test to diagnose endometriosis?

Obstetrician-gynecologists (OB-GYNs) are the type of doctors that commonly treat endometriosis.

Endometriosis can be suspected based on symptoms of pelvic pain and findings during physical examinations. Occasionally, during a rectovaginal exam (one finger in the vagina and one finger in the rectum), the doctor can feel nodules (endometrial implants) behind the uterus and along with the ligaments that attach to the pelvic wall. At other times, no nodules are felt, but the examination itself causes unusual pain or discomfort.

Unfortunately, neither the symptoms nor the physical examinations can be relied upon to conclusively establish the diagnosis of endometriosis. Imaging studies, such as ultrasound, can help rule out other pelvic diseases and may suggest the presence of endometriosis in the vaginal and bladder areas, but they cannot reliably diagnose endometriosis. For an accurate diagnosis, a direct visual inspection inside the pelvis and abdomen, as well as a tissue biopsy of the implants are necessary.

As a result, the only definitive method for diagnosing endometriosis is surgical. This requires either laparoscopy or laparotomy (opening the abdomen using a large incision).

Laparoscopy is the most common surgical procedure commonly employees used for the diagnosis of endometriosis. This is a minor surgical procedure performed under general anesthesia, or in some cases under local anesthesia. It is usually performed as an outpatient procedure (the patient does not stay in the facility overnight). Laparoscopy is performed by first inflating the abdominal cavity with carbon dioxide through a small incision in the navel. A thin, tubular viewing instrument (laparoscope) is then inserted into the inflated abdominal cavity to inspect the abdomen and pelvis. Endometrial implants can then be directly seen.

During laparoscopy, biopsies (removal of tiny tissue samples for examination under a microscope) can also be performed to obtain a tissue diagnosis. Sometimes random biopsies obtained during laparoscopy will show microscopic endometriosis, even though no implants are visualized.

Pelvic ultrasound and laparoscopy are also important in excluding malignancies (such as ovarian cancer) which can cause many of the same symptoms that mimic endometriosis symptoms.

A. Translate the following sentences into Chinese.

1. An ovarian cyst is a fluid-filled sac inside an ovary. Although most ovarian cysts don't cause symptoms, large ovarian cysts can cause abdominal pain and frequent urination if they compress the bladder.

2. Endometriosis occurs when the tissue that lines the inside of your uterus grows on the outside instead. During your menstrual cycle, the tissue thickens and bleeds but becomes trapped in the body, which can cause abdominal pain, especially during your menstrual period.

3. Ectopic pregnancy occurs when a fertilized ovum implants in places other than the uterus. It usually occurs in the fallopian tube, whose function is to connect ovaries to the uterus.

4. Ovarian cysts are common. Most of the time, you have little or no discomfort, and the cysts are harmless. Most cysts go away without treatment within a few months. But sometimes ovarian cysts can become twisted or burst open (rupture). This can cause serious symptoms. To protect your health, get regular pelvic exams and know the symptoms that can signal what might be a serious problem.

5. During laparoscopy, biopsies (removal of tiny tissue samples for examination under a microscope) can also be performed to obtain a tissue diagnosis. Sometimes random biopsies obtained during laparoscopy will show microscopic endometriosis, even though no implants are visualized.

B. Prepare a lecture on abdominal pain in female after doing the further reading above.

扫码获取
提示

Unit 12

Uterine Fibroid

I Warming-up

A. Match the following words and phrases with their Chinese translations.

A	menopause	1	盆腔检查
B	ultrasound and MRI	2	肌瘤切除术
C	pelvic exam	3	排尿
D	uterine fibroid	4	绝经
E	miscarriage	5	便秘
F	urination	6	子宫
G	estrogen	7	子宫肌瘤
H	uterus	8	雌激素
I	constipation	9	流产
J	myomectomy	10	超声和核磁共振成像

B. Complete the sentences with the following words or phrases in their proper forms.

menstrual-related	gynecologist	hormonal imbalance	herbal medicine
infertility	recur to	be secondary to	inactivate

1. A herb is a plant or plant part used for its scent, flavor, or therapeutic properties.

_____ are one type of dietary supplement. They are sold as tablets, capsules, powders, teas, extracts, and fresh or dried plants. People use them to try to maintain or improve their health.

2. A disinfectant is a chemical substance or compound used to _____ or destroy microorganisms on inert surfaces. Disinfection does not necessarily kill all microorganisms, especially resistant bacterial spores; it is less effective than sterilization, which is an extreme physical or chemical process that kills all types of life.

3. Chronic ulcer of skin (CUS), a common clinical disease, can _____ many diseases and be treated difficultly. Collagen metabolism being out of control is an important factor in chronic skin ulcer.

4. Approximately 19% of women aged 18—55 years reported experiencing _____ problems (e. g., heavy bleeding, bothersome cramping, or premenstrual syndrome [PMS]). These women were significantly more likely than those without these problems to report frequent anxiety and depression, insomnia, excessive sleepiness, and pain over the past 12 months.

5. Male _____ can be caused by low sperm production, abnormal sperm function or blockages that prevent the delivery of sperm. Illnesses, injuries, chronic health problems, lifestyle choices and other factors may contribute to it. The inability to conceive a child can be stressful and frustrating, but a number of treatments are available for the problem.

6. However, there are several other reasons why your hormone levels may be irregular at unexpected times. Some of the most common causes of fluctuating or imbalanced hormone levels include stress, certain medications and steroid use. These _____ are more likely to be temporary or fixable with a change in medication or properly managing stress.

7. Symptoms of mania, depression, or mixed state appear in episodes, or distinct periods of time, which typically _____ and become more frequent across the life span. These episodes, especially early in the course of illness, are separated by periods of wellness during which a person suffers few to no symptoms.

8. Abnormal vaginal discharge should absolutely be evaluated by a _____. It may be an indication of a vaginal imbalance, a sexually transmitted infection, and a variety of other issues. Abnormal vaginal discharge can be hard to self-diagnose, so an exam is often indicated.

C. Watch the video *Uterine Fibroids* and answer the questions.

扫码获取视频

1. According to the speaker, what are uterine fibroids?

2. What are the symptoms of uterine fibroids?

3. What are some complications of uterine fibroids?

4. How is someone diagnosed with uterine fibroids?

5. How are uterine fibroids treated?

扫码获取
音频及文本

II Dialogue

 A. Listen to the dialogue for the first time and try to get the general idea.

 B. Listen to the dialogue for the second time and try to answer the following questions.

1. What did the patient complain of?

2. What were the results of the physical examination?

3. What did the gynecological examination suggest?

4. What were the results of the lab examination?

5. What did the doctors finally decide?

C. Choose the following words and/or expressions to complete the sentences in their proper forms.

recurrence rate	复发率	reproductive history	生育史
propose a diagnosis	拟诊断为	anemic	贫血的
holistic approach	整体方法	complain of	主诉
go on with the ward round	继续查房	gynecological check	妇科检查
abortion	堕胎	norm	标准
metabolize	新陈代谢	hypersensitivity	过敏症

1. Many studies have indicated that the abilities of the liver to _____ drugs and of the kidney to excrete drug metabolites decline with the aging process.

2. Periodic and routine _____ as well as B ultrasound examination are significant to the early diagnosis of pelvic tumor after menopause，thus avoiding benign tumors to turn into malignant ones.

3. The goal of this study was to assess whether menopausal symptoms were more common and/or more severe among women with depressive symptoms. Information on demographics，medical and _____，medication use，menopausal experience and

depressive symptoms was collected.

4. The FDA（Food and Drug Administration）approved the ESAs（Erythropoietin stimulating Agents）erythropoietin and darbepoetin in 2003 as a treatment for _____ cancer patients to avoid blood transfusions. However，evidence linking these drugs to a higher risk of death has been mounting. In March 2007，the FDA issued a public health advisory on EPAs，warning of an increased risk of serious and life-threatening side effects.

5. The aim of this systematic review was to identify the stroke _____ for each stroke subtype over time as well as risk factors for recurrent ischemic stroke identified through the currently available literature.

6. Traditional Chinese Medicine（TCM）is an ancient form of healthcare that dates back over 2,500 years and includes natural treatments such as acupuncture，herbal remedies，dietary advice，stress/emotional support，exercise including *taichi* and *qigong* and treatments such as cupping and moxibustion. TCM practitioners look to treat the root cause of disease and take a _____ to helping people experience complete healing without the use of conventional drugs.

7. Because of funding and staffing pressures，experts are now warning that the UK is facing a "crisis point" in _____ provision，with rising demand and restricted access to care in many areas putting unprecedented strain on already struggling NHS services.

8. Clinically，many children have respiratory symptoms，but their causes are different. Numerous studies have found children with family history of asthma or individual history of _____ were more likely to develop respiratory symptoms.

9. Diabetes mellitus type 2（T2DM），formerly known as noninsulin-dependent diabetes mellitus（NIDDM）or adult-onset diabetes is a chronic metabolic disease，which usually occurs after the age of 35 to 40 years，accounting for more than 90% of diabetic patients. Diabetics often _____ peripheral neuropathy，a disorder characterized by numbness of extremities described by patients as "pins and needles" or burning.

10. Contemporary society has placed a great emphasis on the factors that cause or effect psychological disorders in individuals. These are the drivers that affect the behaviorism and understanding of individuals with mental conditions and include platforms such as cultural and social _____ and how they get reception from the general society.

D. Read the dialogue and try to make a conversation with your classmates.

扫码获取
提示

E. Translate the following Chinese into English.

R—Resident   CP—Chief Physician

R：Dr. Wang，this is a patient with uterine fibroids and anemia who may need surgery.

CP：1. 请介绍一下她的情况。

1. _____

R：OK. Patient Wahla，40 years old, complained of menorrhagia for one-year，abdominal mass for six months，and excessive leucorrhea. 6 fetuses, 5 births, 1 abortion. 2. 她上次妊娠5年前,上次月经两周前。

2. _____

_____

CP：What are the results of examinations?

R：Physical examination：moderately anemic appearance, blood pressure 120/80 mmHg, pulse 84/ min, normal heart and lung. The abdomen is soft, the liver and spleen are impalpable, and the margin of the mass can be vaguely palpable on the symphysis pubis. Gynecological check：smooth cervix, hypertrophic uterus, like 3 months of pregnancy; not smooth surface, hard, good movement; 3. 子宫体后壁可扪及肿块,无压痛,附件阴性。Laboratory examination：4. 尿常规阴性,血色素7克,肝肾功能正常。Based on the patient's age, reproductive history and clinical symptoms, combined with gynecological double examination and gynecological ultrasound examination, 5. 拟诊断为子宫肌瘤。

3. _____

_____

4. _____

_____

5. _____

CP：You didn't mention an important point. You said the patient had excessive menstruation. How much more?

R：Oh, I'm sorry, I missed it. 6. 病人主诉一年前月经持续2至3天, using only 2 packs of sanitary pads at a time. In the past year, her menstruation lasted for more than 4 days, and sometimes even up to 7—10 days, using 4 to 5 pack sanitary pads.

6. _____

CP：I agree with you. 7. 什么时候手术?

7. _____

R：The day after tomorrow.

CP：OK. 8. 我们继续查房。

8. _____

III Further Reading：Acupuncture and Herbs for Uterine Fibroids

Have you been recently diagnosed with uterine fibroids and wondering what's the next step?

Susan, an attractive 47-year-old hair-dresser, first came to the TCM Health Center in January 1998. She had been diagnosed with uterine fibroids about seven months previously. By the time of her six-month follow-up with her gynecologist, the tumor had grown so big she could not button her pants, or zip up her skirt. She looked like a five-month-pregnant woman. Her gynecologist suggested an immediate hysterectomy. Susan resisted this, because she felt that losing her uterus would be a traumatic experience for her, and she wanted to explore other possibilities. She saw my article, "Endometriosis：A Natural Option," in a newspaper, and came to my clinic. At point, her hemoglobin was 9.6. She suffered from heavy uterine bleeding, which could be triggered by coughing, squatting, bending over, even walking. She was also exhausted and depressed from loss of blood and constant worry about her condition. After three months of weekly acupuncture treatments and Chinese herbal medicine, she felt her tummy getting smaller and smaller. She could fit into all her favorite clothes again, and the bleeding had totally stopped. I sent her back to her gynecologist to do a follow-up. She did not tell her doctor about the treatment she had from me. She was told the tumor was 50% smaller than it had been three months before. Her doctor was surprised, and asked her what she had done. When Susan told her about her experience with acupuncture, the doctor was very happy to hear about it. The doctor herself had received acupuncture for a sinus problem, and said, "It worked very well for my sinus, but I didn't know it would also be so effective for fibroid tumor." Currently, we are continuing to do treatments in order to shrink the tumor further.

After a few treatments, Susan asked me if her condition could be associated with emotional stress. Before her tumor was diagnosed, there had been a lot of stress at work, and anger with her family. A traditional Chinese medicine diagnosis and treatment can give a clear answer to this question.

Flora came in for what at first she thought was just really bad period cramps. She was in her mid-40's and had started experiencing cramping for the first time in years. The pain was unbearable: she was unable to go to work, it radiated to her back and down into her legs. After she went to the doctor and had an MRI done, they discovered a uterine fibroid measuring close to 6 cm. This was about the size of a lemon!

This wasn't the first time she was diagnosed with fibroids. She had one when she was in her 20's and it was surgically removed. As mentioned before, fibroids have a high rate of recurrence, and this was exactly such an instance. Due to the size of the fibroid and degree of pain, her doctor recommended a surgery. This time, however, the doctor recommended they do a hysterectomy (complete removal of the uterus) to 100% prevent the recurrence of a fibroid. Her surgery was scheduled for two months away.

Flora basically came in to find a way to naturally manage the pain until her surgery. She came in right as her period was beginning and the pain was at its height. We used acupuncture to activate her body's natural painkillers, boost blood flow quality in her uterus, and reduce the pain. After 30 minutes of napping with the acupuncture points in her body, her pain level had reduced from an 8/10 to 0/10. It was an incredible result. The following week she reported that while she would normally have pain for a full week, that she had no more pain in the days following the acupuncture treatment. Instead of 7 days of pain, she only had 1. We repeated this protocol for her next cycle with similar results. Our goal was to keep her out of pain and her body strong going into her surgery. It is an amazing experience to share because even though the fibroid is still there, we were able to modify her body's perception of pain to such an incredible degree!

Uterine fibroids are benign (non-cancerous) growths that occur in the uterus. They are incredibly common amongst women, and many will have the fibroid without even knowing it because they don't show any symptoms.

While finally gaining an answer to what's been causing your symptoms can bring relief, it is often followed with the uncertainty of how to proceed—especially if you're interested in holistically approaching the situation and wanting to shrink fibroids naturally.

We'll take a look at the basics behind uterine fibroids from both a western and Chinese medicine point of view.

Many of the women I see in my clinic with uterine fibroids aren't coming in primarily for the fibroid itself. In fact, a lot of them had no idea they had a fibroid to begin with. They had a persisting menstrual-related issue that was getting worse over time, and when they got it checked out with their gynecologist, it turned out there was also a fibroid. The most common symptoms secondary to fibroids are excessively heavy menstrual bleeding accompanied with anemia, periods that last longer than 7 days, lower abdominal pressure and swelling, menstrual cramps, low back pain and infertility.

Chinese medicine is amazing at working on the above issues while simultaneously working on the fibroid. The reason is simple. Our goal is not to just reduce the fibroid, but to understand the hormonal imbalance causing the fibroid growth. This imbalance is also most likely causing your problem with heavy flow or cramps or infertility.

In the world of Chinese medicine, using acupuncture and herbal medicine to work on uterine fibroids is nothing new. Treatments are most effective at helping with small to medium size fibroids. This means a fibroid up to around 5 cm, which is about the size of a lemon.

If the size of the fibroid is large (upwards of 7 cm and more) and it's causing a lot of pain, having it removed through one of the various surgical treatments seems to be the norm. Another reason to consider immediate surgical removal of the fibroid is if the location of the fibroid is sensitive. For example, the fibroid is pressing on the intestines or bladder causing problems there. Or it may be located in the inside layer of the uterus making it difficult to fall pregnant. In those situations, removing the fibroid would give you a rapid solution and relief.

So the main question here is why take the holistic approach? One of the main reasons to consider a holistic approach to fibroids is their high rate of recurrence. Different studies have shown the recurrence rate to be as high as 30% in some instances. Basically what this means is that simply removing a fibroid doesn't guarantee that it's gone for good. Many women have had their fibroids surgically removed, only to have new ones show up on their ultrasounds a few years later. It is for this reason that women who aren't interested in getting pregnant or are done having kids, are routinely recommended to have a complete removal of their uterus (hysterectomy) to prevent recurrence.

The reason for these recurrences is simple. If you don't change the environment which created the problem in the first place, it is highly likely the issue will recur. When treating fibroids we have to dig deep and understand what environmental and hormonal factors contributed to the creation of this tumor. If we don't remove the environmental toxins and correct the hormonal imbalances, we are not taking care of the situation from all angles.

One of the biggest issues when it comes to fibroids is your exposure to estrogen. It's well established that estrogen can promote fibroid growth. In holistically treating fibroids, we need to understand whether your body's exposure to excess estrogen is caused by outside factors (like foods / chemicals / etc.) or from the body's inability to properly metabolize it.

In Chinese medicine, fibroids are said to be caused by two different imbalances: stagnation of blood in the uterus or an accumulation of dampness. Blood stagnation refers to a lack of smooth blood flow in the pelvis. The flow is so unsmooth that it is causing blockages and obstructions. Think of a freeway where cars begin to drive erratically and chaotically—an accident is bound to happen and once it does, there are major traffic jams. This is the type of environment that engenders fibroids. The fibroid is essentially a more tangible and physical manifestation of these obstructions. It is interesting to note that the blood stagnation imbalance shares many of the same symptoms of estrogen dominance (excess estrogen): painful cramps, PMS symptoms, heavy bleeding. In a sense, they are east-west parallel versions of each other. Dampness refers to impaired fluid metabolism in the body because of poor digestion. In Chinese medicine, the digestive organs are responsible for refining food and drink into nutrition and transporting it to the different parts of the body. When this factory process is messed up, your body produces dampness. When you bloat or feel sluggish after eating even the lightest meals, this is a manifestation of that dampness.

Your intestines play an incredible role in metabolizing estrogen. Excess estrogen in the body is inactivated by the liver and removed from the body via the stool. If your digestive health isn't optimal, it's possible you're holding onto more estrogen than you need, and this can be fueling fibroid growth. It is for this reason that if dampness is a presenting factor in your case, your digestive health must certainly be addressed.

Like we talked about earlier, Chinese medicine views poor blood flow as one of the main causes behind fibroids. The impaired flow eventually leads to blockages and ultimately the growth of fibrous tissues. In such situation, we can try acupuncture and herbal medicine. Both are amazing at promoting blood flow in the uterus and helping to reduce fibroid sizes. We can also apply heat packs to the lower abdomen. Heat helps to promote movement of blood and improve circulation. This is especially effective for women who get menstrual cramp relief from heating pads.

Like we talked about, your liver is responsible for metabolizing and inactivating excess estrogen in the body. If your liver is not happy, you will be holding on to more than you need and this can encourage fibroid growth.

In Chinese medicine, when we treat gynecological issues, one of the most important organs we look at and treat is the liver. It's incredible because the traditional doctors from hundreds of years ago had no idea about the liver's role in estrogen metabolism, and yet, the medicine recognized its importance in menstrual health.

Things you can do to keep your liver happy are to avoid alcohol. Alcohol keeps your liver from functioning optimally. Sub-optimal liver performance puts you at risk for estrogen excess and fibroid growth. Next, avoid excessive medication usage. This is not in reference to medications necessary to manage a health issue. This is more about liberally taking over-the-counter pain killers, cold medicines, acid blockers, etc. Most drugs need to be metabolized by the liver and over time, excessive usage can lead to liver injury and hence, impaired estrogen metabolism. Finally, try to eat REAL food such as fermented foods, fruits, nuts, seeds, cruciferous vegetables, dark leafy greens, good quality protein, wild caught fatty fish are all great foods that support a healthy liver.

Reduce inflammation. Inflammation becomes a problem when it tends to linger on long-term in your body. Short bursts of inflammation to manage acute situations like injuries or infections is normal, but when it keeps going on and on it's going to wreck havoc. For a person with fibroids this is important because chronic inflammation can make your body's estrogen receptors more sensitive to estrogen. This hypersensitivity causes your body to have an extra-strong reaction to even normal amounts of estrogen in the body. This in turn can fuel fibroid growth.

Be honest with your emotions. In Chinese medicine, emotional health can be a big contributing factor in the formation of fibroids. It's not so simple as getting angry will magically make a fibroid grow. Rather, holding on to strong emotions long term like anger or sadness will slowly start to compromise the physical functioning of the body. Intuitively this makes complete sense. Think of people who have lost the will to live and see how soon after they pass. There are very clear connections between the mind and the body.

If you seek Chinese medicine treatments, an integral part of your holistic treatment plan will be Chinese herbs. There is no single herb or collection of herbs that is always used for uterine fibroids. It always depends on your specific constitution and root cause.

Of the many types of herbal formulas that can be used to shrink fibroids, one of the most common formulas are Cinnamon & Poria Pills. Much research has been done on this formula and its effect on uterine tumors over the years. A 2019 research article explored the pharmacological effects of this formula on fibroids and discovered that the possible mechanism by which it works is that it induces apoptosis (the death of cells) within the fibroid tumor. Other studies purport its usefulness in treating fibroids because of its anti-tumor and anti-inflammatory effect.

Beth came in to the clinic because she had extremely heavy periods for the past 3 years. She had always bled on the heavier side, but when it started to get worse, she went to her OBGYN for a check-up and was diagnosed with uterine fibroids via ultrasound. Her heavier bleeds were accompanied with period cramps and low back pain. Since the largest fibroid measured around 4 cm, they decided to wait and see how the fibroids progressed: would they grow or stay the same? The idea was if the discomfort wasn't detrimental, then she could avoid surgery.

Beth's situation is not all that uncommon. While her symptoms weren't detrimental to her daily life, they most definitely affected her quality of life physically and emotionally. Having to use both a pad and tampon for the first few days and changing them almost every 1 hour was incredibly stressful while she was at work. In the nights, the bleeding could be so heavy that she would place towels on the bed for the inevitable leakage that happened while she slept. The cramping and lower back pain left her no choice but to take Advil multiple times a day. She didn't want to have the surgery, but she definitely didn't want to have to keep going through this torture every month.

Based off of her history, constitution and symptoms, we decided to take a two-pronged approach: we needed to improve the poor blood circulation in the pelvic area. This was contributing to the fibroid growth and the pain she was experiencing around her periods. Second, we needed to tackle her digestive health. Her chronic digestive issues were definitely a factor in how her body was poorly metabolizing estrogen. When estrogen metabolism is disrupted, the body can hold on to more estrogen than needed, and this over-accumulation can promote fibroid growth.

We began with a weekly regimen of acupuncture and herbal medicine to enact the approach described above. The first symptoms to improve were her digestive issues: less bloating along with more comfortable and regular bowel movements. Her second period since beginning the acupuncture was when her period symptoms began to improve. The first significant change was a major reduction in her overall pain: no more ovulatory pain, much less period cramping, and no more lower back pain. As the months progressed, the bleeding amount also began to change. No more leakages at night, she could go for 2—3 hours before having to change pads. The biggest change here was that she wasn't feeling incredibly anxious and emotional around her periods. Her overall experience of life surrounding her periods was shifting from something chronically negative to more positive and normal. It is now 1 year since she first came in to our clinic, and we are happy to report that her period bleeds have returned to their normal amount from before the fibroids.

Chinese acupuncture and herbs have turned out to be natural ways to shrink fibroids.

A. Translate the following sentences into Chinese.

1. Chinese medicine is amazing at working on the above issues while simultaneously working on the fibroid. The reason is simple. Our goal is not to just reduce the fibroid, but to understand the hormonal imbalance causing the fibroid growth. This imbalance is also most likely causing your problem with heavy flow or cramps or infertility.

2. For example, the fibroid is pressing on the intestines or bladder causing problems there. Or it may be located in the inside layer of the uterus making it difficult to fall pregnant. In those situations, removing the fibroid would give you a rapid solution and relief.

3. One of the biggest issues when it comes to fibroids is your exposure to estrogen. It's well established that estrogen can promote fibroid growth. In holistically treating fibroids, we need to understand whether your body's exposure to excess estrogen is caused by outside factors (like foods / chemicals / etc.) or from the body's inability to properly metabolize it.

4. The fibroid is essentially a more tangible and physical manifestation of these obstructions. It is interesting to note that the blood stagnation imbalance shares many of the same symptoms of estrogen dominance (excess estrogen): painful cramps, PMP symptoms, heavy bleeding. In a sense, they are east-west parallel versions of each other.

5. Next, avoid excessive medication usage. This is not in reference to medications necessary to manage a health issue. This is more about liberally taking over-the-counter pain killers, cold medicines, acid blockers, etc. Most drugs need to be metabolized by the liver and over time, excessive usage can lead to liver injury and hence, impaired estrogen metabolism.

B. Prepare a lecture on uterine fibroid after doing the further reading above.

扫码获取
提示

Unit 13

Bronchial Asthma

Ⅰ Warming-up

A. Match the following words and phrases with their Chinese translations.

A	bronchiole	1	黏液
B	exacerbation	2	过度充气
C	asthmatic	3	β-受体激动剂
D	mucus	4	刺激物
E	hyperinflation	5	恶化,加剧
F	beta-agonist	6	喘息
G	corticosteroid	7	分泌
H	irritant	8	细支气管
I	wheeze	9	糖皮质激素
J	secrete	10	哮喘病人

B. Complete the sentences with the following words or phrases in their proper forms.

lead to	run out of	worsen	range from ... to
shallow	present	result in	chronical

1. Your breathing speeds up and gets _____ , making you feel short of breath.
2. In people with asthma, the airways are _____ inflamed, which can make them

hyper-responsive to certain triggers.

3. But how exactly do such everyday factors _____ an asthma attack?

4. Simultaneously the trigger _____ inflammation，causing the mucosal lining to become more swollen and secrete more mucus.

5. Smooth muscle constriction _____ the feeling of chest tightness.

6. These symptoms may make a person feel like they're _____ air.

7. One way is to reduce the _____ of triggers.

8. This may be due to reasons _____ exposure _____ additional pollutants and environmental irritants to difficulties in obtaining medical care or treatment.

 C. Watch the video *How Does Asthma Work* and answer the questions.

扫码获取视频

1. What are the common symptoms of an asthma attack?

2. Why do people get asthma and how can this disease be deadly?

3. What may cause the wheezing noise?

4. How do we prevent these uncomfortable and potentially fatal attacks in people who have asthma?

5. What are the possible causes of asthma according to the video?

Ⅱ Dialogue

扫码获取
音频及文本

 A. Listen to the dialogue for the first time and try to get the general idea.

 B. Listen to the dialogue for the second time and try to answer the following questions.

1. What is wrong with the pediatric patient?

2. Why all the medicines taken by the patient only work for a temporary relief?

3. What could be the triggers to the asthma attack?

4. Why is this pediatric patient required to be examined in the allergy clinic?

5. What can be done to bring the asthma

symptoms under well control?

C. Choose the following words and/or expressions to complete the sentences in their proper forms.

bout	发作	for instance	例如
coughing spell	一阵咳嗽	rather than	而不是
severe	十分严重的	bring ... on	使……发生
relationship to	与……的关系	now and then	偶尔,不时
contact with	与接触	allergic to	对……过敏
particular	特定的	prevent ... from	防止……

1. She continued to have _____ stomach cramps, aches, fatigue, and depression.
2. Yet one study after another indicates that _____ nature gives huge benefits to ADHD children.
3. Cases of the bacterial disease pertussis, nicknamed for the "whoop" sufferers sometimes make as they gasp for breath after a long _____, have risen from 1,010 in 1976 to over 25,000 today, according to the CDC.
4. In an actual test, your response would be judged on the quality of your writing and on how well your response presents the points in the lecture and their _____ the reading passage.
5. A person, for example, who is _____ cats would probably never become an animal doctor.
6. A baby may frequently get a _____ of hiccups during or soon after a feeding.
7. South Wales Police decided to learn from last year's experiences and keep a _____ eye on car crime.
8. She had started to devote her energies to teaching _____ performing.
9. The speaker told a joke or story _____ when he gave the talk to keep us interested.
10. The second attack was so serious that his airway swelled, _____ him _____ breathing, his blood pressure dropped suddenly, and his heart stopped for a moment.

D. Read the dialogue and try to make a conversation with your classmates.

扫码获取
提示

E. Translate the following Chinese into English.

P—Patient   D—Doctor

D：1. 你能告诉我孩子何时开始咳嗽的?
    1. _____
P：My baby has been coughing and wheezing for three days. 2. 她晚上总是睡不好觉,吵

得全家都睡不了。
    2. _____
D：Is the cough very bad? Much sputum? Any temperature?
P：3. 一阵阵咳嗽,咳得非常厉害,痰很少,不

发烧。

 3. _____

             _____

D：Has she had any foods like melon seeds or peanuts lately?

P：No，I don't think so. 4. 但她好像呼吸很费力，喉咙里有鸡鸣声。

 4. _____

_____

D：Is it the first time that she has found it difficult to get breath?

P：No，this has happened three times before.

D：Can she lie flat? Do her lips appear blue?

P：5. 在发作厉害时候，她不能平躺。Both her lips and nails appear blue.

 5. _____

D：6. 你有没有注意到她的发作和什么有关

吗？ Cold? Specific foods? Or，contact with some flowers or herbs? Does she have more attacks during a particular season，for instance，in the rainy season rather than in the dry season?

 6. _____

P：Yes，I have，7. 与天气冷有关。

 7. _____

D：Has she had any treatment for this?

P：Yes，she has had some treatment every now and then. 8. 她用过很多药物，比如舒喘宁吸入剂，爱喘乐等，所有的药物都是暂时缓解一下。

 8. _____

_____

Ⅲ Further Reading：Pediatric Asthma

Background

  Asthma is a chronic inflammatory disorder of the airways characterized by an obstruction of airflow，which may be completely or partially reversed with or without specific therapy. Airway inflammation is the result of interactions between various cells，cellular elements，and cytokines. In susceptible individuals，airway inflammation may cause recurrent or persistent bronchospasm，which causes symptoms that include wheezing，breathlessness，chest tightness，and cough，particularly at night（early morning hours）or after exercise.

  Airway inflammation is associated with airway hyperreactivity or bronchial hyperresponsiveness（BHR），which is defined as the inherent tendency of the airways to narrow in response to various stimuli（eg，environmental allergens and irritants）.

  Asthma affects an estimated 300 million individuals worldwide. The prevalence of asthma is increasing，especially in children. Annually，the World Health Organization（WHO）has estimated that 15 million disability-adjusted life-years are lost and 250, 000 asthma deaths are reported worldwide. Approximately 500,000 annual hospitalizations (34.6% in individuals aged 18 or younger) are due to asthma. In the United States, asthma prevalence, having increased from 1980 to 1996, showed a plateau at 9.1% of children (6.7 million) in 2007.

The cost of illness related to asthma is around $6.2 billion. Each year, an estimated 1.81 million people (47.8% in individuals aged 18 y or younger) require treatment in the emergency department. Among children and adolescents aged 5—17 years, asthma accounts for a loss of 10 million school days and costs caretakers $726.1 million because of work absence.

Pathophysiology

Interactions between environmental and genetic factors result in airway inflammation, which limits airflow and leads to functional and structural changes in the airways in the form of bronchospasm, mucosal edema, and mucus plugs.

Airway obstruction causes increased resistance to airflow and decreased expiratory flow rates. These changes lead to a decreased ability to expel air and may result in hyperinflation. The resulting over distention helps maintain airway patency, thereby improving expiratory flow; however, it also alters pulmonary mechanics and increases the work of breathing.

Hyperinflation compensates for the airflow obstruction, but this compensation is limited when the tidal volume approaches the volume of the pulmonary dead space; the result is alveolar hypoventilation. Uneven changes in airflow resistance, the resulting uneven distribution of air, and alterations in circulation from increased intra-alveolar pressure due to hyperinflation all lead to ventilation-perfusion mismatch.

Vasoconstriction due to alveolar hypoxia also contributes to this mismatch. Vasoconstriction is also considered an adaptive response to ventilation/perfusion mismatch.

In the early stages, when ventilation-perfusion mismatch results in hypoxia, hypercarbia is prevented by the ready diffusion of carbon dioxide across alveolar capillary membranes. Thus, patients with asthma who are in the early stages of an acute episode have hypoxemia in the absence of carbon dioxide retention. Hyperventilation triggered by the hypoxic drive also causes a decrease in $PaCO_2$. An increase in alveolar ventilation in the early stages of an acute exacerbation prevents hypercarbia.

With worsening obstruction and increasing ventilation-perfusion mismatch, carbon dioxide retention occurs. In the early stages of an acute episode, respiratory alkalosis results from hyperventilation. Later, the increased work of breathing, increased oxygen consumption, and increased cardiac output result in metabolic acidosis. Respiratory failure leads to respiratory acidosis. Fatigue is also a potential contributor to respiratory acidosis.

Role of inflammation

Chronic inflammation of the airways is associated with increased BHR, which leads to bronchospasm and typical symptoms of wheezing, shortness of breath, and coughing after exposure to allergens, environmental irritants, viruses, cold air, or exercise. In some patients with chronic asthma, airflow limitation may be only partially reversible because of airway remodeling (hypertrophy and hyperplasia of smooth muscle, angiogenesis, and subepithelial fibrosis) that occurs with chronic untreated disease.

New insights in the pathogenesis of asthma suggest that lymphocytes play a role. Airway inflammation in asthma may represent a loss of normal balance between two "opposing" populations of T helper (Th) lymphocytes. Two types of Th lymphocytes have been characterized: Th1 and Th2. Th1 cells produce interleukin (IL)-2 and interferon-α (IFN-α), which are critical in cellular defense mechanisms in response to infection. Th2, in contrast, generates a family of cytokines (interleukin-4 [IL-4], IL-5, IL-6, IL-9, and IL-13) that can mediate allergic inflammation.

The hygiene hypothesis

The current "hygiene hypothesis" of asthma illustrates how this cytokine imbalance may explain some of the dramatic increases in asthma prevalence in Westernized countries. This hypothesis is based on the concept that the immune system of the newborn is skewed toward Th2 cytokine generation (mediators of allergic inflammation). Over time, environmental stimuli such as infections activate Th1 responses and bring the Th1/Th2 relationship to an appropriate balance.

Evidence suggests that the prevalence of asthma is reduced in children who experience the following events:
- Certain infections (Mycobacterium tuberculosis, measles, or hepatitis A)
- Rural living
- Exposure to other children (eg, presence of older siblings and early enrollment in childcare)
- Less frequent use of antibiotics, including in the first week of life
- Early introduction of fish in the diet

Furthermore, the absence of these lifestyle events is associated with the persistence of a Th2 cytokine pattern.

Under these conditions, the genetic background of the child, with a cytokine imbalance toward Th2, sets the stage to promote the production of immunoglobulin E (IgE) antibody to key environmental antigens (eg, dust mites, cockroaches, Alternaria, and possibly cats). Therefore, a gene-by-environment interaction occurs in which the susceptible host is exposed to environmental factors that are capable of generating IgE, and sensitization occurs.

A reciprocal interaction is apparent between the two subpopulations, in which Th1 cytokines can inhibit Th2 generation and vice versa. Allergic inflammation may be the result of an excessive expression of Th2 cytokines. Alternatively, recent studies have suggested the possibility that the loss of normal immune balance arises from a cytokine dysregulation in which Th1 activity in asthma is diminished.

Genetic factors

Some studies highlight the importance of genotypes in contributing to asthma susceptibility and allergic sensitization, as well as response to specific asthma treatments.

Through the use of cluster analysis, an institute identified 5 phenotypes of asthma. Cluster 1 patients have early-onset atopic asthma with normal lung function treated with two or fewer controller medications and minimal health care utilization. Cluster 2 patients have early-onset atopic asthma and preserved lung function but increased medication requirements (29% on three or more medications) and health care utilization.

Cluster 3 comprises mostly older obese women with late-onset nonatopic asthma, moderate reductions in pulmonary function, and frequent oral corticosteroid use to manage exacerbations. Cluster 4 and cluster 5 patients have severe airflow obstruction with bronchodilator responsiveness but differ in to their ability to attain normal lung function, age of asthma onset, atopic status, and use of oral corticosteroids.

A recently reported meta-analysis of genome-wide association studies of asthma in ethnically diverse North American populations identified 5 susceptibility loci. Four were on previously reported loci on 17q21 and a new asthma susceptibility locus at PYHIN1, which is specific to the African American population.

An Australian study identified 2 new loci with genome-wide significant association with asthma risk: rs4129267 in IL6R and rs7130588 on band 11q13.5. The IL6R association supports the hypothesis that cytokine dysregulation affects asthma risk, hence a specific antagonist to IL6R may help. The results for the 11q13.5 locus suggest its association with allergic sensitization and subsequent development of asthma.

Other factors

A study that examined whether the lipid profile is associated with concurrent asthma concluded that the blood lipid profile is associated with asthma, airway obstruction, bronchial responsiveness, and aeroallergen sensitization in 7-year-old children. Caution must be applied before saying that asthma might be a systemic disorder. First, we don't know if the children with the elevated LDL levels were more likely exposed to higher doses of inhaled, or systemic corticosteroids. The authors did find that those with worse lung function had higher LDL levels. However, it could also be that those children exercised less, a potential cause of obesity and abnormal lipid levels. The BMI was also not reported.

A 2012 study reported a significant association between lung function deficit and bronchial responsiveness in the neonatal period with development of asthma by age seven years.

Lemanske et al reported that wheezing illnesses caused by rhinovirus infection during infancy were the strongest predictor of wheezing in the third year of life.

In a study of preschool children with asthma, Guilbert et al found that 2 years of inhaled corticosteroid therapy did not change the asthma symptoms or lung function during a third, treatment-free year. This suggests that no disease-modifying effect of inhaled corticosteroids is present after the treatment is discontinued.

In a study of children in the Cincinnati area, Reponen et al found that a high Environmental Relative Moldiness Index (ERMI) at age 1 year made asthma at age 7 years more likely. The ERMI did not predict specific mold allergies at age 7 years. Air conditioning made asthma less likely. An elevated ERMI at age 7 years had no correlation with current asthma. Seeing or smelling mold in a home inspection at age 1 year did not correlate with the ERMI or with the development of asthma. They also found that black race, having a parent with asthma, and house dust allergy was predictive of a greater likelihood of asthma.

A recent study from Australia reported that obesity is a determinant of asthma control independent of inflammation, lung function, and airway hyperresponsiveness. A similar association between increased risk of worse asthma control and obesity was reported in a recent retrospective study of 32,321 children aged 5—17 years.

A significant inverse relationship between serum vitamin D levels and patient IgE levels, steroid requirements, and in vitro responsiveness to corticosteroids in children has been reported.

Parental cigarette smoking has been shown to increase the likelihood of asthma. This is more true for maternal smoking, though the authors of one study did not correct for primary caretakers. The more cigarettes the mother smoked, the greater the risk of asthma.

A randomized clinical trial by Sheehan et al evaluated the association in children between frequent acetaminophen use and asthma-related complications. The study found that among young children with mild persistent asthma, as-needed use of acetaminophen was not shown to be associated with a higher incidence of asthma exacerbation or worse asthma control than was as-needed use of ibuprofen.

Etiology

In most cases of asthma in children, multiple triggers or precipitants are recognized, and the patterns of reactivity may change with age. Treatment can also change the pattern. Wheeze is common with respiratory syncytial virus (RSV) bronchiolitis and recurrent wheeze may persist up to 3—5 years. However, RSV is unlikely the sole explanation for the development of atopic asthma later in life. On the other hand, infection with human rhinovirus that requires hospitalization has been associated with future development of asthma (age 6 y).

Respiratory infections

Most commonly, these are viral infections. In some patients, fungi (eg, allergic bronchopulmonary aspergillosis), bacteria (eg, Mycoplasma, pertussis), or parasites may be responsible. Most infants and young children who continue to have a persistent wheeze and asthma have high immunoglobulin E (IgE) production and eosinophilic immune responses (in the airways and in circulation) at the time of the first viral upper respiratory tract infection (URTI). They also have early IgE-mediated responses to local aeroallergens.

Allergens and irritants

In patients with asthma, 2 types of bronchoconstrictor responses to allergens are recognized: early and late. Early asthmatic responses occur via IgE-induced mediator release from mast cells within minutes of exposure and last for 20—30 minutes.

Late asthmatic responses occur 4—12 hours after antigen exposure and result in more severe symptoms that can last for hours and contribute to the duration and severity of the disease. Inflammatory cell infiltration and inflammatory mediators play a role in the late asthmatic response. Allergens can be foods, household inhalants (eg, animal allergens, molds, fungi, roach allergens, dust mites), or seasonal outdoor allergens (eg, mold spores, pollens, grass, trees).

Tobacco smoke, cold air, chemicals, perfumes, paint odors, hair sprays, air pollutants, and ozone can initiate BHR by inducing inflammation.

Other factors

Asthma attacks can be related to changes in atmospheric temperature, barometric pressure, and the quality of air (eg, humidity, allergen and irritant content). In some individuals, emotional upsets clearly aggravate asthma.

Exercise can trigger an early asthmatic response. Mechanisms underlying exercise-induced asthmatic response remain somewhat uncertain. Heat and water loss from the airways can increase the osmolarity of the fluid lining the airways and result in mediator release. Cooling of the airways results in congestion and dilatation of bronchial vessels. During the rewarming phase after exercise, the changes are magnified because the ambient air breathed during recovery is warm rather than cool.

The presence of acid in the distal esophagus, mediated via vagal or other neural reflexes, can significantly increase airway resistance and airway reactivity. Inflammatory conditions of the upper airways (eg, allergic rhinitis, sinusitis, or chronic and persistent infections) must be treated before asthmatic symptoms can be completely controlled.

Multiple factors have been proposed to explain nocturnal asthma. Circadian variation in lung function and inflammatory mediator release in the circulation and airways (including parenchyma) have been demonstrated. Other factors, such as allergen exposure and posture-related irritation of airways (eg, gastroesophageal reflux, sinusitis), can also play a role. In some cases, abnormalities in CNS control of the respiratory drive may be present, particularly in patients with a defective hypoxic drive and obstructive sleep apnea.

Children exposed to higher maternal stress during the pre- and postnatal period were reported to be at higher risk for wheeze. This was only true in non-atopic mothers.

A 2012 Danish study reported an association between maternal obesity (BMI$\geqslant$35 and gestational weight gain $\geqslant$ 25 kg) during pregnancy with increased risk of asthma and wheezing in the offspring.

Results of a prospective birth cohort study of 568 pregnant women and their offspring showed that postnatal bisphenol A (BPA) exposure in the first years of a child's life is associated with significantly increased risk for wheeze and asthma. Feeding bottles, sippy cups, or other containers designed for infants may contain it. The study also found, however, that fetal exposure to BPA during the third trimester of pregnancy was inversely associated with risk for wheeze in offspring at age 5 years.

Prognosis

Of infants who wheeze with URTIs, 60% are asymptomatic by age 6 years. However, children who have asthma (recurrent symptoms continuing at age 6 y) have airway reactivity later in childhood. Some findings suggest a poor prognosis if asthma develops in children younger than 3 years, unless it occurs solely in association with viral infections.

Children with mild asthma who are asymptomatic between attacks are likely to improve and be symptom-free later in life.

Children with asthma appear to have less severe symptoms as they enter adolescence, but half of these children continue to have asthma. Asthma has a tendency to remit during puberty, with a somewhat earlier remission in girls. However, compared with men, women have more BHR.

Patient Education

Patient and parent education should include instructions on how to use medications and devices (eg, spacers, nebulizers, metered-dose inhalers [MDIs]). The patient's MDI technique should be assessed on every visit. Discuss the management plan, which includes instructions about the use of medications, precautions with drug and/or device usage, monitoring symptoms and their severity (peak flow meter reading), and identifying potential adverse effects and necessary actions.

Write and discuss in detail a rescue plan for an acute episode. This plan should include instructions for identifying signs of an acute attack, using rescue medications, monitoring, and contacting the asthma care team. Parents should understand that asthma is a chronic disorder with acute exacerbations; hence, continuity of management with active participation by the patient and/or parents and interaction with asthma care medical personnel is important.

A. Translate the following sentences into Chinese.

1. Asthma is a chronic inflammatory disorder of the airways characterized by an obstruction of airflow, which may be completely or partially reversed with or without specific therapy.

2. Interactions between environmental and genetic factors result in airway inflammation, which limits airflow and leads to functional and structural changes in the airways in the form of bronchospasm, mucosal edema, and mucus plugs.

3. A study that examined whether the lipid profile is associated with concurrent asthma concluded that the blood lipid profile is associated with asthma, airway obstruction, bronchial responsiveness, and aeroallergen sensitization in 7-year-old children.

4. The study found that among young children with mild persistent asthma, as-needed use of acetaminophen was not shown to be associated with a higher incidence of asthma exacerbation or worse asthma control than was as-needed use of ibuprofen.

5. Parents should understand that asthma is a chronic disorder with acute exacerbations; hence, continuity of management with active participation by the patient and/or parents and interaction with asthma care medical personnel is important.

B. Prepare a lecture on bronchial asthma after doing the further reading above.

扫码获取
提示

Unit 14

Sickle Cell Anemia

Ⅰ Warming-up

A. Match the following words and phrases with their Chinese translations.

A	anemia	1	分子,少量,微粒
B	complication	2	血红蛋白
C	mutation	3	缺氧的
D	molecule	4	视网膜脱落
E	hemoglobin	5	并发症
F	oxygen-starved	6	孵化器
G	spleen	7	贫血,贫血症
H	retinal detachment	8	突变,变异
I	incubator	9	脾脏
J	hydroxyurea	10	羟基脲

B. Complete the sentences with the following words or phrases in their proper forms.

constant	obstruct	malignant	no longer
play a key role in	from ... to ...	resist	accommodation

1. Sickle cell disease affects the red blood cells, which transport oxygen _____ the lungs _____ all the tissues in the body.

2. These proteins float independently inside the red blood cell's pliable donut like shape，keeping the cells flexible enough to _____ even the tiniest of blood vessels.

3. These red blood cells are harder and stickier and _____ flow smoothly through the blood vessels.

4. And if the _____ vessels supplied the brain，the patient could even suffer a stroke.

5. Worse still，sickle red blood cells also don't survive very long，just 10 or 20 days，versus healthy cells for a month，this short lifespan means that patients live with a _____ depleted supply of red blood cells，a condition called sickle cell anemia.

6. Perhaps what's most surprising about this _____ mutation is that it originally evolved as a beneficial adaptation.

7. And this mutation still _____ Africa，where more than 90% of malaria infections occur worldwide.

8. However，the same structural changes that turn red blood cells into roadblocks also make them more _____ to malaria.

C. Watch the video *What is Sickle Cell Anemia* and answer the questions.

扫码获取视频

1. What helps red blood cells to transport oxygen from the lungs to all the tissues in the body?

2. What are the commonly seen symptoms in sickle cell disease?

3. What is most surprising about this malignant mutation of red blood cells?

4. What are the origins of the sickle cell mutation?

5. What will happen if a child inherits a copy of the mutation from only one parent?

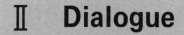

II Dialogue

扫码获取
音频及文本

A. Listen to the dialogue for the first time and try to get the general idea.

B. Listen to the dialogue for the second time and try to answer the following questions.

1. What's wrong with the patient?

2. What diseases did the patient have in the past?

3. Why does the doctor ask if any other kids or relatives in the patient's family have the same things?

4. Why is the patient required to have a routine blood test?

5. What can be done to help the patient with sickle cell anemia?

C. Choose the following words and/or expressions to complete the sentences in their proper forms.

have no clue	毫无头绪	further examination	进一步检查
calcium deficient	缺钙	confirm	确定,确认
compare to	与……相比	sickle cell anemia	镰状细胞性贫血
be more liable to	更容易	hereditary	遗传的
pneumonia	肺炎	alleviate	缓解
what on earth	究竟是什么	blood transfusion	输血

1. I'll be wondering _____ is Pepsi(百事) up to, but that's fine.

2. Some inherited anemias, such as _____, can be serious and lead to life-threatening complications.

3. The company _____ the news and said further investigation was underway.

4. It is considered that the patients with breast cancer _____ develop colon carcinoma. This is thought to be related to high fatty diet, heredity and endocrine factors.

5. Mutations of the BRCA1 and BRCA2 genes have been linked to _____ breast and ovarian cancer.

6. I'll prepare the blood for you in case a _____ is needed. You should be admitted to the hospital immediately.

7. After hours of drinking, he remembers nothing from the incident and _____ whose snake it was.

8. His action plan includes combating corruption, _____ poverty and reinstating salaries to the previous scales for workers.

9. Length of trial and number of measurements did not influence the selection of trials for study. Where indicated, individual patient data were requested for _____.

10. It is known that _____ in human body is related to many diseases such as osteoporosis, arteriosclerosis, cancer, kidney diseases, arthritis, and so on.

D. Read the dialogue and try to make a conversation with your classmates.

E. Translate the following Chinese into English.

P—Patient   D—Doctor

P：1. 医生，麻烦您帮我孩子检查检查。

　　1. _____

D：Is there anything wrong with him?

P：2. 我也不清楚。He is now 3 years old，but he seems smaller compared to his peers and he always cries complaining of leg pain. Is he possibly calcium deficient?

　　2. _____

D：Please place the kid on the couch. I'll have a look at him. 3. 请问孩子过去生过什么病?

　　3. _____

P：4. 我这孩子特别容易生病。He has suffered from pneumonia several times. 5. 好像他的抵抗力特别差。

　　4. _____

　　5. _____

D：6. 您的孩子有贫血，肝脾肿大。Do any other kids or relatives in your family have the same things?

　　6. _____

P：My second kid died of severe anemia when he was 6 months old. 7. 医生，这孩子究竟是什么病?

　　7. _____

D：Your kid is highly likely to suffer from a genetic disease，which should be confirmed by routine blood test. 8. 请您拿上化验单带孩子到检验科去检查一下。

　　8. _____

　　_____

P：OK. I'll come back when the results have come out. Thank you，doctor.

Ⅲ Further Reading：Sickle Cell Disease（SCD）

Background

Carriers of the sickle cell trait（ie，heterozygotes who carry one HbS allele and one normal adult hemoglobin［HbA］allele）have some resistance to the often-fatalmalaria caused by Plasmodium falciparum. This property explains the distribution and persistence of this gene in the population in malaria-endemic areas.

However，in areas such as the United States，where malaria is not a problem，the trait no longer provides a survival advantage. Instead，it poses the threat of SCD，which occurs in children of carriers who inherit the sickle cell gene from both parents(ie，HbSS).

Although carriers of sickle cell trait do not suffer from SCD, individuals with one copy of HbS and one copy of a gene that codes for another abnormal variant of hemoglobin, such as HbC or Hb beta-thalassemia, have a less severe form of the disease.

Genetics

SCD denotes all genotypes containing at least one sickle gene, in which HbS makes up at least half the hemoglobin present. Major sickle genotypes described so far include the following:

- HbSS disease or sickle cell anemia (the most common form)—Homozygote for the S globin with usually a severe or moderately severe phenotype and with the shortest survival
- HbS/b-0 thalassemia—Double heterozygote for HbS and b-0 thalassemia; clinically indistinguishable from sickle cell anemia (SCA)
- HbS/b + thalassemia—Mild-to-moderate severity with variability in different ethnicities
- HbSC disease—Double heterozygote for HbS and HbC characterized by moderate clinical severity
- HbS/hereditary persistence of fetal Hb (S/HPHP)—Very mild or asymptomatic phenotype
- HbS/HbE syndrome—Very rare with a phenotype usually similar to HbS/b+ thalassemia
- Rare combinations of HbS with other abnormal hemoglobins such as HbD Los Angeles, G-Philadelphia, and others

Sickle cell trait or the carrier state is the heterozygous form characterized by the presence of around 40% HbS, absence of anemia, inability to concentrate urine (isosthenuria), and hematuria. Under conditions leading to hypoxia, it may become a pathologic risk factor.

SCD is the most severe and most common form. Affected individuals present with a wide range of clinical problems that result from vascular obstruction and ischemia. Although the disease can be diagnosed at birth, clinical abnormalities usually do not occur before age 6 months, when functional asplenia develops. Functional asplenia results in susceptibility to overwhelming infection with encapsulated bacteria. Subsequently, other organs are damaged. Typical manifestations include recurrent pain and progressive incremental infarction.

Pathophysiology

HbS arises from a mutation substituting thymine for adenine in the sixth codon of the beta-chain gene, GAG to GTG. This causes coding of valine instead of glutamate in position 6 of the Hb beta chain. The resulting Hb has the physical properties of forming polymers under deoxy conditions. It also exhibits changes in solubility and molecular stability. These properties are responsible for the profound clinical expressions of the sickling syndromes.

Under deoxy conditions, HbS undergoes marked decrease in solubility, increased viscosity, and polymer formation at concentrations exceeding 30 g/dL. It forms a gel-like substance containing Hb crystals called tactoids. The gel-like form of Hb is in equilibrium with its liquid-soluble form. A number of factors influence this equilibrium, including oxygen tension, concentration of Hb S, and the presence of other hemoglobins.

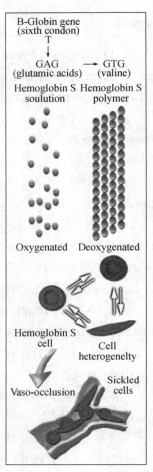

Oxygen tension is a factor in that polymer formation occurs only in the deoxy state. If oxygen is present, the liquid state prevails. Concentration of Hb S is a factor in that gelation of HbS occurs at concentrations greater than 20. 8 g/dL (the normal cellular Hb concentration is 30 g/dL). The presence of other hemoglobins is a factor in that normal adult hemoglobin (HbA) and fetal hemoglobin (HbF) have an inhibitory effect on gelation.

When red blood cells (RBCs) containing homozygous HbS are exposed to deoxy conditions, the sickling process begins. A slow and gradual polymer formation ensues. Electron microscopy reveals a parallel array of filaments. Repeated and prolonged sickling involves the membrane; the RBC assumes the characteristic sickled shape.

Molecular and cellular changes of hemoglobin S.

After recurrent episodes of sickling, membrane damage occurs and the cells are no longer capable of resuming the biconcave shape upon reoxygenation. Thus, they become irreversibly sickled cells (ISCs). From 5%—50% of RBCs permanently remain in the sickled shape.

When RBCs sickle, they gain Na + and lose K + . Membrane permeability to Ca + + increases, possibly due, in part, to impairment in the Ca + + pump that depends on adenosine triphosphatase (ATPase). The intracellular Ca + + concentration rises to 4 times the reference level. The membrane becomes more rigid, possibly due to changes in cytoskeletal protein interactions; however, these changes are not found consistently. In addition, whether calcium is responsible for membrane rigidity is not clear.

Membrane vesicle formation occurs, and the lipid bilayer is perturbed. The outer leaflet has increased amounts of phosphatidyl ethanolamine and contains phosphatidylserine. The latter may play a role as a contributor to thrombosis, acting as a catalyst for plasma clotting factors. Membrane rigidity can be reversed in vitro by replacing HbS with HbA, suggesting that HbS interacts with the cell membrane.

Interactions with vascular endothelium

Complex multifactorial mechanisms involving endothelial dysfunction underlie the acute and chronic manifestations of SCD. A current model proposes that vaso-occlusive crises in SCD result from adhesive interactions of sickle cell RBCs and leukocytes with the endothelium.

In this model, the endothelium becomes activated by sickle cell RBCs, either directly, through adhesion molecules on the RBC surface, or indirectly through plasma proteins (eg, thrombospondin, von Willebrand factor) that act as a soluble bridge molecule. This leads, sequentially, to recruitment of adherent leukocytes, activation of recruited neutrophils and of other leukocytes (eg, monocytes or natural killer T cells), interactions of RBCs with adherent neutrophils, and clogging of the vessel by cell aggregates composed of RBCs, adherent leukocytes, and possibly platelets.

Sickle cells express very late antigen-4 (VLA-4) on the surface. VLA-4 interacts with the endothelial cell adhesive molecule, vascular cell adhesive molecule-1 (VCAM-1). VCAM-1 is upregulated by hypoxia and inhibited by nitric oxide.

Hypoxia also decreases nitric oxide production, thereby adding to the adhesion of sickle cells to the vascular endothelium. Nitric oxide is a vasodilator. Free Hb is an avid scavenger of nitric oxide. Because of the continuing active hemolysis, there is free Hb in the plasma, and it scavenges nitric oxide, thus contributing to vasoconstriction.

In addition to leukocyte recruitment, inflammatory activation of endothelium may have an indispensable role in enhanced sickle RBC—endothelium interactions. Sickle RBC adhesion in postcapillary venules can cause increased microvascular transit times and initiate vaso-occlusion.

Several studies have shown involvement of an array of adhesion molecules expressed on sickle RBCs, including CD36, a-4-β-1 integrin, intercellular cell adhesion molecule-4 (ICAM-4), and basal cell adhesion molecule (B-CAM). Adhesion molecules (ie, P-selectin, VCAM-1, a-V-β-3 integrin) are also expressed on activated endothelium. Finally, plasma factors and adhesive proteins (ie, thrombospondin [TSP], von Willebrand factor [vWf], laminin) play an important role in this interaction.

For example, the induction of VCAM-1 and P-selectin on activated endothelium is known to enhance sickle RBC interactions. In addition, a-V-β-3 integrin is upregulated in activated endothelium in patients with sickle cell disease. a-V-β-3 integrin binds to several adhesive proteins (TSP, vWf, red-cell ICAM-4, and, possibly, soluble laminin) involved in sickle RBC adhesion, and antibodies to this integrin dramatically inhibit sickle RBC adhesion.

In addition, under inflammatory conditions, increased leukocyte recruitment in combination with adhesion of sickle RBCs may further contribute to stasis.

Sickle RBCs adhere to endothelium because of increased stickiness. The endothelium participates in this process, as do neutrophils, which also express increased levels of adhesive molecules.

Deformable sickle cells express CD18 and adhere abnormally to endothelium up to 10 times more than normal cells, while ISCs do not. As paradoxical as it might seem, individuals who produce large numbers of ISCs have fewer vaso-occlusive crises than those with more deformable RBCs.

Other properties of sickle cells

Sickle RBCs also adhere to macrophages. This property may contribute to erythrophagocytosis and the hemolytic process.

The microvascular perfusion at the level of the pre-arterioles is influenced by RBCs containing Hb S polymers. This occurs at arterial oxygen saturation, before any morphologic change is apparent.

Hemolysis is a constant finding in sickle cell syndromes. Approximately one third of RBCs undergo intravascular hemolysis, possibly due to loss of membrane filaments during oxygenation and deoxygenation. The remainder hemolyze by erythrophagocytosis by macrophages. This process can be partially modified by Fc (crystallizable fragment) blockade, suggesting that the process can be mediated by immune mechanisms.

Sickle RBCs have increased immunoglobulin G (IgG) on the cell surface. Vaso-occlusive crisis is often triggered by infection. levels of fibrinogen, fibronectin, and D-dimer are elevated in these patients. Plasma clotting factors likely participate in the microthrombi in the pre-arterioles.

Development of clinical disease

Although hematologic changes indicative of SCD are evident as early as the age of 10 weeks, symptoms usually do not develop until the age of 6—12 months because of high levels of circulating fetal hemoglobin. After infancy, erythrocytes of patients with sickle cell anemia contain approximately 90% hemoglobin S (HbS), 2%—10% hemoglobin F (HbF), and a normal amount of minor fraction of adult hemoglobin (HbA2). Adult hemoglobin (HbA), which usually gains prominence at the age of 3 months, is absent.

The physiological changes in RBCs result in a disease with the following cardinal signs:

1. Hemolytic anemia

2. Painful vaso-occlusive crisis

3. Multiple organ damage from microinfarcts, including heart, skeleton, spleen, and central nervous system

Silent cerebral infarcts are associated with cognitive impairment in SCD. These infarcts tend to be located in the deep white matter where cerebral blood flow is low. However, cognitive impairment, particularly slower processing speed, may occur independent of the presence of infarction and may worsen with age.

Musculoskeletal manifestations

The skeletal manifestations of sickle cell disease result from changes in bone and bone marrow caused by chronic tissue hypoxia, which is exacerbated by episodic occlusion of the microcirculation by the abnormal sickle cells. The main processes that lead to bone and joint destruction in sickle cell disease are as follows:

• Infarction of bone and bone marrow

• Compensatory bone marrow hyperplasia

• Secondary osteomyelitis

• Secondary growth defects

When the rigid erythrocytes jam in the arterial and venous sinusoids of skeletal tissue, the result is intravascular thrombosis, which leads to infarction of bone and bone marrow. Repeated episodes of these crises eventually lead to irreversible bone infarcts and osteonecrosis, especially in weight-bearing areas. These areas of osteonecrosis (avascular necrosis/aseptic necrosis) become radiographically visible as sclerosis of bone with secondary reparative reaction and eventually result in degenerative bone and joint destruction.

Infarction tends to occur in the diaphysis of small tubular bones in children and in the metaphysis and subchondrium of long bones in adults. Because of the anatomic distribution of the blood vessels supplying the vertebrae, infarction affecting the central part of the vertebrae (fed by a spinal artery branch) results in the characteristic H vertebrae of sickle cell disease. The outer portions of the plates are spared because of the numerous apophyseal arteries.

Osteonecrosis of the epiphysis of the femoral head is often bilateral and eventually progresses to collapse of the femoral heads. This same phenomenon is also seen in the humeral head, distal femur, and tibial condyles.

Infarction of bone and bone marrow in patients with sickle cell disease can lead to the following changes:

- Osteolysis (in acute infarction)
- Osteonecrosis (avascular necrosis/aseptic necrosis)
- Articular disintegration
- Myelosclerosis
- Periosteal reaction (unusual in the adult)
- H vertebrae (steplike endplate depression; also known as the Reynold sign or codfish vertebrae)
- Dystrophic medullary calcification
- Bone-within-bone appearance

The shortened survival time of the erythrocytes in sickle cell anemia (10—20 days) leads to a compensatory marrow hyperplasia throughout the skeleton. The bone marrow hyperplasia has the resultant effect of weakening the skeletal tissue by widening the medullary cavities, replacing trabecular bone and thinning cortices.

Deossification due to marrow hyperplasia can bring about the following changes in bone:

- Decreased density of the skull
- Decreased thickness of outer tables of skull due to widening of diploe
- Hair on-end striations of the calvaria
- Osteoporosis sometimes leading to biconcave vertebrae, coarsening of trabeculae in long and flat bones, and pathologic fractures

Patients with sickle cell disease can have a variety of growth defects due to the abnormal maturation of bone. The following growth defects are often seen in sickle cell disease:

- Bone shortening (premature epiphyseal fusion)
- Epiphyseal deformity with cupped metaphysis
- Peg-in-hole defect of distal femur
- Decreased height of vertebrae (short stature and kyphoscoliosis)

Prognosis

Because SCD is a lifelong disease, prognosis is guarded. The goal is to achieve a normal life span with minimal morbidity. As therapy improves, the prognosis also improves. Morbidity is highly variable in patients with SCD, partly depending on the level of HbF. Nearly all individuals with the condition are affected to some degree and experience multiple organ system involvement. Patients with Hb SA are heterozygous carriers and essentially are asymptomatic.

Vaso-occlusive crisis and chronic pain are associated with considerable economic loss and disability. Repeated infarction of joints, bones, and growth plates leads to aseptic necrosis, especially in weight bearing areas such as the femur. This complication is associated with chronic pain and disability and may require changes in employment and lifestyle.

Prognostic factors in SCD

The following prognostic factors have been identified as predictors of an adverse outcome:
- Hand-foot syndrome (dactylitis) in infants younger than 1 year
- Hb level of less than 7 g/dL
- Leukocytosis in the absence of infection

Hand-foot syndrome, which affects children younger than 5 years, has proved a strong predictor of overall severity (ie, death, risk of stroke, high pain rate, recurrent acute chest syndrome). Those that have an episode before age 1 year are at high risk of a severe clinical course. The risk is further increased if the child's baseline hemoglobin level is less than 7 g/dL or the baseline WBC count is elevated.

Patient education

Patients must be educated about the nature of their disease. They must be able to recognize the earliest signs of a vaso-occlusive crisis and seek help, treat all febrile illness promptly, and identify environmental hazards that may precipitate a crisis. Reinforcement should occur incrementally during the course of ongoing care.

Patients or parents should be instructed on how to palpate the abdomen to detect splenic enlargement, and the importance of observation for pallor, jaundice, and fever. Teach patients to seek medical care in certain situations, including the following:
- Persistent fever (>38.3℃)
- Chest pain, shortness of breath, nausea, and vomiting
- Abdominal pain with nausea and vomiting
- Persistent headache not experienced previously

Patients should avoid the following:
- Alcohol
- Nonprescribed prescription drugs
- Cigarettes, marijuana, and cocaine
- Seeking care in multiple institutions

Families should be educated on the importance of hydration, diet, outpatient medications, and immunization protocol. Emphasize the importance of prophylactic penicillin. Patients on hydroxyurea must be educated on the importance of regular follow-up with blood counts.

Patients (including asymptomatic heterozygous carriers) should understand the genetic basis of the disease, be educated about prenatal diagnosis, and know that genetic counseling is available. Genetic testing can identify parents at risk for having a child with sickle cell disease.

If both parents have the sickle cell trait, the chance that a child will have sickle cell disease is 25%. If one parent is carrying the trait and the other actually has disease, the odds increase to 50% that their child will inherit the disease. Screening and genetic counseling theoretically have the potential to drastically reduce the prevalence of SCD. This promise has not been realized. Some authors have recommended emergency department screening or referral for patients unaware of their status as a possible heterozygote.

Families should be encouraged to contact community sickle cell agencies for follow-up information, new drug protocols, and psychosocial support. Families should also follow the advances of gene therapy, bone marrow transplantation, and the usage of cord blood stem cells.

A. Translate the following sentences into Chinese.

1. Affected individuals present with a wide range of clinical problems that result from vascular obstruction and ischemia.

2. They must be able to recognize the earliest signs of a vaso-occlusive crisis and seek help, treat all febrile illness promptly, and identify environmental hazards that may precipitate a crisis.

3. Although hematologic changes indicative of SCD are evident as early as the age of 10 weeks, symptoms usually do not develop until the age of 6—12 months because of high levels of circulating fetal hemoglobin.

4. In addition to leukocyte recruitment, inflammatory activation of endothelium may have an indispensable role in enhanced sickle RBC—endothelium interactions.

5. The bone marrow hyperplasia has the resultant effect of weakening the skeletal tissue by widening the medullary cavities, replacing trabecular bone and thinning cortices.

B. Prepare a lecture on sickle cell anemia after doing the further reading above.

扫码获取
提示

Unit 15

Infantile Diarrhea

Ⅰ Warming-up

A. Match the following words and phrases with their Chinese translations.

A	diarrhea	1	呕吐
B	stomachache	2	肠,肠道
C	nauseous	3	腹痛
D	vomit	4	排便,大便
E	dehydrated	5	胃肠的
F	bowel	6	腹泻
G	motion	7	脱水的
H	gastrointestinal	8	受污染的,弄脏的
I	contaminated	9	消化
J	digestion	10	令人作呕的

B. Complete the sentences with the following words or phrases in their proper forms.

induce	frequent	vary	suffer from
consult	as soon as	full	over-the-counter

1. I think I'm _____ diarrhea again just like I experienced years ago when I was baby.

2. The environment was energetic and the house was filled with _____ food items

which was sweet, salty, and spicy.

3. But shortly after the sweet dream turned into one nightmare, as I started to feel the effect _____ I reached my house, and I began to feel nauseous, followed by vomiting, fever, and severe pain in my stomach.

4. Diarrhea is a condition in which poop is _____ discharged from the bowels in a wet watery sticky form and is commonly known as "loose motions".

5. It is usually caused by gastrointestinal infections _____ by viruses and bacteria, which are often picked up from contaminated food and parasites spread in contaminated water.

6. Hope we gained adequate knowledge about this problem disease that stops us from consuming our favorite food and live our life to the _____.

7. But _____ medications can offer some relief from symptoms to adults.

8. But for children, it's often recommended _____ your doctor before taking any medicines.

C. Watch the video *What Causes Diarrhea* and answer the questions.

扫码获取视频

1. Why did the sweet dream of the happy birthday party turn into one nightmare shortly?

2. What is diarrhea?

3. What do you know can cause infantile diarrhea?

4. How does doctor usually do to treat infantile diarrhea?

5. What is recommended for children with diarrhea?

Ⅱ Dialogue

扫码获取
音频及文本

A. Listen to the dialogue for the first time and try to get the general idea.

B. Listen to the dialogue for the second time and try to answer the following questions.

1. What's wrong with this patient?

2. Is the patient's stool watery?

3. Why the doctor asks the parent to help rip off the patient's clothes?

4. Why should the patient be admitted into the hospital?

5. What medicines should the patient take?

C. Choose the following words and/or expressions to complete the sentences in their proper forms.

vomit	呕吐	complaint	抱怨,埋怨
plenty of	大量	do ... a favor	帮……一个忙
thirsty	口渴的	rip off	扯掉
manage to	设法达成	elastic	有弹性的
unfortunately	不幸地,遗憾地	suffer from	患……病,受……之苦
burst out	突发,爆发	be admitted into	住院

1. So please _____ and let them know how much I appreciate them as well.

2. We reported last week that Helen Keller _____ a strange sickness when she was only nineteen months old.

3. The doctor then was worried inch by inch _____ the gauze(纱布) dressing on his wound.

4. From the flooded depths of the ship, some _____ claw their way up iron ladders to the safety of the upper deck.

5. _____ , this is not favorable to the war we are fighting against the militants and terrorists.

6. Doctors say people with such problems should rest quietly in a cool place and drink _____ water.

7. Her long fair hair was fastened at the nape of her neck by an _____ band.

8. The bankers all _____ laughing after hearing the signature line that earned Gooding an Oscar.

9. He decided I needed surgery and made all the necessary arrangements for me to _____ hospital at the appropriate time, which can take place at any age.

10. Rats can't _____ or burp because of a limiting wall between their two stomachs and their inability to control the diaphragm muscles needed for the action.

D. Read the dialogue and try to make a conversation with your classmates.

扫码获取
提示

E. Translate the following Chinese into English.

P—Patient   D—Doctor

D：1. 您的孩子叫什么名字？

　　1. _____

P：Tom.

D：How old is he?

P：Nine months.

D：What's the matter with him?

P：2. 腹泻已经3天了。

　　2. _____

D：3. 大便一天几次？ The amount? Is the stool watery? Is there any pus or blood or mucus in the stool?

　　3. _____

P：4. 一天10多次。The stool is watery and in large amounts. 5. 绿色或淡黄色，蛋花汤样。There is no pus or blood but some mucus.

　　4. _____

5. _____

D：Does the baby cry when he has a bowel movement?

P：6. 哭，他好像肚子痛。

　　6. _____

D：Has he ever vomited?

P：At the beginning, no. But he vomited 3 times yesterday, though not severely.

D：What did he vomit? Mucus, milk or food? Was there any yellow liquid?

P：7. 吐奶和食物，没有黄水。

　　7. _____

D：Does he have a fever?

P：Yes. I think he is running a fever.

D：Does he drink plenty of water?

P：8. 要喝水，看起来很口渴。

_____

Ⅲ Further Reading：Diarrhea

Background

Acute diarrhea is defined as the abrupt onset of 3 or more loose stools per day. The augmented water content in the stools（above the normal value of approximately 10 mL/kg/d in the infant and young child, or 200 g/d in the teenager and adult）is due to an imbalance in the physiology of the small and large intestinal processes involved in the absorption of ions, organic substrates, and thus water. A common disorder in its acute form, diarrhea has many causes and may be mild to severe.

Childhood acute diarrhea is usually caused by infection of the small and/or large intestine; however, numerous disorders may result in diarrhea, including a malabsorption syndrome and various enteropathies. Acute-onset diarrhea is usually self-limited; however, an acute infection can have a protracted course. By far, the most common complication of acute diarrhea is dehydration.

Although the term "acute gastroenteritis" is commonly used synonymously with "acute diarrhea", the former term is a misnomer. The term gastroenteritis implies inflammation of both the stomach and the small intestine, whereas, in reality, gastric involvement is rarely if ever seen in acute diarrhea (including diarrhea with an infectious origin); in addition, enteritis is also not consistently present. Examples of infectious acute diarrhea syndromes that do not cause enteritis include Vibrio cholerae—induced diarrhea and Shigella-induced diarrhea. Thus, the term acute diarrhea is preferable to acute gastroenteritis.

Diarrheal episodes are classically distinguished into acute and chronic (or persistent) based on their duration. Acute diarrhea is thus defined as an episode that has an acute onset and lasts no longer than 14 days; chronic or persistent diarrhea is defined as an episode that lasts longer than 14 days. The distinction, supported by the World Health Organization (WHO), has implications not only for classification and epidemiological studies but also from a practical standpoint because protracted diarrhea often has a different set of causes, poses different problems of management, and has a different prognosis.

Pathophysiology

Diarrhea is the reversal of the normal net absorptive status of water and electrolyte absorption to secretion. Such a derangement can be the result of either an osmotic force that acts in the lumen to drive water into the gut or the result of an active secretory state induced in the enterocytes. In the former case, diarrhea is osmolar in nature, as is observed after the ingestion of nonabsorbable sugars such as lactulose or lactose in lactose malabsorbers. Instead, in the typical active secretory state, enhanced anion secretion (mostly by the crypt cell compartment) is best exemplified by enterotoxin—induced diarrhea.

In osmotic diarrhea, stool output is proportional to the intake of the unabsorbable substrate and is usually not massive; diarrheal stools promptly regress with discontinuation of the offending nutrient, and the stool ion gap is high, exceeding 100 mOsm/kg. In fact, the fecal osmolality in this circumstance is accounted for not only by the electrolytes but also by the unabsorbed nutrient(s) and their degradation products. The ion gap is obtained by subtracting the concentration of the electrolytes from total osmolality (assumed to be 290 mOsm/kg), according to the formula: ion gap $= 290 - [(Na + K) \times 2]$.

In secretory diarrhea, the epithelial cells' ion transport processes are turned into a state of active secretion. The most common cause of acute-onset secretory diarrhea is a bacterial infection of the gut. Several mechanisms may be at work.

After colonization, enteric pathogens may adhere to or invade the epithelium; they may produce enterotoxins (exotoxins that elicit secretion by increasing an intracellular second messenger) or cytotoxins. They may also trigger release of cytokines attracting inflammatory cells, which, in turn, contribute to the activated secretion by inducing the release of agents such as prostaglandins or platelet-activating factor. Features of secretory diarrhea include a high purging rate, a lack of response to fasting, and a normal stool ion gap (ie, 100 mOsm/kg or less), indicating that nutrient absorption is intact.

Frequency

United States

In the United States, one estimate before the introduction of specific antirotavirus immunization in 2006 assumed a cumulative incidence of 1 hospitalization for diarrhea per 23—27 children by age 5 years, with more than 50,000 hospitalizations. By these estimates, rotavirus was associated with 4%—5% of all childhood hospitalizations and a cost of nearly $ 1 billion. Furthermore, acute diarrhea is responsible for 20% of physician referrals in children younger than 2 years and for 10% in children younger than 3 years.

The impact of vaccination on rotavirus morbidity has been remarkable, with significant reduction of diarrhea-associated hospitalizations and visits to emergency departments in children in the years 2007—2008 compared with the prevaccine period.

A study by Olortegui et al that included 2,082 children reported that 35% of the children experienced astrovirus infections and astrovirus prevalence in diarrheal stools was 5.6%, and severity exceeded all enteropathogens except rotavirus.

International

In developing countries, an average of 3 episodes per child per year in children younger than 5 years is reported; however, some areas report 6—8 episodes per year per child. In these settings, malnutrition is an important additional risk factor for diarrhea, and recurrent episodes of diarrhea lead to growth faltering and substantially increased mortality. Childhood mortality associated with diarrhea has constantly but slowly declined during the past 2 decades, mostly because of the widespread use of oral rehydration solutions; however, it appears to have plateaued over the past several years.

Because the single most common cause of infectious diarrhea worldwide is rotavirus, and because a vaccine has been in use for over 3 years now, a reduction in the overall frequency of diarrheal episodes is hoped for in the near future.

A study by Lübbert et al found the incidence of Clostridium difficile infection in Germany in 2012 to be 83 cases per 100,000 population. The chance of recurrence increased with each relapse; an initial recurrence of the infection was found in 18.2% of patients with index events, with 28.4% of these patients having a second recurrence and 30.2% of second-recurrence patients having a third recurrence.

Mortality/Morbidity

Mortality from acute diarrhea is overall globally declining but remains high. Most estimates have diarrhea as the second cause of childhood mortality, with 18% of the 10.6 million yearly deaths in children younger than age 5 years.

Despite a progressive reduction in global diarrheal disease mortality over the past 2 decades, diarrhea morbidity in published reports from 1990—2000 slightly increased worldwide compared with previous reports. In the United States, an average of 369 diarrhea-associated deaths/year occurred among children aged 1—59 months during 1992—1998 and 2005—2006. The vast majority of diarrhea-associated infant deaths were reported in 2005—2007, with 86% of deaths occurring among low-birthweight ($<$2500 g) infants.

Furthermore, in countries in which the toll of diarrhea is highest, poverty also adds an enormous additional burden, and long-term consequences of the vicious cycle of enteric infections, diarrhea, and malnutrition are devastating.

Sex

Most cases of infectious diarrhea are not sex specific. Females have a higher incidence of Campylobacter species infections and hemolytic uremic syndrome (HUS).

Age

Viral diarrhea is most common in young children. Rotavirus and adenovirus are particularly prevalent in children younger than 2 years. Astrovirus and norovirus usually infect children younger than 5 years. Yersinia enterocolitis typically infects children younger than 1 year, and the Aeromonas organism is a significant cause of diarrhea in young children.

Very young children are particularly susceptible to secondary dehydration and secondary nutrient malabsorption. Age and nutritional status appear to be the most important host factors in determining the severity and the duration of diarrhea. In fact, the younger the child, the higher is the risk for severe, life-threatening dehydration as a result of the high body-water turnover and limited renal compensatory capacity of very young children. Whether younger age also means a risk of running a prolonged course is an unsettled issue. In developing countries, persistent postenteritis diarrhea has a strong inverse correlation with age.

Medical care

In 2003 the Center for Disease Control (CDC) put forth recommendations for the management of acute pediatric diarrhea in both the outpatient and inpatient settings including indication for referral.

Indications for medical evaluation of children with acute diarrhea include the following:

- Younger than 3 months
- Weight of less than 8 kg
- History of premature birth, chronic medical conditions, or concurrent illness
- Fever of 38℃ or higher in infants younger than 3 months or 39℃ or higher in children aged 3—36 months
- Visible blood in the stool
- High-output diarrhea
- Persistent emesis
- Signs of dehydration as reported by caregiver, including sunken eyes, decreased tears, dry mucous membranes, and decreased urine output
- Mental status changes
- Inadequate responses to oral rehydration therapy (ORT) or caregiver unable to administer ORT

The report also includes information on assessment of dehydration and what steps should be taken to adequately treat acute diarrhea.

Treatment of dehydration due to diarrhea includes the following:

- Minimal or no dehydration

-Rehydration therapy—Not applicable

-Replacement of losses

°Less than 10 kg body weight—60—120 mL oral rehydration solution for each diarrhea stool or vomiting episode

°More than 10 kg body weight—120—140 mL oral rehydration solution for each diarrhea stool or vomiting episode

- Mild-to-moderate dehydration

-Rehydration therapy—Oral rehydration solution (50—100 mL/kg over 3—4 h)

-Replacement of losses

°Less than 10 kg body weight—60—120 mL oral rehydration solution for each diarrhea stool or vomiting episode

°More than 10 kg body weight—120—140 mL oral rehydration solution for each diarrhea stool or vomiting episode

- Severe dehydration

-Rehydration therapy—Intravenous lactated Ringer solution or normal saline (20 mL/kg until perfusion and mental status improve), followed by 100 mL/kg oral rehydration solution over 4 hours or 5% dextrose (half normal saline) intravenously at twice maintenance fluid rates

-Replacement of losses

°Less than 10 kg body weight—60—120 mL oral rehydration solution for each diarrhea stool or vomiting episode

°More than 10 kg body weight—120—140 mL oral rehydration solution for each diarrhea stool or vomiting episode

°If unable to drink, administer through nasogastric tube or intravenously administer 5% dextrose (one fourth normal saline) with 20 mEq/L potassium chloride

ORT is the cornerstone of treatment, especially for small-bowel infections that produce a large volume of watery stool output. ORT with a glucose-based oral rehydration syndrome must be viewed as by far the safest, most physiologic, and most effective way to provide rehydration and maintain hydration in children with acute diarrhea worldwide, as recommended by the WHO; by the ad hoc committee of European Society for Pediatric Gastroenterology, Hepatology and Nutrition (ESPGHAN); and by the American Academy of Pediatrics. However, the global use of ORT is still insufficient. Developed countries, in particular the United States, seem to be lagging behind despite studies that demonstrate beyond doubt the efficacy of ORT in emergency care settings, in which intravenous rehydration unduly continues to be widely privileged.

Not all commercial ORT formulas promote optimal absorption of electrolytes, water, and nutrients. The ideal solution has a low osmolarity (210—250) and a sodium content of 50—60 mmol/L. Administer maintenance fluids plus replacement of losses. Educate caregivers in methods necessary to replace this amount of fluid. Administer small amounts of fluid at frequent intervals to minimize discomfort and vomiting. A 5-mL or 10-mL syringe without a needle is a very useful tool. The syringe can be quickly used to place small amounts of fluid in the mouth of a child who is uncooperative. Once the child becomes better hydrated, cooperation improves enough to take small sips from a cup. This method is time intensive and requires a dedicated caregiver. Encouragement from the physician is necessary to promote compliance. Oral rehydration is now universally recommended to be completed within 4 hours.

The addition of zinc to oral rehydration solution has been proven effective in children with acute diarrhea in developing countries and is recommended by the WHO. However, no evidence suggests efficacy in children living in developed countries, in which the prevalence of zinc deficiency is assumed to be extremely low.

The composition of almost all other beverages (carbonated or not) that are commercially available and frequently used in children with diarrhea is completely inadequate for rehydration or for maintaining hydration, considering the sodium content, which is invariably extremely low, and osmolarity that is often dangerously elevated. For instance, Coca-Cola, Pepsi-Cola, and apple juice have an osmolarity of 493, 576, and 694—773, respectively.

However, research conducted in a community clinic in Nicaragua indicated that green tea and pomegranate extract combined with a standard oral rehydration solution help children with diarrhea improve faster. Results showed the average time to achieve a Bristol Stool Scale (BSS) score of 4 or less was significantly shorter in the extract group than in the control group (3.1 vs 9.2 hours, respectively). In addition, a BSS score of 4 or less in the first bowel movement after treatment was achieved by more patients in the extract group than the control group (60% vs 29%, respectively). BSS scores in the extract group were maintained on day 2.

At completion of hydration, resumption of feeding is strongly recommended. In fact, many studies convincingly demonstrate that early refeeding hastens recovery. Also, robust evidence suggests that, in the vast majority of episodes of acute diarrhea, refeeding can be accomplished without the use of any special (eg, lactose-free or soy-based) formulas.

Antimotility agents are not indicated for infectious diarrhea, except for refractory cases of Cryptosporidium infection. Antimicrobial therapy is indicated for some nonviral diarrhea because most is self-limiting and does not require therapy.

Consultations

See the list below:

• Surgeon

-Certain organisms cause abdominal pain and bloody stools.

-Symptoms resembling appendicitis, hemorrhagic colitis, intussusception, or toxic megacolon may be appreciated.

-If the infectious etiology in individuals with such symptoms is not certain, seek consultation with a surgeon.

• Infectious-disease specialist: Consider consultation with an infectious-disease specialist for any patient who is immunocompromised because of HIV infection, chemotherapy, or immunosuppressive drugs because atypical organisms are more likely, and complications can be more serious and fulminate.

Diet

Breastfed infants with acute diarrhea should be continued on breast milk without any need for interruption. In fact, breastfeeding not only has a well-known protective effect against the development of enteritis, it also promotes faster recovery and provides improved nutrition. This is even more important in developing countries, where with-drawal of breastfeeding during diarrhea has been shown to have a deleterious effect on the development of dehydration in infants with acute watery diarrhea.

- Bananas, rice, applesauce, and toast diet

-A banana, rice, applesauce, and toast (BRAT) diet was introduced in the United States in 1926 and has enjoyed vast popularity. However, no evidence shows that this diet is useful, and its poor protein content may be a contraindication; therefore, it is not recommended.

-A strong body of evidence now suggests that resuming the prediarrhea diet is perfectly safe and must be encouraged, obviously respecting any (usually temporary) lack of appetite.

- Lactose ingestion

-Although rotavirus can cause secondary transient lactose intolerance, this finding is believed to be generally not clinically relevant; use lactose-containing formulas in all individuals with diarrhea.

-In an incident of worsening of diarrhea proven to be secondary to a clinically important lactose malabsorption in infants positive for rotavirus, a very transient use of lactose-free formulas (5—6 d) can be considered.

A. Translate the following sentences into Chinese.

1. Childhood acute diarrhea is usually caused by infection of the small and/or large intestine; however, numerous disorders may result in diarrhea, including a malabsorption syndrome and various enteropathies.

2. The impact of vaccination on rotavirus morbidity has been remarkable, with significant reduction of diarrhea-associated hospitalizations and visits to emergency departments in children in the years 2007—2008 compared with the prevaccine period.

3. Childhood mortality associated with diarrhea has constantly but slowly declined during the past 2 decades, mostly because of the widespread use of oral rehydration solutions; however, it appears to have plateaued over the past several years.

4. In fact, the younger the child, the higher is the risk for severe, life-threatening dehydration as a result of the high body-water turnover and limited renal compensatory capacity of very young children.

5. In these settings, malnutrition is an important additional risk factor for diarrhea, and recurrent episodes of diarrhea lead to growth faltering and substantially increased mortality.

B. Prepare a lecture on infantile diarrhea after doing the further reading above.

扫码获取
提示

Unit 16

Cataract

Warming-up

A. Match the following words and phrases with their Chinese translations.

A   metabolic cataract   1   混浊晶状体
B   intraocular lens implantation   2   老年性白内障
C   post cataractous operation   3   角膜主切口
D   opaque lens   4   代谢性白内障
E   blurred vision   5   人工晶体植入
F   main corneal incision   6   先天性白内障
G   ultrasonic emulsification   7   白内障手术后
H   senile cataract   8   皮质混浊
I   opacity of cortex   9   视物模糊
J   congenital cataract   10 超声乳化

B. Complete the sentences with the following words or phrases in their proper forms.

develop	age	disorder	affect
interfere with	right away	make up	pass through

1. But if impaired vision _____ your usual activities, you might need cataract surgery.

2. At first, the cloudiness in your vision caused by a cataract may _____ only a small

part of the eye's lens and you may be unaware of any vision loss.

3. As the cataract grows larger, it clouds more of your lens and distorts the light _____ the lens.

4. Most cataracts _____ when aging or injury changes the tissue that makes up the eye's lens.

5. If you develop sudden vision changes, such as double vision or flashes of light, sudden eye pain, or sudden headache, see your doctor _____.

6. Most cataracts develop when aging or injury changes the tissue that _____ the eye's lens.

7. Some inherited genetic _____ that cause other health problems can increase your risk of cataracts.

8. As you _____, the lenses in your eyes become less flexible, less transparent and thicker.

C. Watch the video *How to Prevent Cataracts* and answer the questions.

扫码获取视频

1. What are the usual causes leading to cataracts?

2. What are the ways of helping people avoid cataracts?

3. Why should people avoid tanning booths, sunlamps, and excessive sun exposure?

4. Do you think that taking food supplements such as vitamins E and C are effective in risk reduction in developing cataracts? Why or why not?

5. What regular eye checkups are you recommended your patients to do?

II Dialogue

扫码获取
音频及文本

A. Listen to the dialogue for the first time and try to get the general idea.

B. Listen to the dialogue for the second time and try to answer the following questions.

1. What is the course of the patient's eye blurring?

2. What other diseases has the patient had?

3. What treatment can be effective to the patient's eye disease?

4. How will the doctor conduct the operation?

5. What should the patient pay attention to after the operation?

C. Choose the following words and/or expressions to complete the sentences in their proper forms.

diabetes	糖尿病	impaired vision	视力下降
disturb	干扰	progression	发展
cloudy lenses	混浊晶状体	retina	视网膜
born with	天生的	break down	发生故障
advanced	发展得快	a variety of	各种各样的
double vision	复视	nearsightedness	近视眼

1. For people who have cataracts, seeing through _____ is a bit like looking through a frosty or fogged-up window.

2. But if _____ interferes with your usual activities, you might need cataract surgery.

3. The cataract in one eye may be more _____ than the other, causing a difference in vision between eyes.

4. Proteins and fibers in the lens begin to _____, causing vision to become hazy or cloudy.

5. Cataracts can also be caused by other eye conditions, past eye surgery or medical conditions such as _____.

6. A cataract scatters and blocks the light as it passes through the lens, preventing a sharply defined image from reaching your _____.

7. A nuclear cataract may at first cause more _____ or even a temporary improvement in your reading vision.

8. Some people are _____ cataracts or develop them during childhood.

9. No studies have proved how to prevent cataracts or slow the _____ of cataracts.

10. Adding _____ colorful fruits and vegetables to your diet ensures that you're getting many vitamins and nutrients.

D. Read the dialogue and try to make a conversation with your classmates.

扫码获取
提示

E. Translate the following Chinese into English.

P—Patient   D—Doctor

D：How old are you?

P：I'm fifty-five years old.

D：1. 你的眼睛有什么不适吗?

  1. _____

P：I can't see clearly.

D：How long has it been like that?

P：It has been so for one year.

D：2. 请详细告诉我你眼睛模糊的过程。

  _____

P：Well，I felt blurring in the left eye one year ago，and eventually the right eye soon after that. I thought it would be better soon，so I didn't see a doctor. But it went from bad to worse recently. 3. 我的左眼已经完全失明,我的右眼也几乎看不见了。

  3. _____

  _____

D：Besides the blurring of your eyes，is there any other discomfort? Say，pain，distention and redness of the eyes and headache，or a history of injury.

P：4. 不,我的两只眼睛除了看东西模糊,从来没有什么不舒服或受到外伤。

  4. _____

D：5. 你有其他疾病吗?

  5. _____

P：Let me see. Oh，I had hypertension in the past.

D：Have you been treated?

P：Yes. I have. The blood pressure returned to normal quickly. I haven't taken any drug since two to three years.

D：Do you have diabetes?

P：Yes，I do，but it is under control.

D：Do you void much urine at other times?

P：Not much.

D：6. 好的,我来给你做个检查。Your eye disease is called cataracts. It is the opacity of the lens in the eye due to protein denaturation caused by metabolic disorders of the lens. It is often associated with risk factors such as diabetes or aging. The cataract in your left eye has already ripened，while the right one is not yet ripe. You need to be hospitalized，and your left eye should be operated on as soon as possible.

  6. _____

P：7. 我可以通过手术治愈吗? 可以通过服药治疗吗?

  7. _____

  _____

D：8. 鉴于你的情况,药物是不起作用的。Only surgery will be. Phacoemulsification is the most widely used cataract surgery，the aim of which is to take out the cataract by implanting an artificial lens.

  8. _____

Ⅲ   Further Reading: Cataracts

Overview

A cataract is a clouding of the normally clear lens of the eye. For people who have cataracts, seeing through cloudy lenses is a bit like looking through a frosty or fogged-up window. Clouded vision caused by cataracts can make it more difficult to read, drive a car (especially at night) or see the expression on a friend's face.

Most cataracts develop slowly and don't disturb your eyesight early on. But with time, cataracts will eventually interfere with your vision.

At first, stronger lighting and eyeglasses can help you deal with cataracts. But if impaired vision interferes with your usual activities, you might need cataract surgery. Fortunately, cataract surgery is generally a safe, effective procedure.

Symptoms

Signs and symptoms of cataracts include:
- Clouded, blurred or dim vision
- Increasing difficulty with vision at night
- Sensitivity to light and glare
- Need for brighter light for reading and other activities
- Seeing "halos" around lights
- Frequent changes in eyeglass or contact lens prescription
- Fading or yellowing of colors
- Double vision in a single eye

At first, the cloudiness in your vision caused by a cataract may affect only a small part of the eye's lens and you may be unaware of any vision loss. As the cataract grows larger, it clouds more of your lens and distorts the light passing through the lens. This may lead to more-noticeable symptoms.

When to see a doctor

Make an appointment for an eye exam if you notice any changes in your vision. If you develop sudden vision changes, such as double vision or flashes of light, sudden eye pain, or sudden headache, see your doctor right away.

Causes

Most cataracts develop when aging or injury changes the tissue that makes up the eye's lens. Proteins and fibers in the lens begin to break down, causing vision to become hazy or cloudy.

Some inherited genetic disorders that cause other health problems can increase your risk of cataracts. Cataracts can also be caused by other eye conditions, past eye surgery or medical conditions such as diabetes. Long-term use of steroid medications, too, can cause cataracts to develop.

How a cataract forms

A cataract is a cloudy lens. The lens is positioned behind the colored part of your eye (iris). The lens focuses light that passes into your eye, producing clear, sharp images on the retina—the light-sensitive membrane in the eye that functions like the film in a camera.

As you age, the lenses in your eyes become less flexible, less transparent and thicker. Age-related and other medical conditions cause proteins and fibers within the lenses to break down and clump together, clouding the lenses.

As the cataract continues to develop, the clouding becomes denser. A cataract scatters and blocks the light as it passes through the lens, preventing a sharply defined image from reaching your retina. As a result, your vision becomes blurred.

Cataracts generally develop in both eyes, but not always at the same rate. The cataract in one eye may be more advanced than the other, causing a difference in vision between eyes.

Types of cataracts

Cataract types include:

Cataracts affecting the center of the lens (nuclear cataracts). A nuclear cataract may at first cause more nearsightedness or even a temporary improvement in your reading vision. But with time, the lens gradually turns more densely yellow and further clouds your vision.

As the cataract slowly progresses, the lens may even turn brown. Advanced yellowing or browning of the lens can lead to difficulty distinguishing between shades of color.

Cataracts that affect the edges of the lens (cortical cataracts). A cortical cataract begins as whitish, wedge-shaped opacities or streaks on the outer edge of the lens cortex. As it slowly progresses, the streaks extend to the center and interfere with light passing through the center of the lens.

Cataracts that affect the back of the lens (posterior subcapsular cataracts). A posterior subcapsular cataract starts as a small, opaque area that usually forms near the back of the lens, right in the path of light. A posterior subcapsular cataract often interferes with your reading vision, reduces your vision in bright light, and causes glare or halos around lights at night. These types of cataracts tend to progress faster than other types do.

Cataracts you're born with (**congenital cataracts**). Some people are born with cataracts or develop them during childhood. These cataracts may be genetic, or associated with an intrauterine infection or trauma.

These cataracts may also be due to certain conditions, such as myotonic dystrophy, galactosemia, neurofibromatosis type 2 or rubella. Congenital cataracts don't always affect vision, but if they do, they're usually removed soon after detection.

Risk factors

Factors that increase your risk of cataracts include:
- Increasing age
- Diabetes
- Excessive exposure to sunlight
- Smoking
- Obesity
- High blood pressure
- Previous eye injury or inflammation
- Previous eye surgery
- Prolonged use of corticosteroid medications
- Drinking excessive amounts of alcohol

Prevention

No studies have proved how to prevent cataracts or slow the progression of cataracts. But doctors think several strategies may be helpful, including:

Have regular eye examinations. Eye examinations can help detect cataracts and other eye problems at their earliest stages. Ask your doctor how often you should have an eye examination.

Quit smoking. Ask your doctor for suggestions about how to stop smoking. Medications, counseling and other strategies are available to help you.

Manage other health problems. Follow your treatment plan if you have diabetes or other medical conditions that can increase your risk of cataracts.

Choose a healthy diet that includes plenty of fruits and vegetables. Adding a variety of colorful fruits and vegetables to your diet ensures that you're getting many vitamins and nutrients. Fruits and vegetables have many antioxidants, which help maintain the health of your eyes.

Studies haven't proved that antioxidants in pill form can prevent cataracts. But a large population study recently showed that a healthy diet rich in vitamins and minerals was associated with a reduced risk of developing cataracts. Fruits and vegetables have many proven health benefits and are a safe way to increase the amount of minerals and vitamins in your diet.

Wear sunglasses. Ultraviolet light from the sun may contribute to the development of cataracts. Wear sunglasses that block ultraviolet B (UVB) rays when you're outdoors.

Reduce alcohol use. Excessive alcohol use can increase the risk of cataracts.

Diagnosis

To determine whether you have a cataract, your doctor will review your medical history and symptoms, and perform an eye examination. Your doctor may conduct several tests, including:

Visual acuity test. A visual acuity test uses an eye chart to measure how well you can read a series of letters. Your eyes are tested one at a time, while the other eye is covered. Using a chart or a viewing device with progressively smaller letters, your eye doctor determines if you have 20/20 vision or if your vision shows signs of impairment.

Slit-lamp examination. A slit lamp allows your eye doctor to see the structures at the front of your eye under magnification. The microscope is called a slit lamp because it uses an intense line of light, a slit, to illuminate your cornea, iris, lens, and the space between your iris and cornea. The slit allows your doctor to view these structures in small sections, which makes it easier to detect any tiny abnormalities.

Retinal exam. To prepare for a retinal exam, your eye doctor puts drops in your eyes to open your pupils wide (dilate). This makes it easier to examine the back of your eyes (retina). Using a slit lamp or a special device called an ophthalmoscope, your eye doctor can examine your lens for signs of a cataract.

Applanation tonometry. This test measures fluid pressure in your eye. There are multiple different devices available to do this.

Treatment

When your prescription glasses can't clear your vision, the only effective treatment for cataracts is surgery.

When to consider cataract surgery

Talk with your eye doctor about whether surgery is right for you. Most eye doctors suggest considering cataract surgery when your cataracts begin to affect your quality of life or interfere with your ability to perform normal daily activities, such as reading or driving at night.

It's up to you and your doctor to decide when cataract surgery is right for you. For most people, there is no rush to remove cataracts because they usually don't harm the eyes. But cataracts can worsen faster in people with certain conditions, including diabetes, high blood pressure or obesity.

Delaying the procedure generally won't affect how well your vision recovers if you later decide to have cataract surgery. Take time to consider the benefits and risks of cataract surgery with your doctor.

If you choose not to undergo cataract surgery now, your eye doctor may recommend periodic follow-up exams to see if your cataracts are progressing. How often you'll see your eye doctor depends on your situation.

What happens during cataract surgery

Cataract surgery involves removing the clouded lens and replacing it with a clear artificial lens. The artificial lens, called an intraocular lens, is positioned in the same place as your natural lens. It remains a permanent part of your eye.

For some people, other eye problems prohibit the use of an artificial lens. In these situations, once the cataract is removed, vision may be corrected with eyeglasses or contact lenses.

Cataract surgery is generally done on an outpatient basis, which means you won't need to stay in a hospital after the surgery. During cataract surgery, your eye doctor uses a local anesthetic to numb the area around your eye, but you usually stay awake during the procedure.

Cataract surgery is generally safe, but it carries a risk of infection and bleeding. Cataract surgery increases the risk of retinal detachment.

After the procedure, you'll have some discomfort for a few days. Healing generally occurs within a few weeks.

If you need cataract surgery in both eyes, your doctor will schedule surgery to remove the cataract in the second eye after you've healed from the first surgery.

Clinical trials

Explore Mayo Clinic studies testing new treatments, interventions and tests as a means to prevent, detect, treat or manage this condition.

Lifestyle and home remedies

To deal with symptoms of cataracts until you decide to have surgery, try to:

• Make sure your eyeglasses or contact lenses are the most accurate prescription possible

　• Use a magnifying glass to read if you need additional help reading

　• Improve the lighting in your home with more or brighter lamps

　• When you go outside during the day, wear sunglasses or a broad-brimmed hat to reduce glare

　• Limit your night driving

Self-care measures may help for a while, but as the cataract progresses, your vision may deteriorate further. When vision loss starts to interfere with your everyday activities, consider cataract surgery.

Preparing for your appointment

Make an appointment with your usual eye care provider if you notice changes in your vision. If your doctor determines that you have cataracts, then you may be referred to an eye specialist who can perform cataract surgery.

Because there's often a lot to talk about, it's a good idea to be well prepared for your appointment so that you can make the most of your time with your doctor. Here's some information to help you get ready.

What you can do

• **List any symptoms you're experiencing,** including any that may seem unrelated to the reason for which you scheduled the appointment.

• **Make a list of all medications,** vitamins or supplements that you're taking.

• **Take a family member or friend along.** Sometimes it can be difficult to absorb all the information provided during an appointment. Someone who accompanies you may remember something that you missed or forgot.

• **List questions to** ask your doctor.

For cataracts, some basic questions to ask your doctor include:

• Are cataracts causing my vision problems?

• What kinds of tests do I need?

• Will cataract surgery correct my vision problems?

• What are the potential risks of cataract surgery? Are there risks in delaying surgery?

• What will cataract surgery cost, and will my insurance cover it?

• How much time will I need to recover from cataract surgery?

• Will any usual activities be restricted after cataract surgery? For how long?

• After cataract surgery, how long should I wait before getting new glasses?

• If I use Medicare, will it cover the cost of cataract surgery? Does Medicare cover the cost of new glasses after surgery?

• If I don't want surgery right now, what else can I do to cope with my vision changes?

• How will I know if my cataracts are getting worse?

• I have these other health conditions. How can I best manage these conditions together?

• Are there any brochures or other printed material that I can take with me? What websites do you recommend?

• In addition to the questions that you've prepared to ask your doctor, don't hesitate to ask questions at any time that you don't understand something.

What to expect from your doctor

Your doctor is likely to ask you a number of questions. Being ready to answer them may allow more time later to cover other points you want to address. Your doctor may ask:

- When did you begin experiencing symptoms?
- Do you have your symptoms all the time or do they come and go?
- Do you experience vision problems in bright light?
- Have your symptoms gotten worse?
- Do your vision problems make it difficult for you to drive?
- Do your vision problems make it difficult to read?
- Do your vision problems make it difficult to do your job?
- Have you ever had an eye injury or eye surgery?
- Have you ever been diagnosed with an eye problem, such as inflammation of your iris (iritis)?
- Have you ever received radiation therapy to your head or neck?

A. Translate the following sentences into Chinese.

1. A cataract is a clouding of the normally clear lens of the eye. For people who have cataracts, seeing through cloudy lenses is a bit like looking through a frosty or fogged-up window. Clouded vision caused by cataracts can make it more difficult to read, drive a car (especially at night) or see the expression on a friend's face.

2. At first, the cloudiness in your vision caused by a cataract may affect only a small part of the eye's lens and you may be unaware of any vision loss. As the cataract grows larger, it clouds more of your lens and distorts the light passing through the lens. This may lead to more-noticeable symptoms.

3. Some inherited genetic disorders that cause other health problems can increase your risk of cataracts. Cataracts can also be caused by other eye conditions, past eye surgery or medical conditions such as diabetes. Long-term use of steroid medications, too, can cause cataracts to develop.

4. As the cataract continues to develop, the clouding becomes denser. A cataract scatters and blocks the light as it passes through the lens, preventing a sharply defined image from reaching your retina. As a result, your vision becomes blurred.

5. Cataract surgery involves removing the clouded lens and replacing it with a clear artificial lens. The artificial lens, called an intraocular lens, is positioned in the same place as your natural lens. It remains a permanent part of your eye.

B. Prepare a lecture on cataract after doing the further reading above.

扫码获取
提示

Unit 17

Glaucoma

I Warming-up

A. Match the following words and phrases with their Chinese translations.

A	secondary glaucoma	1	开角型青光眼
B	anterior chamber	2	眼前房出血
C	intraocular tension	3	继发性青光眼
D	angle-closure glaucoma	4	虹视
E	scieropia	5	眼压
F	optic disk	6	闭角型青光眼
G	intraocular hypertension	7	雾视
H	open-angle glaucoma	8	高眼压症
I	iridescent vision	9	视盘
J	hyphema	10	前房

B. Complete the sentences with the following words or phrases in their proper forms.

for reasons that	gradual	depend on	properly
send ... from ...	check-up	in its early stages	as the result of

1. The optic nerve _____ visual information _____ your eye to your brain and is vital for good vision.

2. The effect of glaucoma is so _____ that you may not notice a change in vision until the condition is in its later stages.

3. _____ doctors don't fully understand, this optic nerve damage is usually related to increased pressure in the eye.

4. Elevated eye pressure happens _____ a buildup of fluid that flows throughout the inside of the eye.

5. When the eye makes too much fluid or the drainage system doesn't work _____, eye pressure may increase.

6. Regular comprehensive eye exams can help detect glaucoma _____, before significant damage occurs.

7. But treatment and regular _____ can help slow or prevent vision loss, especially if you catch the disease in its early stages.

8. _____ how low your eye pressure needs to be, you may be prescribed more than one eye drop.

扫码获取视频

 C. Watch the video *Glaucoma Treatment* and answer the questions.

1. What do eye drops work for glaucoma treatment?

2. As an ophthalmologist, what would you do if the eye drops alone failed to treat glaucoma?

3. What is argon laser trabeculoplasty (ALT)? Can you introduce the surgical procedures of it?

4. What is selective laser trabeculoplasty (SLT)? What is the difference between ALT and SLT?

5. What is iridotomy? Can you introduce the surgical procedures of it?

II Dialogue

扫码获取
音频及文本

 A. Listen to the dialogue for the first time and try to get the general idea.

B. Listen to the dialogue for the second time and try to answer the following questions.

1. What's wrong with the patient's eyes?

2. What's wrong with the patient's father's and younger brother's eyes?

3. By what means is glaucoma treated?

4. Why does the doctor suggest the patient ask his relatives to visit the eye clinic as quickly as possible?

5. What treatment should be done if the pressure remains high?

C. Choose the following words and/or expressions to complete the sentences in their proper forms.

progression	（病情的）发展	a healthy diet	健康饮食
frequent urination	尿频	treatment	治疗
eye pressure	眼压	common	常见的
occur	发生	tear duct	泪腺
acute angle-closure glaucoma		side effects	副作用
	急性闭角型青光眼	helpful	有帮助的
lifelong	终身		

1. If you experience symptoms that come on suddenly, you may have _____.

2. Laser therapy also may be used if medicine hasn't slowed the _____ of your disease.

3. Because some of the eye drop medicine is absorbed into your bloodstream, you may experience some _____ unrelated to your eyes.

4. If you're diagnosed with the acute angle-closure glaucoma, you'll need urgent _____ to reduce the pressure in your eye.

5. Beta blockers reduce the production of fluid in your eye, helping to lower _____.

6. You also may press lightly at the corner of your eyes near your nose to close the _____ for 1 or 2 minutes.

7. Eating _____ can help you maintain your health, but it won't prevent glaucoma from worsening.

8. Possible side effects include _____, tingling in the fingers and toes, depression, stomach upset, and kidney stones.

9. When you receive a diagnosis of glaucoma, you're potentially facing _____ treatment, regular checkups and the possibility of progressive vision loss.

10. Meeting and talking with other people with glaucoma can be very _____, and many support groups exist.

D. Read the dialogue and try to make a conversation with your classmates.

扫码获取
提示

E. Translate the following Chinese into English.

P—Patient   D—Doctor

D：What's wrong with your eyes?

P：I have found that I cannot see things clearly, and things look smaller in their visual field. 1. 有时候, 我感觉眼睛有点肿胀。

1. _____

D：How long has it been like that?

P：It has been so for about a couple of months.

D：2. 还有其他什么不舒服吗? 比如说头疼和眼睛发红?

2. _____

_____

P：So far, I can remember, there is no headache or redness of the eyes. However, when the eyes are strained, they will feel uncomfortably distended.

D：3. 你家里还有其他成员眼睛有问题吗?

3. _____

P：4. 我父亲 60 岁的时候就完全失去视力了。My father completely lost his sight when he was 60 years old. My younger brother also has some troubles with his eyes.

4. _____

D：Do you happen to know what's wrong with them?

P：My father has died, and my younger brother has not seen an eye doctor.

D：Allow me to do an exam for you. 5. 你的右眼内压是 32 毫米汞柱, 左眼内压 28 毫米汞柱。The fundus presents typical glaucomatous damage with the cup-to-disc ratio (C/D) on the right eye 0.9 and left 0.8. Perimetry shows the arcuate scotoma to be linked with the physiologic blind spot, which is a typical glaucomatous visual field loss. Gonioscope also shows that the chamber angle is open, which suggests that you've got primary open-angle glaucoma for both eyes. It's nearing the advanced stage. 6. 青光眼是一种眼内压不断上升的眼部疾病, 它会造成对视神经的损坏。If left untreated, total vision loss will happen and then potentially leading to blindness. You need to be treated at once.

5. _____

6. _____

_____

D：Glaucoma is treated by means of controlling the pressure to prevent the vision nerve from being damaged further. With glaucoma, there's no way we can get back the vision that's been lost, that is to say, what we're doing now is a matter of retaining what vision is left, but we can't bring back your lost vision.

P：I see. I should get it treated as soon as possible by controlling the intraocular pressure before it brings damage to the optic nerves.

D：7. 是的, 你完全正确。I suggest you ask your relatives to visit the eye clinic as quickly as possible because glaucoma is a hereditary disease.

7. _____

P：OK, thank you very much, doctor. What can be done now?

D：8. 我给你开三种眼药水减眼压。You

should use them on time and come back to me in a week to measure the intraocular pressure. If the pressure is well controlled, you carry on with the medicines. However, if the pressure remains high, we need to consider surgery.

8. _____

P: Thank you very much.

Ⅲ Further Reading: Glaucoma

Overview

Glaucoma is a group of eye conditions that damage the optic nerve. The optic nerve sends visual information from your eye to your brain and is vital for good vision. Damage to the optic nerve is often related to high pressure in your eye. But glaucoma can happen even with normal eye pressure.

Glaucoma can occur at any age but is more common in older adults. It is one of the leading causes of blindness for people over the age of 60.

Many forms of glaucoma have no warning signs. The effect is so gradual that you may not notice a change in vision until the condition is in its later stages.

It's important to have regular eye exams that include measurements of your eye pressure. If glaucoma is recognized early, vision loss can be slowed or prevented. If you have glaucoma, you'll need treatment or monitoring for the rest of your life.

Symptoms

The symptoms of glaucoma depend on the type and stage of your condition.

Open-angle glaucoma

• No symptoms in early stages

• Gradually, patchy blind spots in your side vision. Side vision also is known as peripheral vision

• In later stages, difficulty seeing things in your central vision

Acute angle-closure glaucoma

• Severe headache   • Blurred vision

• Severe eye pain   • Halos or colored rings around lights

• Nausea or vomiting   • Eye redness

Normal-tension glaucoma

- No symptoms in early stages
- In later stages, loss of side vision
- Gradually, blurred vision

Glaucoma in children

- A dull or cloudy eye (infants)
- Blurred vision
- Increased blinking (infants)
- Nearsightedness that gets worse
- Tears without crying (infants)
- Headache

Pigmentary glaucoma

- Halos around lights
- Gradual loss of side vision
- Blurred vision with exercise

When to see a doctor

If you experience symptoms that come on suddenly, you may have acute angle-closure glaucoma. Symptoms include severe headache and severe eye pain. You need treatment as soon as possible. Go to an emergency room or call an eye doctor's (ophthalmologist's) office immediately.

Causes

Glaucoma develops when the optic nerve becomes damaged. As this nerve gradually deteriorates, blind spots develop in your vision. For reasons that doctors don't fully understand, this nerve damage is usually related to increased pressure in the eye.

Elevated eye pressure happens as the result of a buildup of fluid that flows throughout the inside of the eye. This fluid also is known as the aqueous humor. It usually drains through a tissue located at the angle where the iris and cornea meet. This tissue also is called the trabecular meshwork. The cornea is important to vision because it lets light into the eye. When the eye makes too much fluid or the drainage system doesn't work properly, eye pressure may increase.

Open-angle glaucoma

This is the most common form of glaucoma. The drainage angle formed by the iris and cornea remains open. But other parts of the drainage system don't drain properly. This may lead to a slow, gradual increase in eye pressure.

Angle-closure glaucoma

This form of glaucoma occurs when the iris bulges. The bulging iris partially or completely blocks the drainage angle. As a result, fluid can't circulate through the eye and pressure increases. Angle-closure glaucoma may occur suddenly or gradually.

Normal-tension glaucoma

No one knows the exact reason why the optic nerve becomes damaged when eye pressure is normal. The optic nerve may be sensitive or experience less blood flow. This limited blood flow may be caused by the buildup of fatty deposits in the arteries or other conditions that damage circulation. The buildup of fatty deposits in the arteries also is known as atherosclerosis.

Glaucoma in children

A child may be born with glaucoma or develop it in the first few years of life. Blocked drainage, injury or an underlying medical condition may cause optic nerve damage.

Pigmentary glaucoma

In pigmentary glaucoma, small pigment granules flake off from the iris and block or slow fluid drainage from the eye. Activities such as jogging sometimes stir up the pigment granules. That leads to a deposit of pigment granules on tissue located at the angle where the iris and cornea meet. The granule deposits cause an increase in pressure.

Glaucoma tends to run in families. In some people, scientists have identified genes related to high eye pressure and optic nerve damage.

Risk factors

Glaucoma can damage vision before you notice any symptoms. So be aware of these risk factors:

- High internal eye pressure, also known as intraocular pressure
- Age over 55
- Black, Asian or Hispanic heritage
- Family history of glaucoma
- Certain medical conditions, such as diabetes, migraines, high blood pressure and sickle cell anemia
- Corneas that are thin in the center
- Extreme nearsightedness or farsightedness
- Eye injury or certain types of eye surgery
- Taking corticosteroid medicines, especially eye drops, for a long time
- Some people have narrow drainage angles, putting them at increased risk of angle-closure glaucoma

Prevention

These steps may help detect and manage glaucoma in its early stages. That may help to prevent vision loss or slow its progress.

Get regular eye examinations. Regular comprehensive eye exams can help detect glaucoma in its early stages, before significant damage occurs. As a general rule, the American Academy of Ophthalmology recommends a comprehensive eye exam every 5 to 10 years if you're under 40 years old; every 2 to 4 years if you're 40 to 54 years old; every 1 to 3 years if you're 55 to 64 years old; and every 1 to 2 years if you're older than 65.

If you're at risk of glaucoma, you'll need more **frequent screening**. Ask your health care provider to recommend the right screening schedule for you.

Know your family's eye health history. Glaucoma tends to run in families. If you're at increased risk, you may need more frequent screening.

Wear eye protection. Serious eye injuries can lead to glaucoma. Wear eye protection when using power tools or playing sports.

Take prescribed eye drops regularly. Glaucoma eye drops can significantly reduce the risk that high eye pressure will progress to glaucoma. Use eye drops as prescribed by your health care provider even if you have no symptoms.

Diagnosis

Your health care provider will review your medical history and conduct a comprehensive eye examination. Your provider may perform several tests, including:
- Measuring intraocular pressure, also called tonometry
- Testing for optic nerve damage with a dilated eye examination and imaging tests
- Checking for areas of vision loss, also known as a visual field test
- Measuring corneal thickness with an exam called pachymetry
- Inspecting the drainage angle, also known as gonioscopy

Treatment

The damage caused by glaucoma can't be reversed. But treatment and regular check-ups can help slow or prevent vision loss, especially if you catch the disease in its early stages.

Glaucoma is treated by lowering intraocular pressure. Treatment options include prescription eye drops, oral medicines, laser treatment, surgery or a combination of approaches.

Eyedrops

Glaucoma treatment often starts with prescription eye drops. Some may decrease eye pressure by improving how fluid drains from your eye. Others decrease the amount of fluid your eye makes. Depending on how low your eye pressure needs to be, you may be prescribed more than one eye drop.

Prescription eye drop medicines include:

Prostaglandins. These increase the outflow of the fluid in your eye, helping to reduce eye pressure. Medicines in this category include latanoprost (Xalatan), travoprost (Travatan Z), tafluprost (Zioptan), bimatoprost (Lumigan) and latanoprostene bunod (Vyzulta).

Possible side effects include mild reddening and stinging of the eyes, darkening of the iris, darkening of the pigment of the eyelashes or eyelid skin, and blurred vision. This class of drug is prescribed for once-a-day use.

Beta blockers. These reduce the production of fluid in your eye, helping to lower eye pressure. Examples include timolol (Betimol, Istalol, Timoptic) and betaxolol (Betoptic S).

Possible side effects include difficulty breathing, slowed heart rate, lower blood pressure, impotence and fatigue. This class of drug can be prescribed for once-or twice-daily use depending on your condition.

Alpha-adrenergic agonists. These reduce the production of the fluid that flows throughout the inside of your eye. They also increase the outflow of fluid in your eye. Examples include apraclonidine (Iopidine) and brimonidine (Alphagan P, Qoliana).

Possible side effects include irregular heart rate, high blood pressure, fatigue, red, itchy or swollen eyes, and dry mouth. This class of drug is usually prescribed for twice-daily use but sometimes can be prescribed for use three times a day.

Carbonic anhydrase inhibitors. These medicines reduce the production of fluid in your eye. Examples include dorzolamide and brinzolamide (Azopt). Possible side effects include a metallic taste, frequent urination, and tingling in the fingers and toes. This class of drug is usually prescribed for twice-daily use but sometimes can be prescribed for use three times a day.

Rho kinase inhibitor. This medicine lowers eye pressure by suppressing the rho kinase enzymes responsible for fluid increase. It is available as netarsudil (Rhopressa) and is prescribed for once-a-day use. Possible side effects include eye redness and eye discomfort.

Miotic or cholinergic agents. These increase the outflow of fluid from your eye. An example is pilocarpine (Isopto Carpine). Side effects include headache, eye ache, smaller pupils, possible blurred or dim vision, and nearsightedness. This class of medicine is usually prescribed to be used up to four times a day. Because of potential side effects and the need for frequent daily use, these medicines are not prescribed very often anymore.

Because some of the eye drop medicine is absorbed into your bloodstream, you may experience some side effects unrelated to your eyes. To minimize this absorption, close your eyes for 1 to 2 minutes after putting the drops in. You also may press lightly at the corner of your eyes near your nose to close the tear duct for 1 or 2 minutes. Wipe off any unused drops from your eyelid.

You may have been prescribed multiple eye drops or need to use artificial tears. Make sure you wait at least five minutes in between using different drops.

Oral medications

Eye drops alone may not bring your eye pressure down to the desired level. So your eye doctor may also prescribe oral medicine. This medicine is usually a carbonic anhydrase inhibitor. Possible side effects include frequent urination, tingling in the fingers and toes, depression, stomach upset, and kidney stones.

Surgery and other therapies

Other treatment options include laser therapy and surgery. The following techniques may help to drain fluid within the eye and lower eye pressure:

Laser therapy. Laser trabeculoplasty is an option if you can't tolerate eye drops. It also may be used if medicine hasn't slowed the progression of your disease. Your eye doctor also may recommend laser surgery before using eye drops. It's done in your eye doctor's office. Your eye doctor uses a small laser to improve the drainage of the tissue located at the angle where the iris and cornea meet. It may take a few weeks before the full effect of this procedure becomes apparent.

Filtering surgery. This is a surgical procedure called a trabeculectomy. The eye surgeon creates an opening in the white of the eye, which also is known as the sclera. The surgery creates another space for fluid to leave the eye.

Drainage tubes. In this procedure, the eye surgeon inserts a small tube in your eye to drain excess fluid to lower eye pressure.

Minimally invasive glaucoma surgery (**MIGS**). Your eye doctor may suggest a MIGS procedure to lower your eye pressure. These procedures generally require less immediate postoperative care and have less risk than trabeculectomy or using a drainage device. They are often combined with cataract surgery. There are a number of MIGS techniques available, and your eye doctor will discuss which procedure may be right for you.

After your procedure, you'll need to see your eye doctor for follow-up exams. And you may eventually need to undergo additional procedures if your eye pressure begins to rise or other changes occur in your eye.

Treating acute angle-closure glaucoma

Acute angle-closure glaucoma is a medical emergency. If you're diagnosed with this condition, you'll need urgent treatment to reduce the pressure in your eye. This generally will require treatment with medicine and laser or surgical procedures.

You may have a procedure called a laser peripheral iridotomy. The doctor creates a small hole in your iris using a laser. This allows fluid to flow through the iris. This helps to open the drainage angle of the eye and relieves eye pressure.

Clinical trials

Explore Mayo Clinic studies testing new treatments, interventions and tests as a means to prevent, detect, treat or manage this condition.

Lifestyle and home remedies

These tips may help you control high eye pressure or promote eye health.

Eat a healthy diet. Eating a healthy diet can help you maintain your health, but it won't prevent glaucoma from worsening. Several vitamins and nutrients are important to eye health, including zinc, copper, selenium and antioxidant vitamins C, E and A.

Exercise safely. Regular exercise may reduce eye pressure. Talk to your health care provider about an appropriate exercise program.

Limit your caffeine. Drinking beverages with large amounts of caffeine may increase your eye pressure.

Sip fluids carefully. Drink moderate amounts of fluids. Drinking a quart or more of any liquid within a short time may temporarily increase eye pressure.

Take prescribed medicine. Using your eye drops or other medicines as prescribed can help you get the best possible result from your treatment. Be sure to use the drops exactly as prescribed. Otherwise, your optic nerve damage could get worse.

Alternative medicine

Some alternative medicine approaches may help your overall health, but none is an effective glaucoma remedy. Talk with your doctor about their possible benefits and risks.

Herbal remedies. Some herbal supplements, such as bilberry extract, have been advertised as glaucoma remedies. But further study is needed to prove their effectiveness. Don't use herbal supplements in place of proven therapies.

Relaxation techniques. Stress may trigger an attack of acute angle-closure glaucoma. Try to find healthy ways to cope with stress. Meditation and other techniques may help.

Marijuana. Research shows that marijuana lowers eye pressure in people with glaucoma, but only for 3 to 4 hours. Other, standard treatments are more effective. The American Academy of Ophthalmology doesn't recommend marijuana for treating glaucoma.

Coping and support. When you receive a diagnosis of glaucoma, you're potentially facing lifelong treatment, regular check-ups and the possibility of progressive vision loss.

Meeting and talking with other people with glaucoma can be very helpful, and many support groups exist. Check with hospitals and eye care centers in your area to find local groups and meeting times. Look for online resources, including support groups.

Preparing for your appointment

You may start by seeing your primary health care provider. Or you may be referred immediately to an eye specialist (ophthalmologist).

Here's some information to help you get ready for your appointment.

What you can do

When you make the appointment, ask if there's anything you need to do in advance, such as fasting before having a specific test. Make a list of:

• Your symptoms, including any that seem unrelated to the reason for your appointment

• Key personal information, including major stresses, recent life changes and family medical history

• All medications, vitamins or other supplements you take, including the doses

• Questions to ask your doctor

• Take a family or friend along, if possible, to help you remember the information you're given

For glaucoma, some basic questions to ask include:

• What's likely causing my symptoms?

• Other than the most likely cause, what are other possible causes for my symptoms?

• What tests do I need?

• Is my condition likely temporary or chronic?

• What's the best course of action?

• What are the alternatives to the primary approach you're suggesting?

• I have these other health conditions. How can I best manage them together?

• Are there restrictions I need to follow?

• What other self-care measures might help me?

• What is the long-term outlook in my case?

• Should I see a specialist?

• Are there brochures or other printed material I can have? What websites do you recommend?

• Don't hesitate to ask other questions.

What to expect from your doctor

• Your doctor is likely to ask you several questions, such as:

• When did your symptoms begin?

• Have your symptoms been continuous or occasional?

• How severe are your symptoms?

- What, if anything, seems to improve your symptoms?
- What, if anything, appears to worsen your symptoms?
- What you can do in the meantime?
- Avoid doing anything that seems to worsen your symptoms.

A. Translate the following sentences into Chinese.

1. Glaucoma is a group of eye conditions that damage the optic nerve. The optic nerve sends visual information from your eye to your brain and is vital for good vision. Damage to the optic nerve is often related to high pressure in your eye. But glaucoma can happen even with normal eye pressure.

2. If you experience symptoms that come on suddenly, you may have acute angle-closure glaucoma. Symptoms include severe headache and severe eye pain. You need treatment as soon as possible. Go to an emergency room or call an eye doctor's (ophthalmologist's) office immediately.

3. Glaucoma develops when the optic nerve becomes damaged. As this nerve gradually deteriorates, blind spots develop in your vision. For reasons that doctors don't fully understand, this nerve damage is usually related to increased pressure in the eye.

4. Regular comprehensive eye exams can help detect glaucoma in its early stages, before significant damage occurs. As a general rule, the American Academy of Ophthalmology recommends a comprehensive eye exam every 5 to 10 years if you're under 40 years old; every 2 to 4 years if you're 40 to 54 years old; every 1 to 3 years if you're 55 to 64 years old; and every 1 to 2 years if you're older than 65.

5. Eye drops alone may not bring your eye pressure down to the desired level. So your eye doctor may also prescribe oral medicine. This medicine is usually a carbonic anhydrase inhibitor. Possible side effects include frequent urination, tingling in the fingers and toes, depression, stomach upset, and kidney stones.

B. Prepare a lecture on glaucoma after doing the further reading above.

扫码获取
提示

Unit 18

Vitreous Retinal Disease

I Warming-up

A. Match the following words and phrases with their Chinese translations.

A	diabetic retinopathy	1	视网膜脱离
B	optic neuritis	2	视网膜中央静脉阻塞
C	macular degeneration	3	玻璃体混浊
D	obstruction of central retinal artery	4	糖尿病视网膜病变
E	central retinal vein occlusion	5	黄斑前膜
F	macular hole	6	黄斑变性
G	retinal tear	7	视神经炎
H	retinal detachment	8	黄斑裂孔
I	epiretinal membranes	9	视网膜中央动脉阻塞
J	vitreous opacity	10	视网膜裂孔

B. Complete the sentences with the following words or phrases in their proper forms.

such as	pay attention to	millions of	in many cases
sometimes	vary	look for	progression

1. Retinal diseases _____ widely, but most of them cause visual symptoms.
2. The retina contains _____ light-sensitive cells (rods and cones) and other nerve cells

that receive and organize visual information.

3. It's important to _____ any changes in your vision and find care quickly.

4. To make a diagnosis, your ophthalmologist conducts a thorough eye exam and _____ abnormalities anywhere in the eye.

5. It's often accompanied by the sudden onset of symptoms _____ floaters and flashing lights.

6. The main goals of treatment are to stop or slow disease _____ and preserve, improve or restore your vision.

7. _____, damage that has already occurred can't be reversed, making early detection important.

8. Treatment of retinal disease may be complex and _____ urgent.

 C. Watch the video *How Does a Retinal Specialist Diagnose a Patient with a Retinal Disease* **and answer the questions.**

扫码获取视频

1. What questions would you ask to your patient even with the best examination techniques?

2. Why does doctor ask questions about patient's family?

3. What is the purpose for visual field testing?

4. What is the purpose for electro-retinographic testing (ERG) and optical coherence tomography testing (OCT)?

5. Don't you think that genetic testing is necessary for degenerative retinal diseases?

Ⅱ Dialogue

扫码获取
音频及文本

 A. Listen to the dialogue for the first time and try to get the general idea.

 B. Listen to the dialogue for the second time and try to answer the following questions.

1. What's the problem with the patient's eyes?

2. What other diseases does the patient have?

3. How did the doctor examine the patient's vision?

4. What does the type B ultrasound report say about patient's eye disease?

5. Why did the doctor refer the patient to an endocrinologist?

C. **Choose the following words and/or expressions to complete the sentences in their proper forms.**

on top of	在……的上面	tiny blood vessels	毛细血管
central vision	中央视觉	clarity	清晰度
cause	造成	preserve	保护
in the center of	在……的中心	abnormalities	异常情况
optic nerve	视神经	blindness	失明
essential	必不可少的	vision loss	视力丧失

1. Your retina sends this information to your brain through your _____, enabling you to see.

2. Depending on your condition, treatment goals may be to stop or slow the disease and _____, improve or restore your vision.

3. Untreated, some retinal diseases can cause severe _____ or blindness.

4. If you have diabetes, the _____ (capillaries) in the back of your eye can deteriorate and leak fluid into and under the retina.

5. Epiretinal membrane is a delicate tissue-like scar or membrane that looks like crinkled cellophane lying _____ the retina.

6. A macular hole is a small defect _____ the retina at the back of your eye (macula).

7. Macular degeneration causes symptoms such as blurred _____ or a blind spot in the center of the visual field.

8. To make a diagnosis, your ophthalmologist conducts a thorough eye exam and looks for _____ anywhere in the eye.

9. Your doctor may use an Amsler grid to test the _____ of your central vision.

10. The retina is the light-detecting layer at the back of the eye that is _____ for vision.

D. **Read the dialogue and try to make a conversation with your classmates.**

扫码获取
提示

E. **Translate the following Chinese into English.**

D—Doctor　　P—Patient

D: What's the problem with your eyes?

P: 1. 嗯,我的右眼看不见东西一个星期了,而且我的左眼感觉模糊。

1. _____

_____

D: Do you have pain or redness in your eyes?

P：No.

D：Have your eyes been injured?

P：No.

D：2.你有糖尿病或高血压吗?

2. _____

P：I have had diabetes for more than 10 years. My blood pressure is a little bit higher than normal.

D：How is your blood glucose?

P：It's not very steady.

D：Well，let me examine your vision. Your vision is OD HM/30cm；OS 20/200. 3. 现在我给你加一滴溶液放大你的瞳孔。You can go for a type B ultrasound of your eyes first and come back in about half an hour for a further examination after dilation.

3. _____

P：OK，thank you，doctor.

D：4. 我来看一下你的 B 超报告。You have a great number of vitreous opacities in your right eye，nevertheless，the retina is flat. No vitreous opacities were found in your left eye. 5. 请和我到裂隙灯前来。Sit down，please. I'll do an examination. Now，please keep looking forward. Now，please look upward，left upward，left，left downward，downward，right downward，right，right upward. Fine. Thank you for your cooperation.

4. _____

5. _____

P：Thank you，doctor.

D：You have vitreous hemorrhage in your right eye，which is a manifestation of diabetic proliferative retinal disease. In your left eye，hemorrhage and exudation were also found in the retina，and the macular area is edematous as well，which accounts for the poor sight in your left eye.

P：Is it serious?

D：This disease can lead to blindness，and some patients may further develop neovascular glaucoma （NVG） after the blindness，in which pains may occur in the eyes.

P：What can be done now?

D：6. 最重要的事是你要严格控制你的血糖。That's why I'll refer you to an endocrinologist for a better plan to help control your blood glucose. 7. 你的左眼要尽快进行激光治疗,总的来说一周3—4次。The purpose of doing so is to let the diseased retina scar to prevent further bleeding. As for your right eye，we need to observe it further for two weeks. If the blood absorption doesn't occur, vitrectomy will be done to clear up the blood，and at the same time，laser treatment will be performed at the fundus. 8. 如果必要的话,我们将给你进行硅酮油填充或空气注射。

6. _____

7. _____

_____

8. _____

_____

P：I see，thank you，doctor.

Ⅲ Further Reading：Retinal Diseases

Text A

Overview

Retinal diseases vary widely, but most of them cause visual symptoms. Retinal diseases can affect any part of your retina, a thin layer of tissue on the inside back wall of your eye.

The retina contains millions of light-sensitive cells (rods and cones) and other nerve cells that receive and organize visual information. Your retina sends this information to your brain through your optic nerve, enabling you to see.

Treatment is available for some retinal diseases. Depending on your condition, treatment goals may be to stop or slow the disease and preserve, improve or restore your vision. Untreated, some retinal diseases can cause severe vision loss or blindness.

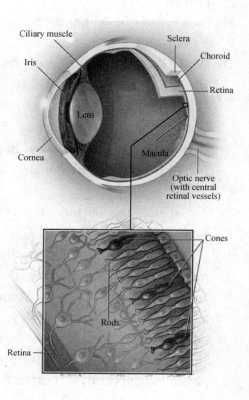

Types

Common retinal diseases and conditions include:

Retinal tear. A retinal tear occurs when the clear, gel-like substance in the center of your eye (vitreous) shrinks and tugs on the thin layer of tissue lining the back of your eye (retina) with enough traction to cause a break in the tissue. It's often accompanied by the sudden onset of symptoms such as floaters and flashing lights.

Retinal detachment. A retinal detachment is defined by the presence of fluid under the retina. This usually occurs when fluid passes through a retinal tear, causing the retina to lift away from the underlying tissue layers.

Diabetic retinopathy. If you have diabetes, the tiny blood vessels (capillaries) in the back of your eye can deteriorate and leak fluid into and under the retina. This causes the retina to swell, which may blur or distort your vision.

Or you may develop new, abnormal capillaries that break and bleed. This also worsens your vision.

Epiretinal membrane. Epiretinal membrane is a delicate tissue-like scar or membrane that looks like crinkled cellophane lying on top of the retina. This membrane pulls up on the retina, which distorts your vision. Objects may appear blurred or crooked.

Macular hole. A macular hole is a small defect in the center of the retina at the back of your eye (macula). The hole may develop from abnormal traction between the retina and the vitreous, or it may follow an injury to the eye.

Macular degeneration. In macular degeneration, the center of your retina begins to deteriorate. This causes symptoms such as blurred central vision or a blind spot in the center of the visual field. There are two types—wet macular degeneration and dry macular degeneration. Many people will first have the dry form, which can progress to the wet form in one or both eyes.

Retinitis pigmentosa. Retinitis pigmentosa is an inherited degenerative disease. It slowly affects the retina and causes loss of night and side vision.

Symptoms

Many retinal diseases share some common signs and symptoms. These may include:
- Seeing floating specks or cobwebs
- Blurred or distorted (straight lines look wavy) vision
- Defects in the side vision
- Lost vision

You may need to try looking with each eye alone to notice these.

When to see a doctor

It's important to pay attention to any changes in your vision and find care quickly. Seek immediate medical attention if you suddenly have floaters, flashes or reduced vision. These are warning signs of potentially serious retinal disease.

Risk factors

Risk factors for retinal diseases might include:
- Aging
- Smoking
- Being obese
- Having diabetes or other diseases
- Eye trauma
- A family history of retinal diseases

Diagnosis

To make a diagnosis, your ophthalmologist conducts a thorough eye exam and looks for abnormalities anywhere in the eye.

The following tests may be done to determine the location and extent of the disease:

Amsler grid test. Your doctor may use an Amsler grid to test the clarity of your central vision. He or she will ask you if the lines of the grid seem faded, broken or distorted and will note where the distortion occurs on the grid to better understand the extent of retinal damage. If you have macular degeneration, he or she might also ask you to use this test to self-monitor your condition at home.

Optical coherence tomography (OCT). This test is an excellent technique for capturing precise images of the retina to diagnose epiretinal membranes, macular holes and macular swelling (edema), to monitor the extent of age-related wet macular degeneration, and to monitor responses to treatment.

Fundus autofluorescence (FAF). FAF may be used to determine the advancement of retinal diseases, including macular degeneration. FAF highlights a retinal pigment (lipofuscin) that increases with retinal damage or dysfunction.

Fluorescein angiography. This test uses a dye that causes blood vessels in the retina to stand out under a special light. This helps to exactly identify closed blood vessels, leaking blood vessels, new abnormal blood vessels and subtle changes in the back of the eye.

Indocyanine green angiography. This test uses a dye that lights up when exposed to infrared light. The resulting images show retinal blood vessels and the deeper, harder-to-see blood vessels behind the retina in a tissue called the choroid.

Ultrasound. This test uses high-frequency sound waves (ultrasonography) to help view the retina and other structures in the eye. It can also identify certain tissue characteristics that can help in the diagnosis and treatment of eye tumors.

CT and MRI. In rare instances, these imaging methods can be used to help evaluate eye injuries or tumors.

Treatment

The main goals of treatment are to stop or slow disease progression and preserve, improve or restore your vision. In many cases, damage that has already occurred can't be reversed, making early detection important. Your doctor will work with you to determine the best treatment.

Treatment of retinal disease may be complex and sometimes urgent. Options include:

Using a laser. Laser surgery can repair a retinal tear or hole. Your surgeon uses a laser to heat small pinpoints on the retina. This creates scarring that usually binds (welds) the retina to the underlying tissue. Immediate laser treatment of a new retinal tear can decrease the chance of it causing a retinal detachment.

Shrinking abnormal blood vessels. Your doctor may use a technique called scatter laser photocoagulation to shrink abnormal new blood vessels that are bleeding or threatening to bleed into the eye. This treatment may help people with diabetic retinopathy. Extensive use of this treatment may cause the loss of some side (peripheral) or night vision.

Freezing. In this process, called cryopexy, your surgeon applies a freezing probe to the external wall of the eye to treat a retinal tear. Intense cold reaches the inside of the eye and freezes the retina. The treated area will later scar and secure the retina to the eye wall.

Injecting air or gas into your eye. This technique, called pneumatic retinopexy, is used to help repair certain types of retinal detachment. It can be used in combination with cryopexy or laser photocoagulation.

Indenting the surface of your eye. This surgery, called scleral buckling, is used to repair a retinal detachment. Your surgeon sews a small piece of silicone material to the outside eye surface (sclera). This indents the sclera and relieves some of the force caused by the vitreous tugging on the retina and reattaches the retina. This technique may be used with other treatments.

Evacuating and replacing the fluid in the eye. In this procedure, called vitrectomy, your surgeon removes the gel-like fluid that fills the inside of your eye (vitreous). He or she then injects air, gas or liquid into the space.

Vitrectomy may be used if bleeding or inflammation clouds the vitreous and obstructs the surgeon's view of the retina. This technique may be part of the treatment for people with a retinal tear, diabetic retinopathy, a macular hole, epiretinal membrane, an infection, eye trauma or a retinal detachment.

Injecting medicine into the eye. Your doctor may suggest injecting medication into the vitreous in the eye. This technique may be effective in treating people with wet macular degeneration, diabetic retinopathy or broken blood vessels within the eye.

Implanting a retinal prosthesis. People who have severe vision loss or blindness owing to certain inherited retinal disease may need surgery. A tiny electrode chip is implanted in the retina that receives input from a video camera on a pair of eyeglasses. The electrode picks up and relays visual information that the damaged retina can no longer process.

Clinical trials

Explore Mayo Clinic studies testing new treatments, interventions and tests as a means to prevent, detect, treat or manage this condition.

Coping and support

Vision loss from retinal disease can affect your ability to do things such as read, recognize faces and drive. These tips may help you cope with your changing vision:

Ask your eye doctor to check your eyeglasses. If you wear contacts or glasses, be sure your prescription is up to date and at maximum strength. If a stronger pair of glasses doesn't help, ask for a referral to a low-vision specialist.

Use prescribed magnifiers. A variety of magnifying devices prescribed by a low-vision specialist can help you with reading and close-up work, such as sewing. Such devices include hand-held lenses or magnifying lenses you wear like glasses. You may also use a closed-circuit television system that uses a video camera to magnify reading material and project it on a video screen. Over-the-counter magnifiers may not work as well.

Change your computer display and add audio systems. Adjust the font size and monitor contrast in your computer's settings. Consider adding speech-output systems or other technologies to your computer.

Use electronic reading aids and voice interface. Try talking watches, clocks and calculators, large-print books, tablet computers, and audio books. Some tablet and smartphone apps are designed to help people with low vision. And many of these devices now come with a voice recognition feature.

Select special appliances made for low vision. Some clocks, radios, telephones and other appliances have extra-large numbers. You may find it easier to watch a television with a larger high-definition screen, or you may want to sit closer to the screen.

Use brighter lights in your home. Better lighting helps with reading and other daily activities, and it may also reduce the risk of falling.

Consider your transportation options. If you drive, check with your doctor to see if it's safe to continue doing so. Be extra cautious in certain situations, such as driving at night, in heavy traffic or in bad weather. Use public transportation or ask a friend or family member to help. Make arrangements to use local van or shuttle services, volunteer driving networks, or ride-shares.

Get support. Having a retinal condition can be difficult, and you may need to make changes in your life. You may go through many emotions as you adjust. Consider talking to a counselor or joining a support group. Spend time with supportive family members and friends.

Preparing for your appointment

To check for retinal disease, a dilated eye exam is usually necessary. Make an appointment with a doctor who specializes in eye care—an optometrist or an ophthalmologist. He or she can perform a complete eye exam.

What you can do

Before your appointment:

• When you make the appointment, ask if you need to do anything to prepare.

• List any symptoms you're experiencing, including those that seem unrelated to your vision problem.

• List all medications, vitamins and supplements you take, including doses.

• Ask a family member or friend to accompany you. Having your pupils dilated for the eye exam will affect your vision for a time afterward, so you may need someone to drive or accompany you after your appointment. List questions to ask your doctor.

For retinal disease, questions to ask your doctor include:

• How advanced is my condition?

• Is it safe for me to drive?

• Will I experience further vision loss?

• Can my condition be treated?

• Will taking a vitamin or mineral supplement help prevent further vision loss?

• What's the best way to monitor my vision for any changes?

• What changes in my symptoms warrant calling you?

• What low-vision aids might be helpful to me?

• What lifestyle changes can I make to protect my vision?

What to expect from your doctor

Your doctor is likely to ask you a number of questions, such as:

• When did you first notice your vision problem?

• Does the condition affect one or both eyes?

• Do you have trouble seeing things near you, at a distance or both?

• Do you smoke or did you ever smoke? If so, how much?

• Do you have other medical problems, such as high cholesterol, high blood pressure or diabetes?

• Do you have a family history of retinal disease?

• Have you experienced an injury to your eye?

Text B 7 types of retinal eye disease

Maintaining eye health is top of mind for many. The retina plays an important role in how well your eyes work. The retina is the light-detecting layer at the back of the eye that is essential for vision. Some retinal conditions are more common with aging or diabetes. Others are hereditary, such as retinitis pigmentosa, or have genetic risk factors.

Keeping your vision safe from retinal disease is important. This article will explore symptoms, types of retinal disease, risk factors, prevention, and when to get an eye examination.

Symptoms

With retinal disease, any part of the retina can be affected. If you don't take steps to treat it, vision loss can be extreme and, in some cases, may ultimately cause blindness. But if you get proper treatment promptly, it's possible to restore vision in some cases or slow down vision loss, sometimes indefinitely.

Early signs

While vision loss can be the first sign that something is wrong with your retina, there may be other clues. These can include:
- Noticing flashes of light
- The sudden appearance of floaters drifting across the eye
- Blurred vision (especially central vision)
- Difficulty seeing in dim light
- Color vision that's muted
- Straight lines that appear wavy

If you contact your eye-care professional promptly, you will likely find the cause of your symptoms and get effective treatment.

Retinal diseases

There is a variety of conditions that can cause retinal issues. Anything that affects the retina should be taken seriously since vision cannot be restored once it's lost here.

Conditions that can cause retinal damage include diabetic retinopathy, retinal tears, retinal detachment, glaucoma, retinitis pigmentosa, and vein occlusion. All can threaten your sight if ignored. Here's what to know:

Diabetic retinopathy

Diabetic retinopathy affects 1 in 3 people with diabetes. High blood sugar in diabetes impacts blood vessels throughout the body, including the small ones that feed the retina. Damage causes the small vessels to leak blood and other fluid into the retina.

Retinal swelling that then occurs can cause blurred or cloudy vision. What's more, new abnormal blood vessels start to grow here. These are less resilient than the normal ones and leak even more easily.

Diabetes prevalence

Surveys show that 10.5% of people in the United States have diabetes. Of those, over 22% have not yet been diagnosed.

Retinal tear

A retinal tear is what it sounds like—a rip or hole in the retina. It can occur when something attached to the retina tugs too hard. This can happen when there's a common posterior vitreous detachment.

With a posterior vitreous detachment, the gel inside the eye shrinks and separates from the sides, including the retina. Sometimes, it tightly sticks to the retina and, in separating, it can rip a hole there, causing a retinal tear.

Fluid can then leak behind the retina and build up, causing the retina to detach. If this is not promptly treated, vision loss can occur.

Retinal detachment

A retinal detachment is when the retina pulls away from the tissues that nourish it. Without the needed blood supply, the retina no longer works as it should. The three causes are:

Rhegmatogenous: This is linked to retinal tears and is the most common type of retinal detachment. Such tears can be caused by aging, being nearsighted, having an injury, or having had eye surgery.

Tractional: Scar tissue formed when blood vessels feeding the retina are damaged pulls the retina away, causing a detachment. This usually happens in cases of diabetic retinopathy.

Exudative: This can result from many conditions, including inflammatory eye diseases, age-related macular degeneration, certain cancers of the eye, and some systemic (body-wide) conditions. It happens if fluid collects behind the retina to the point in which it pushes on the retina and causes it to detach.

Macular degeneration

With age-related macular degeneration, fine central vision (what you see at the center of your visual field) is generally lost over time, but peripheral vision (what you see at the sides of your visual field) is maintained. It is unusual for someone to go completely blind from this. But for those over age 50, this is the most common type of severe vision loss. There are two types of macular degeneration—dry and wet.

Most people with macular degeneration have the dry form. With this, the macula (the oval spot in the retina responsible for central vision) slowly breaks down. It is unclear exactly what causes this. It's believed that the supporting membrane for the macula gradually breaks down.

With wet macular degeneration, there tends to be more severe vision loss. This occurs when abnormal, leaky blood vessels begin to form underneath the retina. These then can leak fluid onto the retina and may damage this, causing vision loss.

Epiretinal membrane

Also known as macular pucker, epiretinal membrane involves a delicate, semitranslucent membrane that can form on the retina's inner surface. It has no blood vessels to leak. But, over time, it can pull on the retina as it contracts. Epiretinal membrane can cause visual distortions, such as crooked lines or blurred vision.

The occurrence of an epiretinal membrane usually happens because of a posterior vitreous detachment. It can also form for other reasons, including retinal detachment, eye surgery, diabetic retinopathy, and eye trauma.

Branch retinal occlusion

With a branch retinal occlusion, the blood flow to the retina can become blocked due to a clot. This can damage the retina, which needs a constant supply of oxygen and nutrients. It can lead to a sudden loss of vision. But if this vision loss is not in the center of the retina, it may go unnoticed.

Also, if a retinal vein is blocked, blood may not drain from the retina, which can cause blocked blood vessels to begin to bleed and leak fluid.

The two types of retinal vein occlusion are:

• **Central retinal vein occlusion**, in which the main retinal vein becomes blocked

• **Branch retinal vein occlusion**, when a smaller vein in the branch becomes blocked

Retinitis pigmentosa

This is a hereditary eye disease in which photoreceptors (light-detecting cells) on the retina begin to degenerate and cause a gradual decline in vision. The degeneration occurs specifically in the retinal photoreceptor cells called rods or cones. It can affect either rods or cones, or both. These cells are situated mainly on the outer layer of the retina.

Risk factors

While every retinal condition is unique, some risk factors to be on alert for include the following:

- Age
- Family history
- Diabetes
- High blood pressure
- Injury
- Smoking
- Obesity

Prevention

While there is currently no medication you can take to keep retinal disorders at bay, there are steps that can help reduce the chances of developing one of these conditions. These include:

- Stopping smoking
- Wearing sunglasses
- Eating antioxidant-rich foods like leafy green vegetables
- Keeping blood pressure and weight in a healthy range
- Maintaining good control of blood sugar if you have diabetes
- Taking multivitamins and other supplements
- Going for routine eye visits and checking your vision with a tool called an Amsler grid

When to get an eye exam

If you see any changes in your vision, it's a good idea to schedule an eye exam. If you see flashes of light or specks in your vision, known as floaters, you may have a retinal detachment and you should immediately see an eye health professional.

An ophthalmologist (medical doctor specializing in eye disorders) is needed to treat retinal conditions.

Summary

Several conditions can affect your vision due to damage to your retina, the light-sensing layer at the back of your eye. Changes in vision such as flashes of light, a sudden increase of floaters, blurred central vision, or vision loss are signs of retinal disorders. You should seek immediate eye care if any of these occur.

Diabetic retinopathy, age-related macular degeneration, retinal tears, and retinal detachment are some of the most common retinal disorders. Risk factors, some of which are preventable, include age, diabetes, high blood pressure, smoking, and injury.

A word from verywell

Preserving your vision means not only keeping retinal symptoms in mind but also being aware of conditions that can threaten retinal health and risk factors for these conditions. The good news is that visiting your eye practitioner at the earliest sign of trouble can go a long way toward maintaining vision.

A. Translate the following sentences into Chinese.

1. Maintaining eye health is top of mind for many. The retina plays an important role in how well your eyes work. The retina is the light-detecting layer at the back of the eye that is essential for vision. Some retinal conditions are more common with aging or diabetes. Others are hereditary, such as retinitis pigmentosa, or have genetic risk factors.

2. With retinal disease, any part of the retina can be affected. If you don't take steps to treat it, vision loss can be extreme and, in some cases, may ultimately cause blindness. But if you get proper treatment promptly, it's possible to restore vision in some cases or slow down vision loss, sometimes indefinitely.

3. There is a variety of conditions that can cause retinal issues. Anything that affects the retina should be taken seriously since vision cannot be restored once it's lost here. Conditions that can cause retinal damage include diabetic retinopathy, retinal tears, retinal detachment, glaucoma, retinitis pigmentosa, and vein occlusion. All can threaten your sight if ignored.

4. Diabetic retinopathy affects 1 in 3 people with diabetes. High blood sugar in diabetes impacts blood vessels throughout the body, including the small ones that feed the retina. Damage causes the small vessels to leak blood and other fluid into the retina.

5. A retinal detachment is when the retina pulls away from the tissues that nourish it. Without the needed blood supply, the retina no longer works as it should.

B. Prepare a lecture on retinal disease after doing the further reading above.

扫码获取
提示

Unit 19

Dental Caries

Ⅰ Warming-up

A. Match the following words and phrases with their Chinese translations.

A	enamel	1	牙本质
B	drill	2	牙釉质
C	fluoride	3	摄入
D	dentin	4	卫生
E	filling	5	（用牙线）清洁牙齿
F	carbohydrate	6	乳酸
G	hygiene	7	填充物
H	floss	8	钻头
I	lactic acid	9	氟化物
J	intake	10	碳水化合物

B. Complete the sentences with the following words or phrases in their proper forms.

indulge in	smooth out	wear down	enclose
be resistant to	be susceptible to	close off	erupt

1. Blood vessels and nerves in our teeth are _____ deep within the dentin.
2. We use tooth fillings to fill and _____ the infected area, preventing them from

getting worse.

3. As our teeth _____, microbes that picked up as babies from our mothers' mouths naturally begin to accumulate communities of bacteria.

4. Those cavemen would hardly have _____ sugar treats, however, so what caused their cavities?

5. Ancient humans even made rudimentary drills to _____ the rough holes left behind and beeswax to plug cavities like modern-day fillings.

6. Some people are _____ cavities due to genes that may cause certain weaknesses, like softer enamel, but for most high sugar consumption is to blame.

7. Mutant streptococci are _____ this acid, but unfortunately our teeth aren't.

8. Enamel is no match for acid. That degrades the armor over time, leaching away its calcium minerals. Gradually, acid _____ a pathway for bacteria into the tooth's secondary layer called the dentin.

扫码获取视频

C. Watch the video *What Causes Cavities* and answer the questions.

1. What did a team of archaeologists recently discover?

2. What caused the teeth cavities of those cavemen?

3. How does a cavity form?

4. What's the function of fluoride?

5. How does the doctor do to prevent cavities?

II Dialogue

扫码获取
音频及文本

A. Listen to the dialogue for the first time and try to get the general idea.

B. Listen to the dialogue for the second time and try to answer the following questions.

1. When does the first patient's toothache occur?

2. Can his tooth be filled? Why?

3. Why should the second patient receive root-canal treatment?

4. What is the first step of root-canal treatment?

5. What is the post-operative instruction for extraction?

C. **Choose the following words and/or expressions to complete the sentences in their proper forms.**

fill the cavity	填补蛀牙	empty stomach	空腹
tap on	敲击	rinse the mouth	漱口
take a dental X-ray	拍牙齿 X 光片	chew on	咀嚼
root-canal treatment	根管治疗	reservation form	预约单
pulp tissue	牙神经	chronic medication	长期服药
anesthesia	麻醉	tooth extraction	拔牙

1. When patients come into our office for the first time，we'll often have to _____ of their teeth if they show signs of decay.

2. _____ is needed when the blood or nerve supply of the tooth（called the "pulp"）is infected through decay or injury.

3. Your dentist might need to apply dental local _____ to numb an area of your mouth while performing certain procedures.

4. _____ usually occurs when there's too much damage to a tooth and can't be repaired.

5. We would normally perform a root-canal treatment in which we remove the _____ and fill the empty pulp chamber and root canals.

6. The American Dental Association（ADA）recommends that people gently _____ with a warm saltwater solution after having a dental procedure.

7. When I _____ tooth number 32，the patient experienced exquisite pain.

8. You should take care not to bite or _____ the tooth before it has been restored with a filling put in place.

9. Before _____，your dentist will numb your teeth，gums and surrounding skin to avoid and lessen discomfort during the procedure.

10. Taking medication on a（n）_____ does not usually mean that a meal has to be skipped. The medication is instead taken before breakfast，lunch or dinner.

D. **Read the dialogue and try to make a conversation with your classmates.**

扫码获取
提示

E. Translate the following Chinese into English.

P—Patient   D—Doctor

P: There's a hole in my back tooth.

D: Is it on the left or right? Upper or lower?

P: 1. 在右边下面。

    1. _____

D: 2. 这颗牙平时有什么不适感或者疼痛吗？

    2. _____

P: It hurts a little.

D: In what condition does it hurt? Does it hurt when you drink hot or cold water?

P: 3. 喝冷水或用冷水刷牙的时候会疼。It doesn't hurt when eating hot food.

    3. _____

D: How long does the pain usually last?

P: It lasts for a few seconds, and then it goes away.

D: 4. 牙齿会不会突然开始疼痛或晚上睡觉的时候疼？

    4. _____

    _____

P: No.

D: OK, let me check. Please open your mouth. I can see a cavity in the lower right back tooth. I will check it with a probe. Raise your hand if it hurts, but please do not move your head.

P: Ouch (Raise hand to indicate).

D: OK, 5. 您现在需要拍一张牙片检查一下龋坏的深度。6. 这颗牙还没有坏到牙髓神经,可以补。7. 我需要把龋坏的部分清理干净。It may feel a little sore. Please raise your hand if it hurts. Then the tooth can be filled after cleaning. It has been filled now. Please bite. 8. 您咬合的时候有不适感吗？

    5. _____

    6. _____

    7. _____

    8. _____

P: It feels like the filling is taller than my teeth.

D: Okay, I will adjust for you. How do you feel now?

P: OK. It's all right. Thank you!

III Further Reading: Tooth Decay

How can hidden tooth decay affect your teeth and body?

If your enamel looks almost perfect with no signs of tooth decay, you might think it's okay to put off your dental appointments. Even if you think your teeth are healthy, cavities can show up in places you can't see with the naked eye. If you don't find and treat the decay, it can potentially cause lifelong problems for you, including pain and infection.

Here are things to know about hidden tooth decay and what you can do to detect it and protect your teeth from having problems.

Where does hidden tooth decay form?

Dentists generally advise patients to brush their teeth twice a day to prevent cavities. Adults should also floss between their teeth at least once a day. However, many adult men and women don't follow their dentist's advice as much as they should. A lack of home and professional dental care potentially leads to hidden cavities.

Hidden cavities can form anywhere in the mouth, including between the deep grooves and crevices of your back teeth, along the sharp edges of your canines, and on the smooth surfaces behind your incisors and bicuspids. Some decay can form above the gumline and on the thick roots of your teeth.

The cavities might not cause any issues right away. In many cases, cavities take some time to create problems for you. But once the decay does cause you problems, the results can be painful.

Tooth decay can eventually spread to the soft and hard tissues inside your teeth. If the decay spreads to the nerves and blood inside the tooth, the decay can lead to an infection. The infection gradually travels down the roots of the tooth until it forms a small pocket of pus called an abscess.

Abscesses can enlarge enough to press against the nerves running through your jawbone. The pain experienced from the compressed nerves can be excruciating for some individuals. If the abscess ruptures, pus can leak out and spread bacteria to other locations in the mouth, face, and jaw.

Ruptured tooth abscesses can potentially release bacteria into your bloodstream. The germs can lead to a dangerous condition called sepsis, or blood poisoning, in some individuals. Sepsis can affect multiple major organs if you don't treat it immediately, including your lungs, kidneys, and heart.

Unless you seek professional dental care regularly, you may not find the decay in time to keep it from permanently damaging your teeth and affecting your health.

How do you detect and treat hidden cavities?

Detection is one of the best ways to keep your teeth and body safe from tooth decay. You can do so by seeing a dentist for a laser cavity detection exam. The exam uses the latest technology in dentistry to locate and diagnose the initial signs of tooth decay. Early detection and treatment keep the decay from spreading further into the tooth.

In addition to the diagnostic test above, a dentist can visually inspect your teeth for decay. The visual exam may include checking your gumline for plaque buildup. The bacteria inside plaque can cause tooth decay when they feed. The feeding germs produce a strong acid that gradually dissolves the minerals inside your enamel.

If a dentist finds decay in your teeth during the exams above, they'll repair them with restorations. Restorations keep cavities from spreading deeper into the crowns of your teeth. Decay found in the roots of your teeth may require more advanced treatment, such as root canal therapy and crowns.

If time permits, a dentist may clean your teeth. The cleaning not only removes plaque from the services of your teeth, it can also remove germs from above and below your gumline. A dental provider may apply sealants to the bite surfaces of your molars to keep bacteria and plaque from settling on them.

A dentist may ask about your diet during the final stages of your visit. Some of the items you consume may contain sugar and acids, which can dissolve or weaken your tooth enamel over time. Weakened tooth enamel can eventually crack or chip from pressure. A dentist may counsel you about the importance of good nutrition for your teeth.

After treatment, keep your teeth healthy by seeing a dentist every six months for exam and cleaning. A dental provider may take X-rays of your teeth during the visits. Along with laser cavity detection exams, X-rays can detect cavities, gum disease, and infection of the jawbone.

If something does show up in the diagnostic tests, a dentist can schedule the treatments you need to correct them, including dental crowns, porcelain veneers, and periodontal treatment. These types of treatments can occur alone or together, depending on the extent of your problems.

A. Translate the following sentences into Chinese.

1. Hidden cavities can form anywhere in the mouth, including between the deep grooves and crevices of your back teeth, along the sharp edges of your canines, and on the smooth surfaces behind your incisors and bicuspids. Some decay can form above the gumline and on the thick roots of your teeth.

2. Abscesses can enlarge enough to press against the nerves running through your jawbone. The pain experienced from the compressed nerves can be excruciating for some individuals. If the abscess ruptures, pus can leak out and spread bacteria to other locations in the mouth, face, and jaw.

3. Ruptured tooth abscesses can potentially release bacteria into your bloodstream. The germs can lead to a dangerous condition called sepsis, or blood poisoning, in some individuals. Sepsis can affect multiple major organs if you don't treat it immediately, including your lungs, kidneys, and heart.

4. A dental provider may apply sealants to the bite surfaces of your molars to keep bacteria and plaque from settling on them.

5. Some of the items you consume may contain sugar and acids, which can dissolve or weaken your tooth enamel over time. Weakened tooth enamel can eventually crack or chip from pressure.

B. Prepare a lecture on tooth decay after doing the further reading above.

扫码获取
提示

Unit 20

Maxillofacial Infection

I Warming-up

A. Match the following words and phrases with their Chinese translations.

A	gum tissue	1	发炎
B	trauma	2	牙龈组织
C	ulceration	3	牙菌斑
D	inflammation	4	智齿冠周炎
E	mouth rinse	5	肿胀的
F	plaque	6	坏死组织
G	gum flap	7	溃疡
H	necrotic tissue	8	龈瓣
I	pericoronitis	9	漱口水
J	swollen	10	外伤

B. Complete the sentences with the following words or phrases in their proper forms.

cut through	on and off	gum flap	get wedged
flush away	pull all the way back	as a general rule of thumb	be triggered by

1. Much like with a teething baby，"cutting" wisdom teeth is a painful experience and it's often a process that will give your teeth _____ discomfort through a period of

several months. This can cause a lot of pressure and pain both in the erupting teeth and neighboring ones as well. It's also common for the gum tissue to be swollen and sore.

2. If you have no room in your mouth to support incoming wisdom teeth, then your dentist may recommend a tooth extraction. If your jaw ridge is large enough to support the incoming tooth, then your dentist might just remove the _____, which could allow the tooth to fully erupt.

3. First step to treat your pericoronitis is to clean out that infected area and _____ all those loose debris. Then, the dentist will prescribe a course of oral antibiotics to clear up the infection. He or she will also recommend an antibacterial oral rinse that you can use to clear the infected area.

4. If you are between the ages of 16 and 30, "Are My Wisdom Teeth Coming In?" is a question that may have crossed your mind once or twice. Just as babies have pain when their teeth begin to _____ the gums, as wisdom teeth develop, they often cause pain and discomfort in adults.

5. Flossing is a great way to reach the areas between your teeth where plaque, bacteria and food can _____. When particles are large and a bit painful, you may want to rip the dental floss through your teeth to find relief. However, doing this could push the particle farther into the crevice or deeper into your gum line.

6. As a result, the gums don't _____ from the chewing surface. You're essentially left with a partially erupted tooth and a flap of gum tissue that's still covering part of or the majority of your wisdom tooth. This flap is called the "operculum."

7. Gum disease (also known as periodontal disease or periodontitis) is a progressive inflammatory infection that can _____ poor oral health habits, genetics, hormonal changes, and inadequate nutrition. Untreated gum disease can potentially lead to these four detrimental effects: bad breath, speech impairment, worsened general wellness and decreased confidence.

8. _____, losing more than 5% of your weight over 6 to 12 months may indicate a problem. If you're an older adult with other medical conditions and health issues, even a smaller amount of weight loss may be significant.

 C. Watch the video *What Does This SWOLLEN Gum Flap Mean*? and answer the questions.

扫码获取视频

1. Why does the wisdom tooth sometimes partially erupt?

2. What are the differences between a wisdom tooth infection (pericoronitis) and normal wisdom tooth eruption ("teething") pain?

3. What are the causes of pericoronitis?

4. What are the two options if you want to fully treat pericoronitis?

5. What is the peak age for the occurrence of pericoronitis?

扫码获取
音频及文本

II Dialogue

 A. Listen to the dialogue for the first time and try to get the general idea.

 B. Listen to the dialogue for the second time and try to answer the following questions.

1. What's wrong with this patient? What was the diagnosis of toothache last time?

2. Why is this patient asked to take blood routine test and panoramic X-ray film?

3. What is the cause of his pericoronitis?

4. What symptoms of maxillofacial infection may be present?

5. How can a doctor identify a skin abscess?

C. Choose the following words and/or expressions to complete the sentences in their proper forms.

periodontal pocket	牙周袋	abscess	脓肿
swallow	吞咽	make an incision	切开（脓肿）
swollen	肿胀的	drain the pus	排脓
blood routine	血常规	subside	消退
throbbing pain	一跳一跳的痛	loss of appetite	没胃口
palpation	触诊	fatigue	乏力的

1. Pain is a common experience that nearly every person will confront in their lifetime. For some, it will be brief and the pain will _____ within seconds or minutes. Other times, the pain may last a bit longer before resolving on its own.

2. _____ requires you to touch the patient with different parts of your hands, using varying degrees of pressure.

3. In order to permanently get rid of a _____ face from a tooth infection, you must treat the source of the infection in addition to the facial swelling. This usually requires a combination of draining the abscess, taking antibiotics, and also getting either a root canal or tooth extraction.

4. Providers should ask their patients for a detailed history of symptoms. If the pain is sharp and of short duration, it could indicate a loose filling or cracked tooth. Sharp,

222 English For Clinical Doctors

_____ that lingers may indicate pulpal inflammation or necrosis.

5. _____ are spaces or openings surrounding the teeth under the gum line. These pockets can become filled with infection-causing bacteria. They are a symptom of periodontitis（gum disease），a serious oral infection and can be treated and reversed with good oral hygiene or with dental treatment. But when left untreated, periodontal pockets can lead to tooth loss.

6. Along with detailed personal, travel and epidemiological history, the patient must be asked about respiratory symptoms such as cough or shortness of breath or fever, if any. Fever and _____ could also be caused by acute dental infection; therefore, the etiology should be confirmed.

7. A typical _____ test is the complete blood count, also called CBC, to count your red and white blood cells as well as measure your hemoglobin levels and other blood components. This test can uncover anemia, infection, and even cancer of the blood.

8. Draining the _____ is done by making a cut in the lining and providing an escape route for the pus, either through a drainage tube or by leaving the cavity open to the skin. The area around it will be numbed before draining. Most people feel immediately better after the draining.

9. Sometimes a dental abscess can be treated with antibiotics, but the real cause of the problem（the tooth）often needs to be addressed too. Sometimes it is necessary to _____ in the abscess to allow the pus to drain off or to pull the tooth.

10. An abscessed tooth is typically darker than the surrounding teeth. If pain is present, it is often worse when pressing on the affected tooth. Swelling and pus collection within the gum tissue can be present. Swelling may spread to the jaw or face. If the infection has spread to deeper tissues, symptoms such as difficulty in _____ and pain when opening the mouth may be present.

D. Read the dialogue and try to make a conversation with your classmates.

扫码获取
提示

E. Translate the following Chinese into English.

P—Patient   D—Doctor

P：Doctor，1. 我右边脸和脖子肿起来了，而且很疼，持续了差不多有 5 天。

1. _____

_____

D：It's seriously swollen. Did you have a toothache before the swollen face?

P：Yes. 2. 我最开始是右侧下面最后一颗牙上面的牙龈有点疼，然后咽口水的时候疼得更

厉害。Later, the pain worsened followed by serious swelling in the face and neck.

2. _____

_____

D：Did you have such a toothache before?

P：Yes, I had. 3. 医生说是右下最后一颗智齿发炎了，要我尽快把它拔掉，但我口服了一些抗生素，后来就慢慢不疼了。However, this time, I began to take antibiotics orally 3 days ago, but it does not seem to work and is getting more and more serious.

3. _____

_____

_____

D：4. 全身有没有其他不舒服？

4. _____

P：I've got a fever，fatigue and loss of appetite.

D：I'll take your temperature，and write you a slip for blood routine and panoramic X-ray film. Your temperature is indeed very high，38.5 degrees Celsius. The results show that the white cell count is very high. Sit in the chair, please. I'll do an examination. Please open your mouth as wide as possible and tell me the place where it hurts the most when I press.

P：I can't open my mouth wide，but it's the last tooth on the lower right side that hurts the most at first，and I can feel significant throbbing pain. Now the area under my right earlobe hurts most when you press.

D：5. 从检查结果看,你右下有一个阻生齿,没有完全长出来,细菌堆积在这个牙齿和牙龈

之间的牙周袋里。It presented as pericoronitis at first，but because the inflammation is not controlled timely，it developed into an infection in the masseteric and submandibular space in the right face. 6. 我通过触诊发现有明显的波动感,说明已经形成了脓肿。

5. _____

_____

6. _____

_____

P：That's too bad. Please do something on it.

D：OK，7. 我现在给你做脓肿切开引流术。It's already done. I'll prescribe you some antibiotics. Remember to come back tomorrow to the clinic. 8. 等感染控制后,嘴巴能正常张开了,尽早拔除智齿以防再次发生感染。

7. _____

8. _____

_____

P：Thank you，doctor. I'm feeling quite better now. I'll do as you say. See you tomorrow.

III Further Reading：Periodontal Abscess

A periodontal abscess（also termed lateral abscess，or parietal abscess），is a localized collection of pus（i. e. an abscess）within the tissues of the periodontium. It is a type of dental abscess. A periodontal abscess occurs alongside a tooth，and is different from the more common periapical abscess，which represents the spread of infection from a dead tooth（i. e. which has undergone pulpal necrosis）. To reflect this，sometimes the term "lateral（periodontal）abscess" is used. In contrast to a periapical abscess，periodontal abscesses are usually associated with a vital（living）tooth. Abscesses of the periodontium are acute bacterial infections classified primarily by location.

Signs and symptoms

The main symptom is pain, which often suddenly appears, and is made worse by biting on the involved tooth, which may feel raised and prominent in the bite. The tooth may be mobile, and the lesion may contribute to destruction of the periodontal ligament and alveolar bone. The pain is deep and throbbing. The oral mucosa covering an early periodontal abscess appears erythematous (red), swollen and painful to touch. The surface may be shiny due to stretching of the mucosa over the abscess. Before pus has formed, the lesion will not be fluctuant, and there will be no purulent discharge. There may be regional lymphadenitis.

When pus forms, the pressure increases, with increasing pain, until it spontaneously drains and relieves the pain. When pus drains into the mouth, a bad taste and smell are perceived. Usually drainage occurs via the periodontal pocket, or else the infection may spread as a cellulitis or a purulent odontogenic infection. Local anatomic factors determine the direction of spread. There may be systemic upset, with an onset of pain and fever.

Causes

A periodontal abscess most commonly occurs as a complication of advanced periodontal disease (which is normally painless). A periodontal pocket contains dental plaque, bacteria and subgingival calculus. Periodontal pathogens continually find their way into the soft tissues, but normally they are held in check by the immune system. A periodontal abscess represents a change in this balance, related to decreased local or systemic resistance of the host. An inflammatory response occurs when bacteria invade and multiply within the soft tissue of the gingival crevice/periodontal pocket. A pus-filled abscess forms when the immune system responds and attempts to isolate the infection from spreading.

Communication with the oral environment is maintained via the opening of the periodontal pocket. However, if the opening of a periodontal pocket becomes obstructed, as may occur if the pocket has become very deep (e. g. with furcation involvement), then plaque and calculus are trapped inside. Food packing may also obstruct a periodontal pocket. Food packing is usually caused by failure to accurately reproduce the contact points when dental restorations are placed on the interproximal surfaces of teeth. Another potential cause occurs when a periodontal pocket is scaled incompletely. Following this procedure, the gingival cuff tightens around the tooth, which may be enough to trap the bacteria left in the pocket. A gingival retraction cord which is accidentally left in situ is an occasional cause of a periodontal abscess.

Penetrating injury to the gingival — for example, with a toothbrush bristle, fishbone, toothpick or periodontal instrument—may inoculate bacteria into the tissues. Trauma to the tissues, such as serious impact on a tooth or excessive pressure exerted on teeth during orthodontic treatment, can be a possible cause as well. Occlusal overload may also be involved in the development of a periodontal abscess, but this is rare and usually occurs in combination with other factors. Bruxism is a common cause of excessive occlusal forces.

Systemic immune factors such as diabetes can predispose a person to the formation of periodontal abscesses.

Perforation of a root canal during endodontic therapy can also lead to a periodontal abscess which if left untreated could become "prolonged" ultimately rupture then enter the blood stream and could lead to serious situations such as endocarditis.

Diagnosis

Periodontal abscesses may be difficult to distinguish from periapical abscesses. Since the management of a periodontal abscess is different from a periapical abscess, this differentiation is important to make. For example, root canal therapy is unnecessary and has no impact on pain in a periodontal abscess.

Classification

There are four types of abscesses that can involve the periodontal tissues:
1. Gingival abscess—a localized, purulent infection involves only the soft gum tissue near the marginal gingiva or the interdental papilla.
2. Periodontal abscess—a localized, purulent infection involving a greater dimension of the gum tissue, extending apically and adjacent to a periodontal pocket.
3. Pericoronal abscess—a localized, purulent infection within the gum tissue surrounding the crown of a partially or fully erupted tooth. Usually associated with an acute episode of pericoronitis around a partially erupted and impacted mandibular third molar (lower wisdom tooth).
4. Combined periodontal/endodontic abscess.

Treatment

An important factor is whether the involved tooth is to be extracted or retained. Although the pulp is usually still vital, a history of recurrent periodontal abscesses and significantly compromised periodontal support indicate that the prognosis for the tooth is poor and it should be removed.

The initial management of a periodontal abscess involves pain relief and control of the infection. The pus needs to be drained, which helps both of these aims. If the tooth is to be removed, drainage will occur via the socket. Otherwise, if pus is already discharging from the periodontal pocket, this can be encouraged by gentle irrigation and scaling of the pocket whilst massaging the soft tissues. If this does not work, incision and drainage is required.

Antibiotics are of secondary importance to drainage, which if satisfactory renders antibiotics unnecessary. Antibiotics are generally reserved for severe infections, in which there is facial swelling, systemic upset and elevated temperature. Since periodontal abscesses frequently involve anaerobic bacteria, oral antibiotics such as amoxicillin, clindamycin (in penicillin allergy or pregnancy) and/or metronidazole are given (although metronidazole should be used in conjunction with a penicillin given its lack of aerobic gram positive coverage). Ideally, the choice of antibiotic is dictated by the results of microbiological culture and sensitivity testing of a sample of the pus aspirated at the start of any treatment, but this rarely occurs outside the hospital setting.

Other measures that are taken during management of the acute phase might include reducing the height of the tooth with a dental drill, so it no longer contacts the opposing tooth when biting down; and regular use of hot salt water mouth washes (antiseptic) that encourages further drainage of the infection.

The management following the acute phase involves removing any residual infection, and correcting the factors that lead to the formation of the periodontal abscess. Usually, this will be therapy for periodontal disease, such as oral hygiene instruction and periodontal scaling.

A. Translate the following sentences into Chinese.

1. A periodontal abscess occurs alongside a tooth, and is different from the more common periapical abscess, which represents the spread of infection from a dead tooth (i. e. which has undergone pulpal necrosis). To reflect this, sometimes the term "lateral (periodontal) abscess" is used. In contrast to a periapical abscess, periodontal abscesses are usually associated with a vital (living) tooth. Abscesses of the periodontium are acute bacterial infections classified primarily by location.

2. The main symptom is pain, which often suddenly appears, and is made worse by biting on the involved tooth, which may feel raised and prominent in the bite. The tooth may be mobile, and the lesion may contribute to destruction of the periodontal ligament and alveolar bone. The pain is deep and throbbing.

3. An inflammatory response occurs when bacteria invade and multiply within the soft tissue of the gingival crevice/periodontal pocket. A pus-filled abscess forms when the immune system responds and attempts to isolate the infection from spreading.

4. Food packing is usually caused by failure to accurately reproduce the contact points when dental restorations are placed on the interproximal surfaces of teeth. Another potential cause occurs when a periodontal pocket is scaled incompletely.

5. If the tooth is to be removed, drainage will occur via the socket. Otherwise, if pus is already discharging from the periodontal pocket, this can be encouraged by gentle irrigation and scaling of the pocket whilst massaging the soft tissues. If this does not work, incision and drainage is required.

B. Prepare a lecture on periodontal abscess after doing the further reading above.

扫码获取
提示

Unit 21

Maxillofacial Tumor（Tongue Cancer）

Ⅰ Warming-up

A. Match the following words and phrases with their Chinese translations.

A	incisional biopsy		1	肿块
B	screen		2	肠道
C	lumps and bumps		3	切口活检
D	kidney		4	喉的
E	gut		5	扁桃体
F	precancerous		6	咀嚼
G	laryngeal		7	肾脏
H	tonsil		8	咽部的
I	chew		9	癌症前期的
J	pharyngeal		10	检查,筛查

B. Complete the sentences with the following words or phrases in their proper forms.

go away	of concern	swab test	be diagnosed with
a great majority of	develop oral cancer	in advanced stage	in the practice

1. Men are more than twice as likely as women to _____, according to new figures released by an institute.

2. None of these symptoms, on their own, means that you necessarily have oral cancer, but if we detect anything that may be _____, we may recommend that you have it checked by your GP.

3. Most of the cases of oral cancer presented _____. At the time of presentation 66.3% were in stages Ⅲ and Ⅳ.

4. _____ of clinical medicine and in all health-related tasks, the diagnostic process is critical. A correct diagnostic evaluation is essential for the effectiveness of disease therapy.

5. If you have any signs and symptoms that don't _____ or get worse, you should see a doctor to find out what's causing them.

6. Obviously, saliva testing involves a much less uncomfortable method of collecting a fluid sample than nasal _____. And ultimately, saliva testing could be a game-changer, in that it allows more people to be tested, while simultaneously keeping health care professionals safer.

7. Close to 54,000 Americans will _____ oral or oropharyngeal cancer this year. It will cause over 9,750 deaths, killing roughly 1 person per hour, 24 hours per day.

8. Overall, _____ dentists (95.8%) recognized tobacco use and alcohol consumption as very important risk factors for oral cancer occurrence.

C. Watch the video *Oral Cancer Risk Factors and Symptoms* and answer the questions.

扫码获取视频

1. Why does the American Dental Association ask dentists to do oral cancer screenings during the month of April?

2. What are the commonly seen symptoms in oral cancer?

3. What are the risk factors of oral cancer?

4. How do we screen the oral cancer?

5. How can we get free oral cancer screening?

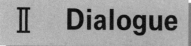

Ⅱ Dialogue

扫码获取
音频及文本

 A. Listen to the dialogue for the first time and try to get the general idea.

B. Listen to the dialogue for the second time and try to answer the following questions.

1. What's the cause of the patient's ulcer?

2. What can clinical examination help the doctor find out?

3. Why should the patient take pathological

examination?

4. What is the treatment of squamous cell carcinoma?

5. What should be done before operation?

C. Choose the following words and/or expressions to complete the sentences in their proper forms.

assist with	辅助	lingual margin	舌缘
pronounced	明显的	clinical examination	临床检查
operate on	给……做手术	cauliflower-like hyperplasia	
register at the admission office			菜花状增生
	办理住院手续	lymph node	淋巴结
get aggravated	加重,恶化	pathological examination	病理检查
stick out	伸出	neck dissection	颈淋巴清扫术

1. _____ is a major surgery done to remove lymph nodes that contain cancer.

2. The gesture of _____ one's tongue can have multiple meanings. It can be an act of rudeness, disgust, playfulness …

3. I have an ulcer on the right side of my tongue that has been hurting for four months and the pain has become more _____ in the recent two weeks.

4. Minimally Invasive or Least Invasive Neck Dissection is the most modern and less painful surgery used to remove a tumor from the neck area. It is sometimes _____ radiotherapy which can be started early as compared to open surgery which helps in providing better results.

5. Occasionally, the clinical and radiological appearances may not be entirely typical or explainable as one of these common cysts, and _____ of the tissue is essential.

6. In robotic surgery, the surgeon can sit at a console and operate these instruments via magnification. Then, the surgeon can precisely remove the cancer tissue only where it was previously difficult to reach or _____ accurately.

7. Cancer can _____ at any age, depending on the kind of atmosphere you're exposed to and the kind of lifestyle you lead.

8. There is a 2-cm ulcer across on the _____ on the right side. The base is fairly hard, with some cauliflower-like hyperplasia on the surface.

9. A _____ comprises three components: the history, the examination, and the explanation, where the doctor discusses the nature and implications of the clinical

findings.

10. Your _____ play a vital role in your body's ability to fight off infections.

D. Read the dialogue and try to make a conversation with your classmates.

扫码获取
提示

E. Translate the following Chinese into English.

P—Patient   D—Doctor

P：Doctor，1. 我右边舌头长了个溃疡 that has been hurting for four months and the pain has become more pronounced in the recent two weeks.

1. _____

D：What do you think has caused the lingual ulceration?

P：Because the back tooth on the lower right side is decayed，the decayed tooth usually grinds on my tongue when I eat. It first happened two years ago，but it got better later. This time，however，it has not recovered since the abrasion，and the ulceration is becoming more severe. Pain has worsened in the last two weeks，which has made me unable to eat.

D：Have you been to the hospital since this abrasion?

P：I had it examined 10 days ago in the local hospital，where the doctor told me that it is oral ulcer and 2. 给我开了一些抗生素口服和漱口水漱口，3. 但是没有效果，反而症状越来越重了。

2. _____

3. _____

D：Please open your mouth wide and stick out your tongue. 4. 你右侧舌缘确实有一个 2 cm 直径的溃疡。The base is fairly hard，with some cauliflower-like hyperplasia on the surface；an enlarged lymph node，about 1.5 cm across，is also found in the lower jaw on the right side. The primary clinical examination suggests that you may have tongue cancer on the right，but a pathological examination is required to confirm the diagnosis. 5. 现在，我要从你的破溃处做切取活检。Don't worry, you won't feel anything because I'll administer a local anesthetic.

4. _____

5. _____

The operation is finished. You can take some semi-liquid food these few days；you should gargle after a meal and try not to talk too much to reduce the movement of the tongue in order to promote healing. Come back in a week when your report is ready.

P：Doctor，is my report ready?

D：Yes，I'm sorry to say that you are confirmed with squamous cell carcinoma on the right side.

P：Oh ... How can it be? Can it be cured?

D：You don't need to be frustrated. We will do our best. First，we will operate on you to remove the lesion on your tongue，6. 还要做同侧的颈淋巴清扫术。

6. _____

P：Sounds really horrible. Does it affect speaking and eating after the tongue is removed?

D：Definitely it will have some effect，but don't worry. Only part of your tongue and some surrounding tissues will be removed. We will use tissues from your thigh or arm to repair the defects using "microvascular free flap reconstruction technique", 7. 尽量减少手术创伤对于面型和功能的影响。 If the condition permits, 8. 手术后再辅助进行放疗和化疗,治疗的远期效果会更好。

7. _____

8. _____

_____

P：I feel relieved after hearing what you said.

When will the operation be?

D：I'll write you a slip for admission. You should register at the admission office as soon as possible. A thorough physical check-up will be done before the operation. If everything is normal, we'll operate on you as soon as we can.

P：OK. I'll register at the admission office right now.

Ⅲ Further Reading：Oral and Oropharyngeal Cancer and Its Diagnosis

Doctors use many tests to find, or diagnose, cancer. They also do tests to learn if cancer has spread to another part of the body from where it started. If this happens, it is called metastasis. For example, imaging tests can show if the cancer has spread. Imaging tests show pictures of the inside of the body. Doctors may also do tests to learn which treatments could work best.

For most types of cancer, a biopsy is the only sure way for the doctor to know if an area of the body has cancer. In a biopsy, the doctor takes a small sample of tissue for testing in a laboratory. If a biopsy is not possible, the doctor may suggest other tests that will help make a diagnosis.

How oral or oropharyngeal cancer is diagnosed

There are many tests used for diagnosing oral or oropharyngeal cancer. Not all tests described here will be used for every person. Your doctor may consider these factors when choosing a diagnostic test：

- The type of cancer suspected
- Your signs and symptoms
- Your age and general health
- The results of earlier medical tests

The following tests may be used to diagnose oral or oropharyngeal cancer：

- **Physical examination.** Dentists and doctors often find lip and oral cavity cancers during routine checkups. If a person shows signs of oral or oropharyngeal cancer, the doctor will take a complete medical history, asking about the patient's symptoms and risk factors. The doctor will feel for any lumps on the neck, lips, gums, and cheeks. Because people with oral or oropharyngeal cancer have a higher risk of other cancers elsewhere in the head and neck region, the doctor will examine the area behind the nose, the larynx (voice box), and the lymph nodes of the neck.

• **Endoscopy.** An endoscopy allows the doctor to see inside the mouth and throat. Typically, a thin, flexible tube with an attached light and view lens, called an endoscope, is inserted through the nose to examine the head and neck areas. Sometimes, a rigid endoscope, which is a hollow tube with a light and view lens, is placed into the back of the mouth to see the back of the throat in more detail.

Endoscopic examinations have different names depending on the area of the body that is examined, such as laryngoscopy to view the larynx, pharyngoscopy to view the pharynx, or nasopharyngoscopy to view the nasopharynx. To make the patient more comfortable, these examinations are performed using an anesthetic spray to numb the area. If an area looks suspicious, the doctor will take a biopsy (see below). Tests are often done in the doctor's office. However, sometimes an endoscopy must be performed in an operating room at a hospital using general anesthesia, which blocks the awareness of pain.

• **Biopsy.** A biopsy is the removal of a small amount of tissue for examination under a microscope. Other tests can suggest that cancer is present, but only a biopsy can make a definite diagnosis. The type of biopsy performed will depend on the location of the cancer. During a fine needle aspiration biopsy, cells are removed using a thin needle inserted directly into the suspicious area. A pathologist then analyzes the cells. A pathologist is a doctor who specializes in interpreting laboratory tests and evaluating cells, tissues, and organs to diagnose disease.

• **Oral brush biopsy.** During routine dental examinations, some dentists are using a newer, simple technique to detect oral cancer in which the dentist uses a small brush to gather cell samples of a suspicious area. The specimen is then sent to a laboratory for analysis. This procedure can be done in the dentist's chair with very little or no pain. If cancer is found using this method, a traditional biopsy is recommended to confirm the results.

• **HPV testing.** HPV testing may be done on a sample of the tumor removed during the biopsy. As described in Risk Factors and Prevention, HPV has been linked to a higher risk of oropharyngeal cancer. Knowing if a person has HPV can help determine the cancer's stage and the treatment options that are likely to be most effective. ASCO recommends that HPV testing is done for all patients newly diagnosed with oropharyngeal squamous cell carcinoma. This is a type of oropharyngeal cancer that starts in flat, scale-like cells called squamous cells. Testing is not usually recommended for oropharyngeal cancer that starts in other types of cells or for other types of head and neck cancer.

• **X-ray.** An X-ray is a way to create a picture of the structures inside of the body, using a small amount of radiation. X-rays may be recommended by your dentist or doctor to look for abnormal findings in the mouth or neck.

• **Barium swallow/modified barium swallow.** There are 2 barium swallow tests that are generally used to look at the oropharynx and to check a patient's swallowing. The first is a traditional barium swallow. During an X-ray exam, the patient is asked to swallow liquid barium. This lets the doctor look for any changes in the structure of the oral cavity and throat and see whether the liquid passes easily to the stomach. A modified barium swallow, or video fluoroscopy, may be used to evaluate difficulties with swallowing.

• **Computed tomography (CT or CAT) scan.** A CT scan takes pictures of the inside of the body using X-rays taken from different angles. A computer combines these pictures into a detailed, 3-dimensional image that shows any abnormalities or tumors. A CT scan can be used to measure the tumor's size, help the doctor decide whether the tumor can be surgically removed, and show whether the cancer has spread to lymph nodes in the neck or lower jawbone. Sometimes, a special dye called a contrast medium is given before the scan to provide better detail on the image. This dye can be injected into a patient's vein or given as a pill or liquid to swallow.

• **Magnetic resonance imaging (MRI).** An MRI uses magnetic fields, not X-rays, to produce detailed images of the body, especially images of soft tissue, such as the tonsils and the base of the tongue. MRI can be used to measure the tumor's size. A special dye called a contrast medium is given before the scan to create a clearer picture. This dye can be injected into a patient's vein or given as a pill or liquid to swallow.

• **Ultrasound.** An ultrasound uses sound waves to create a picture of the internal organs. This test can detect the spread of cancer to the lymph nodes in the neck, which doctors also call the "cervical lymph nodes."

• **Positron emission tomography (PET) or PET-CT scan.** A PET scan is usually combined with a CT scan (see above), called a PET-CT scan. However, you may hear your doctor refer to this procedure just as a PET scan. A PET scan is a way to create pictures of organs and tissues inside the body. A small amount of a radioactive sugar substance is injected into the patient's body. This sugar substance is taken up by cells that use the most energy. Because cancer tends to use energy actively, it absorbs more of the radioactive substance. However, the amount of radiation in the substance is too low to be harmful. A scanner then detects this substance to produce images of the inside of the body.

After diagnostic tests are done, your doctor will review the results with you. If the diagnosis is cancer, these results also help the doctor describe the cancer.

A. **Translate the following sentences into Chinese.**

1. Doctors use many tests to find, or diagnose, cancer. They also do tests to learn if cancer has spread to another part of the body from where it started. If this happens, it is called metastasis.

2. If a person shows signs of oral or oropharyngeal cancer, the doctor will take a complete medical history, asking about the patient's symptoms and risk factors. The doctor will feel for any lumps on the neck, lips, gums, and cheeks.

3. However, sometimes an endoscopy must be performed in an operating room at a hospital using general anesthesia, which blocks the awareness of pain.

4. A biopsy is the removal of a small amount of tissue for examination under a microscope. Other tests can suggest that cancer is present, but only a biopsy can make a definite diagnosis.

5. A PET scan is a way to create pictures of organs and tissues inside the body. A small amount of a radioactive sugar substance is injected into the patient's body. This sugar substance is taken up by cells that use the most energy. Because cancer tends to use energy actively, it absorbs more of the radioactive substance. However, the amount of radiation in the substance is too low to be harmful. A scanner then detects this substance to produce images of the inside of the body.

B. **Prepare a lecture on oral cancer after doing the further reading above.**

扫码获取
提示

Unit 22

Acute Purulent Otitis Media

I Warming-up

A. Match the following words and phrases with their Chinese translations.

A	Eustachian tube	1	鼻咽管
B	etiology	2	特征
C	audiometry	3	鼓膜
D	otoscopy	4	胆脂瘤
E	tympanostomy	5	测听法
F	tympanic membrane	6	观察
G	hallmark	7	耳镜检查
H	watchful waiting	8	病因学
I	cholesteatoma	9	咽鼓管
J	nasopharynx	10	鼓膜造孔术

B. Complete the sentences with the following words or phrases in their proper forms.

perforate	drain	granulate	culture
diminish	irritable	suspect	recur

1. A five-year-old boy was admitted into hospital because of his increasing _____ and fever.

2. The purpose of this study was to investigate the etiology, clinic feature, and therapy of _____ suppurative otitis media.

3. Chronic otitis media is a scenario that's involved a _____ of the tympanic membrane.

4. Samuel estimated that it would take about seventy-two hours for the _____ of bacteria to develop in Ferd.

5. Both the negative pressure _____ vessel and the drop stitch are easier to cause infection.

6. Within 24 hours, _____ tissue forms to fill in areas damaged or removed from the body.

7. Doctors _____ he may have a chronic otitis media.

8. Any sleep disturbance will _____ mental performance.

 C. Watch the video *Otitis Media* and answer the questions.

扫码获取视频

1. Why does acute otitis media happen more on infants and children than adult?

2. What are the most commonly bacterial causes for otitis media?

3. What are the symptoms of otitis media?

4. What does tympanostomy do if the antibiotic does not work?

5. Why the most appropriate next step is giving antibiotics for the first case?

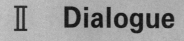 **II Dialogue**

扫码获取
音频及文本

 A. Listen to the dialogue for the first time and try to get the general idea.

 B. Listen to the dialogue for the second time and try to answer the following questions.

1. Why was the patient brought to see ENT doctor?

2. What physical examinations were made by the doctor?

238 English For Clinical Doctors

3. In addition to the physical examination, what other examinations do you think should be made for the patient?

4. What is more important for the patient to be aware of if otitis media is diagnosed?

5. What ENT doctor could do for the patient if his/her hearing was damaged?

C. Choose the following words and/or expressions to complete the sentences in their proper forms.

either ... or ...	要么……要么……	discharge	排出；出院
go from bad to worse	越来越糟	relapse	复发
suppurate	化脓	affect	影响
onset	起病	over-strain	过度紧张
hydrogen peroxide	过氧化氢	depend	取决于
ossicle	听骨	apply	应用

1. The cause of Acute Otitis Media is related to childhood anatomy and immune function. _____ bacteria _____ viruses may be involved.

2. In the most severe cases, the ossicle might be damaged and the hearing will _____.

3. _____ 5 to 7 drops of 0.3% Ofloxacin ear drops and hold there for about 10 minutes, 2 to 3 times a day.

4. Don't _____ yourself and pay attention not to catch cold and keep your ear canal dry and clean.

5. It can heal eventually if you keep the ear dry and prevent it from _____.

6. Chronic _____ otitis media（CSOM）is middle ear inflammation that results in discharge from the ear for more than three months.

7. How students ultimately handle stress may _____ on their personal test-taking abilities.

8. Did you have a cold and cough before the _____ of illness?

9. If your _____ ear suppurates again and again, the perforation will be larger and larger.

10. After the child had been treated, and was being prepared for _____, Dr. Myer talked to the parents about how they should care for the child at home.

D. Read the dialogue and try to make a conversation with your classmates.

扫码获取
提示

E. Translate the following Chinese into English.

D—Doctor   P—Patient

D：How long have you had these troubles? 1.

耳朵痛不痛？

1. _____

P：Three days now. The earache was severe

before suppuration. Now it's better.

D：2. 流出的分泌物是什么样的?

2. ＿＿＿＿＿＿＿＿＿＿＿＿＿＿＿＿＿＿＿

P：It's purulent.

D：Did you have a cold and cough before the onset of illness?

P：Yes，I did. I had a cold one week ago，but it's better now.

D：Let me examine your ears. Does it hurt when I pull your ears? 3. 当我按这儿时你感觉怎样?

3. ＿＿＿＿＿＿＿＿＿＿＿＿＿＿＿＿＿

P：No，it doesn't hurt.

D：Your ear drum has perforated. You are suffering from acute purulent otitis media.

P：Can it be cured?

D：Oh，definitely，but you should take some antibiotics for a week. I'll write you

Ampicillin. 4. 另外,用双氧水先洗干净耳道内分泌物,然后患耳朝上。5. 滴入 5～7 滴 0.3% 氧氟沙星滴耳剂,保持 10 分钟左右,一天两到三次。6. 注意清洁耳道很重要,不然会降低疗效。7. 记住,一周后来复诊。

4. ＿＿＿＿＿＿＿＿＿＿＿＿＿＿＿＿＿

＿＿＿＿＿＿＿＿＿＿＿＿＿＿＿＿＿＿＿

5. ＿＿＿＿＿＿＿＿＿＿＿＿＿＿＿＿＿

＿＿＿＿＿＿＿＿＿＿＿＿＿＿＿＿＿＿＿

6. ＿＿＿＿＿＿＿＿＿＿＿＿＿＿＿＿＿

＿＿＿＿＿＿＿＿＿＿＿＿＿＿＿＿＿＿＿

7. ＿＿＿＿＿＿＿＿＿＿＿＿＿＿＿＿＿

P：Can the perforation heal?

D：8. 如果你能使患耳不反复发作,一直保持干燥,那么鼓膜上的穿孔会长好的。

8. ＿＿＿＿＿＿＿＿＿＿＿＿＿＿＿＿＿

Ⅲ Further Reading：Otitis Media

Otitis media is a group of inflammatory diseases of the middle ear. One of the two main types is acute otitis media（AOM），an infection of rapid onset that usually presents with ear pain. In young children this may result in pulling at the ear，increased crying，and poor sleep. Decreased eating and a fever may also be present. The other main type is otitis media with effusion（OME），typically not associated with symptoms，although occasionally a feeling of fullness is described；it is defined as the presence of non-infectious fluid in the middle ear for more than three months. Chronic suppurative otitis media（CSOM）is middle ear inflammation that results in discharge from the ear for more than three months. It may be a complication of acute otitis media. Pain is rarely present. All three types of otitis media may be associated with hearing loss. The hearing loss in OME，due to its chronic nature，may affect a child's ability to learn.

The cause of AOM is related to childhood anatomy and immune function. Either bacteria or viruses may be involved. Risk factors include exposure to smoke，use of pacifiers，and attending daycare. It occurs more commonly among indigenous peoples and those who have cleft lip and palate or Down Syndrome. OME frequently occurs following AOM and may be related to viral upper respiratory infections, irritants such as smoke, or allergies. Looking at the eardrum is important for making the correct diagnosis. Signs of AOM include bulging or a lack of movement of the tympanic membrane from a puff of air. New discharge not related to otitis externa also indicates the diagnosis.

A number of measures decrease the risk of otitis media including pneumococcal and influenza vaccination, breastfeeding, and avoiding tobacco smoke. The use of pain medications for AOM is important. This may include paracetamol (acetaminophen), ibuprofen, benzocaine ear drops, or opioids. In AOM, antibiotics may speed recovery but may result in side effects. Antibiotics are often recommended in those with severe disease or under two years old. In those with less severe disease they may only be recommended in those who do not improve after two or three days. The initial antibiotic of choice is typically amoxicillin. In those with frequent infections tympanostomy tubes may decrease recurrence. In children with otitis media with effusion antibiotics may increase resolution of symptoms, but may cause diarrhoea, vomiting and skin rash.

Worldwide AOM affects about 11% of people a year (about 325 to 710 million cases). Half the cases involve children less than five years of age and it is more common among males. Of those affected about 4.8% or 31 million develop chronic suppurative otitis media. The total number of people with CSOM is estimated at 65—330 million people. Before the age of ten OME affects about 80% of children at some point. Otitis media resulted in 3,200 deaths in 2015— down from 4,900 deaths in 1990.

Otitis Media

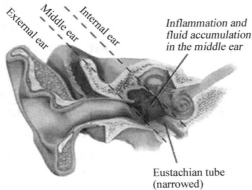

Inflammation and fluid accumulation in the middle ear

Eustachian tube (narrowed)

Signs and symptoms

The primary symptom of acute otitis media is ear pain; other possible symptoms include fever, reduced hearing during periods of illness, tenderness on touch of the skin above the ear, purulent discharge from the ears, irritability, and diarrhea (in infants). Since an episode of otitis media is usually precipitated by an upper respiratory tract infection (URTI), there are often accompanying symptoms like a cough and nasal discharge. One might also experience a feeling of fullness in the ear.

Discharge from the ear can be caused by acute otitis media with perforation of the eardrum, chronic suppurative otitis media, tympanostomy tube otorrhea, or acute otitis externa. Trauma, such as a basilar skull fracture, can also lead to cerebrospinal fluid otorrhea (discharge of CSF from the ear) due to cerebral spinal drainage from the brain and its covering (meninges).

Causes

The common cause of all forms of otitis media is dysfunction of the Eustachian tube. This is usually due to inflammation of the mucous membranes in the nasopharynx, which can be caused by a viral upper respiratory tract infection (URTI), strep throat, or possibly by allergies.

By reflux or aspiration of unwanted secretions from the nasopharynx into the normally sterile middle-ear space, the fluid may then become infected— usually with bacteria. The virus that caused the initial upper respiratory infection can itself be identified as the pathogen causing the infection.

Diagnosis

As its typical symptoms overlap with other conditions, such as acute external otitis, symptoms alone are not sufficient to predict whether acute otitis media is present; it has to be complemented by visualization of the tympanic membrane. Examiners may use a pneumatic otoscope with a rubber bulb attached to assess the mobility of the tympanic membrane. Other methods to diagnose otitis media is with a tympanometry, reflectometry or hearing test.

In more severe cases, such as those with associated hearing loss or high fever, audiometry, tympanogram, temporal bone CT and MRI can be used to assess for associated complications, such as mastoid effusion, subperiosteal abscess formation, bony destruction, venous thrombosis or meningitis.

Acute otitis media in children with moderate to severe bulging of the tympanic membrane or new onset of otorrhea (drainage) is not due to external otitis. Also, the diagnosis may be made in children who have mild bulging of the ear drum and recent onset of ear pain (less than 48 hours) or intense erythema (redness) of the ear drum.

To confirm the diagnosis, middle-ear effusion and inflammation of the eardrum have to be identified; signs of these are fullness, bulging, cloudiness and redness of the eardrum. It is important to attempt to differentiate between acute otitis media and otitis media with effusion (OME), as antibiotics are not recommended for OME. It has been suggested that bulging of the tympanic membrane is the best sign to differentiate AOM from OME, with a bulging of the membrane suggesting AOM rather than OME.

Viral otitis may result in blisters on the external side of the tympanic membrane, which is called bullous myringitis (myringa being Latin for "eardrum").

However, sometimes even examination of the eardrum may not be able to confirm the diagnosis, especially if the canal is small. If wax in the ear canal obscures a clear view of the eardrum it should be removed using a blunt cerumen curette or a wire loop. Also, an upset young child's crying can cause the eardrum to look inflamed due to distension of the small blood vessels on it, mimicking the redness associated with otitis media.

Chronic suppurative otitis media

Chronic suppurative otitis media (CSOM) is a chronic inflammation of the middle ear and mastoid cavity that is characterized by discharge from the middle ear through a perforated tympanic membrane for at least 6 weeks. CSOM occurs following an upperrespiratory tract infection that has led to acute otitis media. This progresses to a prolonged inflammatory response causing mucosal (middle ear) oedema, ulceration and perforation. The middle ear attempts to resolve this ulceration by production of granulation tissue and polyp formation. This can lead to increased discharge and failure to arrest the inflammation, and to development of CSOM, which is also often associated with cholesteatoma. There may be enough pus that it drains to the outside of the ear (otorrhea), or the pus may be minimal enough to be seen only on examination with an otoscope or binocular microscope. Hearing impairment often accompanies this disease. People are at increased risk of developing CSOM when they have poor eustachian tube function, a history of multiple episodes of acute otitis media, live in crowded conditions, and attend pediatric day care facilities. Those with craniofacial malformations such as cleft lip and palate, Down syndrome, and microcephaly are at higher risk.

Worldwide approximately 11% of the human population is affected by AOM every year, or 709 million cases. About 4.4% of the population develop CSOM.

According to the World Health Organization, CSOM is a primary cause of hearing loss in children. Adults with recurrent episodes of CSOM have a higher risk of developing permanent conductive and sensorineural hearing loss.

In Britain, 0.9% of children and 0.5% of adults have CSOM, with no difference between the sexes. The incidence of CSOM across the world varies dramatically where high income countries have a relatively low prevalence while in low income countries the prevalence may be up to three times as great. Each year 21,000 people worldwide die due to complications of CSOM.

Prevention

AOM is far less common in breastfed infants than in formula-fed infants, and the greatest protection is associated with exclusive breastfeeding (no formula use) for the first six months of life. A longer duration of breastfeeding is correlated with a longer protective effect.

Pneumococcal conjugate vaccines (PCV) in early infancy decrease the risk of acute otitis media in healthy infants. PCV is recommended for all children, and, if implemented broadly, PCV would have a significant public health benefit. Influenza vaccination in children appears to reduce rates of AOM by 4% and the use of antibiotics by 11% over 6 months. However, the vaccine resulted in increased adverse-effects such as fever and runny nose. The small reduction in AOM may not justify the side effects and inconvenience of influenza vaccination every year for this purpose alone. PCV does not appear to decrease the risk of otitis media when given to high-risk infants or for older children who have previously experienced otitis media.

Risk factors such as season, allergy predisposition and presence of older siblings are known to be determinants of recurrent otitis media and persistent middle-ear effusions (MEE). History of recurrence, environmental exposure to tobacco smoke, use of daycare, and lack of breastfeeding have all been associated with increased risk of development, recurrence, and persistent MEE. Pacifier use has been associated with more frequent episodes of AOM.

Long-term antibiotics, while they decrease rates of infection during treatment, have an unknown effect on long-term outcomes such as hearing loss. This method of prevention has been associated with emergence of antibiotic-resistant otitic bacteria. They are thus not recommended.

There is moderate evidence that the sugar substitute xylitol may reduce infection rates in those who go to daycare.

Evidence does not support zinc supplementation as an effort to reduce otitis rates except maybe in those with severe malnutrition such as marasmus.

Probiotics do not show evidence of preventing acute otitis media in children.

Management

Oral and topical pain killers are effective to treat the pain caused by otitis media. Oral agents include ibuprofen, paracetamol (acetaminophen), and opiates. Evidence for the combination over single agents is lacking. Topical agents shown to be effective include antipyrine and benzocaine ear drops. Decongestants and antihistamines, either nasal or oral, are not recommended due to the lack of benefit and concerns regarding side effects. Half of cases of ear pain in children resolve without treatment in three days and 90% resolve in seven or eight days. The use of steroids is not supported by the evidence for acute otitis media.

Antibiotics: It is important to weigh the benefits and harms before using antibiotics for acute otitis media. As over 82% of acute episodes settle without treatment, about 20 children must be treated to prevent one case of ear pain, 33 children to prevent one perforation, and 11 children to prevent one opposite-side ear infection. For every 14 children treated with antibiotics, one child has an episode of either vomiting, diarrhea or a rash. If pain is present, pain medications may be used. For people requiring surgery to treat otitis media with effusion, preventative antibiotics may not help reduce the risk of post-surgical complications.

For bilateral acute otitis media in infants younger than 24 months of age, there is evidence that the benefits of antibiotics outweigh the harms. A 2015 Cochrane review concluded that watchful waiting is the preferred approach for children over six months with non-severe acute otitis media.

Most children older than 6 months of age who have acute otitis media do not benefit from treatment with antibiotics. If antibiotics are used, a narrow-spectrum antibiotic like amoxicillin is generally recommended, as broad-spectrum antibiotics may be associated with more adverse events. If there is resistance or use of amoxicillin in the last 30 days then amoxicillin-clavulanate or another penicillin derivative plus beta lactamase inhibitor is recommended. Taking amoxicillin once a day may be as effective as twice or three times a day. While less than 7 days of antibiotics have fewer side effects, more than seven days appear to be more effective. If there is no improvement after 2—3 days of treatment a change in therapy may be considered. Azithromycin appears to have less side effects than either high dose amoxicillin or amoxicillin/clavulanate.

Tympanostomy tube: Tympanostomy tubes (also called "grommets") are recommended with three or more episodes of acute otitis media in 6 months or four or more in a year, with at least one episode or more attacks in the preceding 6 months. There is tentative evidence that children with recurrent acute otitis media (AOM) who receive tubes have a modest improvement in the number of further AOM episodes (around one fewer episode at six months and less of an improvement at 12 months following the tubes being inserted). Evidence does not support an effect on long-term hearing or language development. A common complication of having a tympanostomy tube is otorrhea, which is a discharge from the ear. The risk of persistent tympanic membrane perforation after children have grommets inserted may be low. It is still uncertain whether or not grommets are more effective than a course of antibiotics.

Oral antibiotics should not be used to treat uncomplicated acute tympanostomy tube otorrhea. They are not sufficient for the bacteria that cause this condition and have side effects including increased risk of opportunistic infection. In contrast, topical antibiotic eardrops are useful.

Outcomes

Complications of acute otitis media consists of perforation of the ear drum, infection of the mastoid space behind the ear (mastoiditis), and more rarely intracranial complications can occur, such as bacterial meningitis, brain abscess, or dural sinus thrombosis. It is estimated that each year 21,000 people die due to complications of otitis media.

Membrane rupture: In severe or untreated cases, the tympanic membrane may perforate, allowing the pus in the middle-ear space to drain into the ear canal. If there is enough, this drainage may be obvious. Even though the perforation of the tympanic membrane suggests a highly painful and traumatic process, it is almost always associated with a dramatic relief of pressure and pain. In a simple case of acute otitis media in an otherwise healthy person, the body's defenses are likely to resolve the infection and the ear drum nearly always heals. An option for severe acute otitis media in which analgesics are not controlling ear pain is to perform a tympanocentesis, i. e., needle aspiration through the tympanic membrane to relieve the ear pain and to identify the causative organism(s).

Hearing loss: Children with recurrent episodes of acute otitis media and those with otitis media with effusion or chronic suppurative otitis media have higher risks of developing conductive and sensorineural hearing loss. Globally approximately 141 million people have mild hearing loss due to otitis media (2.1% of the population). This is more common in males (2.3%) than females (1.8%).

This hearing loss is mainly due to fluid in the middle ear or rupture of the tympanic membrane. Prolonged duration of otitis media is associated with ossicular complications and, together with persistent tympanic membrane perforation, contributes to the severity of the disease and hearing loss. When a cholesteatoma or granulation tissue is present in the middle ear, the degree of hearing loss and ossicular destruction is even greater.

Periods of conductive hearing loss from otitis media may have a detrimental effect on speech development in children. Some studies have linked otitis media to learning problems, attention disorders, and problems with social adaptation. Furthermore, it has been demonstrated that patients with otitis media have more depression/anxiety-related disorders compared to individuals with normal hearing. Once the infections resolve and hearing thresholds return to normal, childhood otitis media may still cause minor and irreversible damage to the middle ear and cochlea. More research on the importance of screening all children under 4 years old for otitis media with effusion needs to be performed.

A. Translate the following sentences into Chinese.

1. Otitis media is a group of inflammatory diseases of the middle ear. One of the two main types is acute otitis media (AOM), an infection of rapid onset that usually presents with ear pain. In young children this may result in pulling at the ear, increased crying, and poor sleep. Decreased eating and a fever may also be present. The other main type is otitis media with effusion (OME), typically not associated with symptoms, although occasionally a feeling of fullness is described; it is defined as the presence of non-infectious fluid in the middle ear for more than three months.

2. The primary symptom of acute otitis media is ear pain; other possible symptoms include fever, reduced hearing during periods of illness, tenderness on touch of the skin above the ear, purulent discharge from the ears, irritability, and diarrhea (in infants). Since an episode of otitis media is usually precipitated by an upper respiratory tract infection (URTI), there are often accompanying symptoms like a cough and nasal discharge. One might also experience a feeling of fullness in the ear.

3. The common cause of all forms of otitis media is dysfunction of the Eustachian tube. This is usually due to inflammation of the mucous membranes in the nasopharynx, which can be caused by a viral upper respiratory tract infection (URTI), strep throat, or possibly by allergies. By reflux or aspiration of unwanted secretions from the nasopharynx into the normally sterile middle-ear space, the fluid may then become infected—usually with bacteria. The virus that caused the initial upper respiratory infection can itself be identified as the pathogen causing the infection.

4. To confirm the diagnosis, middle-ear effusion and inflammation of the eardrum have to be identified; signs of these are fullness, bulging, cloudiness and redness of the eardrum. It is important to attempt to differentiate between acute otitis media and otitis media with effusion (OME), as antibiotics are not recommended for OME. It has been suggested that bulging of the tympanic membrane is the best sign to differentiate AOM

from OME, with a bulging of the membrane suggesting AOM rather than OME.

5. Periods of conductive hearing loss from otitis media may have a detrimental effect on speech development in children. Some studies have linked otitis media to learning problems, attention disorders, and problems with social adaptation. Furthermore, it has been demonstrated that patients with otitis media have more depression/anxiety-related disorders compared to individuals with normal hearing. Once the infections resolve and hearing thresholds return to normal, childhood otitis media may still cause minor and irreversible damage to the middle ear and cochlea. More research on the importance of screening all children under 4 years old for otitis media with effusion needs to be performed.

B. Prepare a lecture on otitis media after doing the further reading above.

扫码获取
提示

Esophageal Foreign Body

Ⅰ Warming-up

A. Match the following words and phrases with their Chinese translations.

A	impaction	1	食道镜
B	latex protector hood	2	气管插管
C	stricture	3	误吸
D	extraction	4	反胃
E	sedation	5	食道胃十二指肠镜
F	endotracheal intubation	6	取出
G	aspiration	7	嵌入
H	EGD	8	狭窄
I	retch	9	乳胶保护罩
J	esophagoscope	10	镇静

B. Complete the sentences with the following words or phrases in their proper forms.

inability	get stuck	prompt	blockage
underlie	undergo	reevaluate	minimal

1. Do not _____ on words you are having a hard time translating.

2. When someone neglects to brush their teeth, flush the toilet or wash their hands, a

speaker can _____ them to do so.

3. Rats can't vomit or burp because of a limiting wall between their two stomachs and their _____ to control the diaphragm muscles needed for the action.

4. TCM's complexity and _____ conceptual foundations present challenges for researchers seeking evidence on how it works.

5. Over time, the buildup of plaque deposits can rupture and cause total _____ of the blood flow to the heart.

6. In addition, researchers should _____ the effects of all medications on men versus women.

7. The rare disorder, in which one side of the brain grows substantially larger than the other, occurs when neurons in the abnormal hemisphere _____ too many cell divisions before they mature.

8. It had _____ effect on biodiversity, and any pollution it caused was typically localized.

 C. Watch the video *Esophageal Foreign Body* and answer the questions.

扫码获取视频

1. What is esophageal foreign body according to the speaker?

2. Under what condition should you be prompted to go to emergency room for further evaluation of suspected foreign body in gullet?

3. What are the causes of esophageal obstruction?

4. What treatment is the specialist usually taking to treat esophageal foreign body in most cases?

5. What procedural sedation is ENT doctor going to use to remove the foreign body in esophagus?

II Dialogue

扫码获取
音频及文本

A. Listen to the dialogue for the first time and try to get the general idea.

B. Listen to the dialogue for the second time and try to answer the following questions.

1. What has happened on the patient according to the dialogue?

2. If you are stuck by a fish bone, what do you think should you do?

3. If the foreign body is at the upper end of the esophagus, what examination is usually needed?

4. What was the doctor going to do for the patient to remove the fishbone?

5. If a kid is found to be stuck by a coin, as the person nearest to the kid, what should you do to help?

C. Choose the following words and/or expressions to complete the sentences in their proper forms.

surface anesthesia	表麻	sedate	镇静
get stuck	卡住	similar	与……相似
inform	了解	ingest	摄入
miniature	微缩	in addition	此外
pyriform sinus	梨状窝	expertise	专长
insert	插入	early cancer	早癌

1. Upper endoscopy is more accurate than X rays for detecting inflammation, ulcers, or tumors. It is used to diagnose _____ and can frequently determine whether a growth is benign (not cancerous) or malignant (cancerous).

2. When treating conditions in the upper gastrointestinal tract, small instruments are passed through the endoscope that can stretch narrowed areas (strictures), or remove swallowed objects (such as coins or pins). _____, bleeding from ulcers or vessels can be treated by a number of endoscopic techniques.

3. Patients should inquire as to the doctor's _____ with these procedures, especially when therapy is the main goal.

4. As I told you, the operation will be done under anesthesia. Besides, we will give you a _____ injection.

5. I will _____ an esophagoscope into your esophagus while your throat is under surface anesthesia, and then I'll try to remove the foreign body.

6. The doctor should be _____ of any allergies, medication use, and medical problems.

7. But vitamins are essential nutrients that people _____ in their daily diets; there is no way to withhold them altogether from research subjects.

8. Doctor, I might have _____ a fishbone _____ in my throat because my throat hurts after eating fish. Can you please help me?

9. A button battery, which can be a very _____ size to a coin, generates hydroxide

ions at the anode and causes a chemical burn in two hours.

10. Some futurists envision nanotechnology also being used to explore the deep sea in small submarine, or even to launch finger-sized rockets packed with micro _____ instruments.

D. Read the dialogue and try to make a conversation with your classmates.

扫码获取
提示

E. Translate the following Chinese into English.

D—Doctor   P—Patient

P：Doctor, I might have gotten a fishbone stuck in my throat because my throat hurts after eating fish. Can you please help me?

D：Take a seat. 1. 是什么时候发生的？

　　1. _____

P：Yesterday evening.

D：2. 现在什么部位感到痛？

　　2. _____

P：At first, it was in the upper part of my throat. 3. 我试着咽些食物把它带下去，结果喉咙下面也开始疼了。I even spit some blood this morning.

　　3. _____

　　_____

D：4. 其他地方还有什么不舒服的吗？

　　4. _____

P：No, only the pain is so severe that I have

difficulty swallowing even my saliva.

D：Please spit out your saliva. 5. 我要检查你的喉咙。Open your mouth and say "Ah—". Okay, now stick out your tongue and say "Yee—" after me. I can't see the bone, but there is some fluid in your pyriform sinus.

　　5. _____

P：That's the right place where the pain is severe.

D：6. 看上去异物很可能在食道里。

　　6. _____

P：What can be done?

D：7. 马上到放射科去拍张片子。8. 鱼刺确实在那儿的话，就要动手术取出来。

　　7. _____

　　8. _____

Ⅲ Further Reading：Foreign Body, Esophagogastroduodenoscopy, and Heimlich Maneuver

A foreign body（FB）is any object originating outside the body of an organism. Foreign bodies can be inert or irritating. If they irritate they will cause inflammation and scarring. They can bring infection into the body or acquire infectious agents and protect them from the body's immune defenses. They can obstruct passageways either by their size or by the scarring they cause. Some can be toxic or generate toxic chemicals from reactions with chemicals produced by the body, as is the case with many examples of ingested metal objects.

Foreign body in gastrointestinal tract

One of the most common locations for a foreign body is the alimentary tract.

Both children and adults experience problems caused by foreign objects becoming lodged within their bodies. Young children, in particular, are naturally curious and may intentionally put shiny objects, such as coins or button batteries, into their mouths. They also like to insert objects into their ear canals and nostrils. The severity of a foreign body can range from unconcerning to a life-threatening emergency. For example, a coin causes local pressure on the tissue but generally is not a medical emergency to remove. A button battery, which can be a very similar size to a coin, generates hydroxide ions at the anode and causes a chemical burn in two hours. An ingested button battery that is stuck in the esophagus is a medical emergency.

Esophagogastroduodenoscopy

Definition

An endoscope as used in the field of gastroenterology is a thin, flexible tube that uses a lens or miniature camera to view various areas of the gastrointestinal tract. When the procedure is limited to the examination of the inside of the gastrointestinal tract's upper portion, it is called upper endoscopy or esphagogastroduodenoscopy (EGD). With the endoscope, the esophagus (swallowing tube), stomach, and duodenum (first portion of the small intestine) can be easily examined, and abnormalities frequently treated. Patients are usually sedated during the exam.

Purpose

EGD is performed to evaluate or treat symptoms relating to the upper gastrointestinal tract, such as:
- upper abdominal or chest pain
- nausea or vomiting
- difficulty swallowing (dysphagia)
- bleeding from the upper intestinal tract
- anemia (low blood count)

EGD can be used to treat certain conditions, such as an area of narrowing or bleeding in the upper gastrointestinal tract.

Upper endoscopy is more accurate than X rays for detecting inflammation, ulcers, or tumors. It is used to diagnose early cancer and can frequently determine whether a growth is benign (not cancerous) or malignant (cancerous).

Biopsies (small tissue samples) of inflamed or "suspicious" areas can be obtained and examined by a pathologist. Cell scrapings can also be taken by the introduction of a small brush; this helps in the diagnosis of cancer or infections.

When treating conditions in the upper gastrointestinal tract, small instruments are passed through the endoscope that can stretch narrowed areas (strictures), or remove swallowed objects (such as coins or pins). In addition, bleeding from ulcers or vessels can be treated by a number of endoscopic techniques.

Recent studies have shown the usefulness of endoscopic removal of early tumors of the esophagus or stomach. This is done either with injection of certain materials (like alcohol), or with the use of instruments (like lasers) that burn the tumor. Other techniques combining medications and lasers also show promise.

Precautions

Patients should inquire as to the doctor's expertise with these procedures, especially when therapy is the main goal. The doctor should be informed of any allergies, medication use, and medical problems.

Description

First, a "topical" (local) medication to numb the gag reflex is given either by spray or is gargled. Patients are usually sedated for the procedure (though not always) by injection of medications into a vein. The endoscopist then has the patient swallow the scope, which is passed through the upper gastrointestinal tract. The lens or camera at the end of the instrument allows the endoscopist to examine each portion of the upper gastrointestinal tract; photos can be taken for reference. Air is pumped in through the instrument to allow proper observation. Biopsies and other procedures can be performed without any significant discomfort.

Preparation

The upper intestinal tract must be empty for the procedure, so it is necessary NOT to eat or drink for at least 6—12 hours before the exam. Patients need to inquire about taking their medications before the procedure.

Foreign body in airways and heimlich maneuver

It is possible for a foreign body to enter the airways and cause choking.

In one study, peanuts were the most common obstruction. In addition to peanuts, hot dogs, grapes, and latex balloons are also serious choking hazards in children that can result in death. A latex balloon will conform to the shape of the trachea, blocking the airway and making it difficult to expel with the Heimlich maneuver.

Foreign body in the bronchi can also present as chronic cough.

Definition

The Heimlich maneuver is an emergency procedure for removing a foreign object lodged in the airway that is preventing a person from breathing.

Description

The Heimlich maneuver can be performed on all people. Modifications are necessary if the choking victim is very obese, pregnant, a child, or an infant.

Indications that a person's airway is blocked include:

- The person can not speak or cry out.
- The person's face turns blue from lack of oxygen.
- The person desperately grabs at his or her throat.
- The person has a weak cough, and labored breathing produces a high-pitched noise.
- The person does all of the above, then becomes unconscious.

Performing the Heimlich maneuver on adults

To perform the Heimlich maneuver on a conscious adult, the rescuer stands behind the victim. The victim may either be sitting or standing. The rescuer makes a fist with one hand, and places it, thumb toward the victim, below the rib cage and above the waist. The rescuer encircles the victim's waist, placing his other hand on top of the fist.

In a series of 6—10 sharp and distinct thrusts upward and inward, the rescuer attempts to develop enough pressure to force the foreign object back up the trachea. If the maneuver fails, it is repeated. It is important not to give up if the first attempt fails. As the victim is deprived of oxygen, the muscles of the trachea relax slightly. Because of this loosening, it is possible that the foreign object may be expelled on a second or third attempt.

If the victim is unconscious, the rescuer should lay him or her on the floor, bend the chin forward, make sure the tongue is not blocking the airway, and feel in the mouth for foreign objects, being careful not to push any farther into the airway. The rescuer kneels astride the victim's thighs and places his fists between the bottom of the victim's breastbone and the navel. The rescuer then executes a series of 6—10 sharp compressions by pushing inward and upward.

After the abdominal thrusts, the rescuer repeats the process of lifting the chin, moving the tongue, feeling for and possibly removing the foreign material. If the airway is not clear, the rescuer repeats the abdominal thrusts as often as necessary. If the foreign object has been removed, but the victim is not breathing, the rescuer starts CPR.

Performing the Heimlich maneuver under special circumstances

Children

The technique in children over one year of age is the same as in adults, except that the amount of force used is less than that used with adults in order to avoid damaging the child's ribs, breastbone, and internal organs.

Infants under one year old

The rescuer sits down and lays the infant along his or her forearm with the infant's face pointed toward the floor. The rescuer's hand supports the infant's head, and his or her forearm rests on his or her own thigh for additional support. Using the heel of the other hand, the rescuer administers four or five rapid blows to the infant's back between the shoulder blades.

After administering the back blows, the rescuer sandwiches the infant between his or her arms, and turns the infant over so that the infant is lying face up supported by the opposite arm. Using the free hand, the rescuer places the index and middle finger on the center of the breastbone and makes four sharp chest thrusts. This series of back blows and chest thrusts is alternated until the foreign object is expelled.

Self-administration of the Heimlich maneuver

To apply the Heimlich maneuver to oneself, one should make a fist with one hand and place it in the middle of the body at a spot above the navel and below the breastbone, then grasp the fist with the other hand and push sharply inward and upward. If this fails, the victim should press the upper abdomen over the back of a chair, edge of a table, porch railing or something similar, and thrust up and inward until the object is dislodged.

A. Translate the following sentences into Chinese.

1. A foreign body (FB) is any object originating outside the body of an organism. Foreign bodies can be inert or irritating. If they irritate they will cause inflammation and scarring. They can bring infection into the body or acquire infectious agents and protect them from the body's immune defenses. They can obstruct passageways either by their size or by the scarring they cause. Some can be toxic or generate toxic chemicals from reactions with chemicals produced by the body, as is the case with many examples of ingested metal objects.

2. Young children, in particular, are naturally curious and may intentionally put shiny objects, such as coins or button batteries, into their mouths. They also like to insert

objects into their ear canals and nostrils. The severity of a foreign body can range from unconcerning to a life-threatening emergency. For example, a coin causes local pressure on the tissue but generally is not a medical emergency to remove. A button battery, which can be a very similar size to a coin, generates hydroxide ions at the anode and causes a chemical burn in two hours. An ingested button battery that is stuck in the esophagus is a medical emergency.

3. Upper endoscopy is more accurate than X rays for detecting inflammation, ulcers, or tumors. It is used to diagnose early cancer and can frequently determine whether a growth is benign (not cancerous) or malignant (cancerous).
Biopsies (small tissue samples) of inflamed or "suspicious" areas can be obtained and examined by a pathologist. Cell scrapings can also be taken by the introduction of a small brush; this helps in the diagnosis of cancer or infections. When treating conditions in the upper gastrointestinal tract, small instruments are passed through the endoscope that can stretch narrowed areas (strictures), or remove swallowed objects (such as coins or pins).

4. First, a "topical" (local) medication to numb the gag reflex is given either by spray or is gargled. Patients are usually sedated for the procedure (though not always) by injection of medications into a vein. The endoscopist then has the patient swallow the scope, which is passed through the upper gastrointestinal tract. The lens or camera at the end of the instrument allows the endoscopist to examine each portion of the upper gastrointestinal tract; photos can be taken for reference. Air is pumped in through the instrument to allow proper observation. Biopsies and other procedures can be performed without any significant discomfort.

5. To perform the Heimlich maneuver on a conscious adult, the rescuer stands behind the victim. The victim may either be sitting or standing. The rescuer makes a fist with one hand, and places it, thumb toward the victim, below the rib cage and above the waist. The rescuer encircles the victim's waist, placing his other hand on top of the fist.
In a series of 6—10 sharp and distinct thrusts upward and inward, the rescuer attempts to develop enough pressure to force the foreign object back up the trachea.

B. Prepare a lecture on foreign body after doing the further reading above.

扫码获取
提示

Vertigo Syndrome

I Warming-up

A. Match the following words and phrases with their Chinese translations.

A	Ménière's disease	1	良性阵发性位置性眩晕
B	episodic	2	前庭眼球反射
C	superior canal dehiscence syndrome	3	眼震电流描记法
D	vestibular disorder	4	眼球震颤
E	the Epley maneuver	5	假性眩晕
F	benign paroxysmal positional vertigo	6	梅尼埃病
G	pseudo vertigo	7	耳石复位法
H	electronystagmography	8	偶发的
I	vestibulo-ocular reflex	9	前庭障碍
J	nystagmus	10	前半规管裂综合征

B. Complete the sentences with the following words or phrases in their proper forms.

persistent	provoke	modify	hypothesize
abbreviate	stimulate	embed	idiopathic

1. Some scientists _____ that the monkeys rub their bodies with the millipedes because doing so helps protect them from mosquitoes.

2. Patients are taught how to _____ their diet and their lifestyle.

3. Benign paroxysmal positional vertigo，which is _____ as BPPV，is the most common inner ear problem and cause of vertigo or false sense of spinning.

4. Dairy products may _____ allergic reactions in some people.

5. A 22-year-old Chinese woman who suffered from a _____ cough was shocked to learn that she had a piece of chicken bone lodged in her lung.

6. To study the efficacy and safety of endoscopic endonasal optic nerve fenestration for the management of _____ intracranial hypertension（IIH）.

7. According to a new study from Cornell University's Food and Brand Lab，small non-food rewards—like the toys in McDonald's Happy Meals—_____ the same reward centers in the brain as food does.

8. Head movement causes relative movement of the endolymph in the semicircular canal which bends the cupula and the _____ hairs of the hair cells and cause stimulation of the relevant vestibular nerve.

扫码获取视频

 C. **Watch the video** *BPPV* **and answer the questions.**

1. What is the video going to talk about?

2. According to the video，what is the cause of BPPV?

3. What does the modified Epley maneuver do to help the patient of BPPV?

4. What measures should be taken when you do the Epley maneuver for the patient? And why?

5. If the patient's Dix-Hallpike test is positive in the right posterior semicircular canal，which side should you start to do the Epley maneuver?

II Dialogue

扫码获取
音频及文本

 A. **Listen to the dialogue for the first time and try to get the general idea.**

B. Listen to the dialogue for the second time and try to answer the following questions.

1. Why did the secretary of the U. S. Consulate in China call Dr. Wang, an ENT doctor?

2. For a patient who complained of dizziness and nausea, what examinations are needed for doctor to make the diagnosis?

3. If the patient is diagnosed of as Meniere's disease, what treatment should be given to?

4. If the patient is diagnosed of as benign paroxysmal positional vertigo, what treatment should be given to?

5. As an ENT doctor, how can you differentiate benign paroxysmal positional vertigo from Meniere's disease?

C. Choose the following words and/or expressions to complete the sentences in their proper forms.

dizzy	眩晕	approximately	大约
engage	占用	classify	分类
distend	膨胀	imbalance	失衡
stable	稳定的	prolong	延长
sway	摇摆	semicircular canal	半规管
expose	暴露	stationary object	静物

1. Physiologic vertigo may occur following being exposed to motion for a _____ period such as when on a ship or simply following spinning with the eyes closed.

2. She said one of her ears was ringing and _____ and could not hear well.

3. You could come right now if you wish. I'm not _____.

4. Vertigo accounts for _____ 2%—3% of emergency department visits in the developed world.

5. Vertigo is _____ into either peripheral or central, depending on the location of the dysfunction of the vestibular pathway, although it can also be caused by psychological factors.

6. This may be associated with nausea, vomiting, sweating, or difficulties walking. It is typically worse when the head is moved. Vertigo is the most common type of _____.

7. Other causes of physiologic vertigo may include toxin _____ such as to carbon monoxide, alcohol, or aspirin.

8. Vertigo is a condition where a person has the sensation of moving or of surrounding objects moving when they are not. Often it feels like a spinning or _____ movement.

9. Regulate _____ of dynamic equilibrium of neck soft tissue and treat the anterior arcuation of cervical vertebrae by acupotomy.

10. We have the confidence，conditions and ability to _____ the overall price level.

D. Read the dialogue and try to make a conversation with your classmates.

扫码获取提示

E. Translate the following Chinese into English.

D—Doctor   S—Secretary

D：Hello，Wang，an ENT doctor speaking.

S：This is Smith speaking. I am the secretary with the U.S. Consulate. 1. 我们有一位工作人员头晕，I wonder when we can see you.

1. _____

D：You could come right now if you wish. 2. 我有空。

2. _____

S：Thank you.

...

D：Come in. Sit down please. 3. 什么时候开始的？

3. _____

S：Just now while she was working.

D：Has the dizziness lasted till now?

S：No. It lasted only a few minutes. 4. 她说头晕，恶心。

4. _____

D：Did she vomit?

S：No.

D：5. 当时她是不是感到东西在她面前旋转？

5. _____

S：She said yes.

D：Any other complaints?

S：6. 她说还有一边耳朵响，有些发胀，听不清楚。

6. _____
_____

D：7. 请告诉病人头不要动。Look at my finger ... Mm，there is no nystagmus. According to her case history and my exam，I think she is suffering from Meniere's disease. It is an inner ear disease. 8. 我将收她住院治疗，OK？

7. _____

8. _____

S：OK. Thank you，doctor.

D：Don't mention it.

Ⅲ Further Reading：Vertigo

Vertigo is a condition where a person has the sensation of moving or of surrounding objects moving when they are not. Often it feels like a spinning or swaying movement. This may be associated with nausea，vomiting，sweating，or difficulties walking. It is typically worse when the head is moved. Vertigo is the most common type of dizziness.

The most common disorders that result in vertigo are benign paroxysmal positional vertigo (BPPV), Ménière's disease, and labyrinthitis. Less common causes include stroke, brain tumors, brain injury, multiple sclerosis, migraines, trauma, and uneven pressures between the middle ears. Physiologic vertigo may occur following being exposed to motion for a prolonged period such as when on a ship or simply following spinning with the eyes closed. Other causes may include toxin exposures such as to carbon monoxide, alcohol, or aspirin. Vertigo typically indicates a problem in a part of the vestibular system. Other causes of dizziness include presyncope, disequilibrium, and non-specific dizziness.

Benign paroxysmal positional vertigo is more likely in someone who gets repeated episodes of vertigo with movement and is otherwise normal between these episodes. The episodes of vertigo should last less than one minute. The Dix-Hallpike test typically produces a period of rapid eye movements known as nystagmus in this condition. In Ménière's disease there is often ringing in the ears, hearing loss, and the attacks of vertigo last more than twenty minutes. In labyrinthitis the onset of vertigo is sudden and the nystagmus occurs without movement. In this condition vertigo can last for days. More severe causes should also be considered. This is especially true if other problems such as weakness, headache, double vision, or numbness occur.

Dizziness affects approximately 20%—40% of people at some point in time, while about 7.5%—10% have vertigo. About 5% have vertigo in a given year. It becomes more common with age and affects women two to three times more often than men. Vertigo accounts for about 2%—3% of emergency department visits in the developed world.

Classification

Vertigo is classified into either peripheral or central, depending on the location of the dysfunction of the vestibular pathway, although it can also be caused by psychological factors.

Vertigo can also be classified into objective, subjective, and pseudo vertigo. Objective vertigo describes when the person has the sensation that stationary objects in the environment are moving. Subjective vertigo refers to when the person feels as if they are moving. The third type is known as pseudo vertigo, an intensive sensation of rotation inside the person's head. While this classification appears in textbooks, it is unclear what relation it has to the pathophysiology or treatment of vertigo.

Peripheral

Vertigo that is caused by problems with the inner ear or vestibular system, which is composed of the semicircular canals, the vestibule (utricle and saccule), and the vestibular nerve is called "peripheral", "otologic", or "vestibular" vertigo. The most common cause is benign paroxysmal positional vertigo (BPPV), which accounts for 32% of all peripheral vertigo. Other causes include Ménière's disease (12%), superior canal dehiscence syndrome, labyrinthitis, and visual vertigo. Any cause of inflammation such as common cold, influenza, and bacterial infections may cause transient vertigo if it involves the inner ear, as may chemical insults (e. g., aminoglycosides) or physical trauma (e.g., skull fractures). Motion sickness is sometimes classified as a cause of peripheral vertigo.

People with peripheral vertigo typically present with mild to moderate imbalance, nausea, vomiting, hearing loss, tinnitus, fullness, and pain in the ear. In addition, lesions of the internal auditory canal may be associated with facial weakness on the same side. Due to a rapid compensation process, acute vertigo as a result of a peripheral lesion tends to improve in a short period of time (days to weeks).

Central

Vertigo that arises from injury to the balance centers of the central nervous system (CNS), often from a lesion in the brainstem or cerebellum, is called "central" vertigo and is generally associated with less prominent movement illusion and nausea than vertigo of peripheral origin. Central vertigo may have accompanying neurologic deficits (such as slurred speech and double vision), and pathologic nystagmus (which is pure vertical/torsional). Central pathology can cause disequilibrium, which is the sensation of being off balance. The balance disorder associated with central lesions causing vertigo is often so severe that many people are unable to stand or walk.

A number of conditions that involve the central nervous system may lead to vertigo including: lesions caused by infarctions or hemorrhage, tumors present in the cerebellopontine angle such as a vestibular schwannoma or cerebellar tumors, epilepsy, cervical spine disorders such as cervical spondylosis, degenerative ataxia disorders, migraine headaches, lateral medullary syndrome, Chiari malformation, multiple sclerosis, parkinsonism, as well as cerebral dysfunction. Central vertigo may not improve or may do so more slowly than vertigo caused by disturbance to peripheral structures. Alcohol can result in positional alcohol nystagmus (PAN).

Signs and symptoms

Vertigo is a sensation of spinning while stationary. It is commonly associated with nausea or vomiting, unsteadiness (postural instability), falls, changes to a person's thoughts, and difficulties in walking. Recurrent episodes in those with vertigo are common and frequently impair the quality of life.

Blurred vision, difficulty in speaking, a lowered level of consciousness, and hearing loss may also occur. The signs and symptoms of vertigo can present as a persistent (insidious) onset or an episodic (sudden) onset.

Persistent onset vertigo is characterized by symptoms lasting for longer than one day and is caused by degenerative changes that affect balance as people age. Naturally, the nerve conduction slows with aging and a decreased vibratory sensation is common. Additionally, there is a degeneration of the ampulla and otolith organs with an increase in age. Persistent onset is commonly paired with central vertigo signs and symptoms.

The characteristics of an episodic onset vertigo are indicated by symptoms lasting for a smaller, more memorable amount of time, typically lasting for only seconds to minutes.

Pathophysiology

The neurochemistry of vertigo includes six primary neurotransmitters that have been identified between the three-neuron arc that drives the vestibulo-ocular reflex (VOR). Glutamate maintains the resting discharge of the central vestibular neurons and may modulate synaptic transmission in all three neurons of the VOR arc. Acetylcholine appears to function as an excitatory neurotransmitter in both the peripheral and central synapses. Gamma-Aminobutyric acid (GABA) is thought to be inhibitory for the commissures of the medial vestibular nucleus, the connections among the cerebellar Purkinje cells, the lateral vestibular nucleus, and the vertical VOR.

Three other neurotransmitters work centrally. Dopamine may accelerate vestibular compensation. Norepinephrine modulates the intensity of central reactions to vestibular stimulation and facilitates compensation. Histamine is present only centrally, but its role is unclear. Dopamine, histamine, serotonin, and acetylcholine are neurotransmitters thought to produce vomiting. It is known that centrally acting antihistamines modulate the symptoms of acute symptomatic vertigo.

Diagnosis

Tests for vertigo often attempt to elicit nystagmus and to differentiate vertigo from other causes of dizziness such as presyncope, hyperventilation syndrome, disequilibrium, or psychiatric causes of lightheadedness. Tests of vestibular system (balance) function include electronystagmography (ENG), Dix-Hallpike maneuver, rotation tests, head-thrust test, caloric reflex test, and computerized dynamic posturography (CDP).

The HINTS test, which is a combination of three physical examination tests that may be performed by physicians at the bedside, has been deemed helpful in differentiating between central and peripheral causes of vertigo. The HINTS test involves the horizontal head impulse test, observation of nystagmus on primary gaze, and the test of skew. CT scans or MRIs are sometimes used by physicians when diagnosing vertigo.

Tests of auditory system (hearing) function include pure tone audiometry, speech audiometry, acoustic reflex, electrocochleography (ECoG), otoacoustic emissions (OAE), and the auditory brainstem response test.

A number of specific conditions can cause vertigo. In the elderly, however, the condition is often multifactorial.

A recent history of underwater diving can indicate a possibility of barotrauma or decompression sickness involvement, but does not exclude all other possibilities. The dive profile (which is frequently recorded by dive computer) can be useful to assess a probability for decompression sickness, which can be confirmed by therapeutic recompression.

Benign paroxysmal positional vertigo

Benign paroxysmal positional vertigo (BPPV) is the most common vestibular disorder and occurs when loose calcium carbonate debris has broken off of the otoconial membrane and enters a semicircular canal thereby creating the sensation of motion. People with BPPV may experience brief periods of vertigo, usually under a minute, which occur with change in the position.

This is the most common cause of vertigo. It occurs in 0.6% of the population yearly with 10% having an attack during their lifetime. It is believed to be due to a mechanical malfunction of the inner ear. BPPV may be diagnosed with the Dix-Hallpike test and can be effectively treated with repositioning movements such as the Epley maneuver.

Ménière's disease

Ménière's disease is an inner ear disorder of unknown origin, but is thought to be caused by an increase in the amount of endolymphatic fluid present in the inner ear (endolymphatic hydrops). However, this idea has not been directly confirmed with histopathologic studies, but electrophysiologic studies have been suggestive of this mechanism. Ménière's disease frequently presents with recurrent, spontaneous attacks of severe vertigo in combination with ringing in the ears (tinnitus), a feeling of pressure or fullness in the ear (aural fullness), severe nausea or vomiting, imbalance, and hearing loss. As the disease worsens, hearing loss will progress.

Labyrinthitis

Labyrinthitis presents with severe vertigo with associated nausea, vomiting, and generalized imbalance and is believed to be caused by a viral infection of the inner ear, although several theories have been put forward and the cause remains uncertain. Individuals with vestibular neuritis do not typically have auditory symptoms, but may experience a sensation of aural fullness or tinnitus. Persisting balance problems may remain in 30% of people affected.

Vestibular migraine

Vestibular migraine is the association of vertigo and migraines and is one of the most common causes of recurrent, spontaneous episodes of vertigo. The cause of vestibular migraines is currently unclear; however, one hypothesized cause is that the stimulation of the trigeminal nerve leads to nystagmus in individuals suffering from migraines.

Other suggested causes of vestibular migraines include the following: unilateral neuronal instability of the vestibular nerve, idiopathic asymmetric activation of the vestibular nuclei in the brainstem, and vasospasm of the blood vessels supplying the labyrinth or central vestibular pathways resulting in ischemia to these structures. Vestibular migraines are estimated to affect 1%—3% of the general population and may affect 10% of people with migraine. Additionally, vestibular migraines tend to occur more often in women and rarely affect individuals after the sixth decade of life.

Motion sickness

Motion sickness is common and is related to vestibular migraine. It is nausea and vomiting in response to motion and is typically worse if the journey is on a winding road or involves many stops and starts, or if the person is reading in a moving car. It is caused by a mismatch between visual input and vestibular sensation. For example, the person is reading a book that is stationary in relation to the body, but the vestibular system senses that the car, and thus the body, is moving.

Alternobaric vertigo

Alternobaric vertigo is caused by a pressure difference between the middle ear cavities, usually due to blockage or partial blockage of one eustachian tube, usually when flying or diving underwater. It is most pronounced when the diver is in the vertical position; the spinning is toward the ear with the higher pressure and tends to develop when the pressures differ by 60 cm of water or more.

Decompression sickness

Vertigo is recorded as a symptom of decompression sickness in 5.3% of cases by the U. S. Navy as reported by Powell, 2008. It includes isobaric decompression sickness.

Decompression sickness can also be caused at a constant ambient pressure when switching between gas mixtures containing different proportions of inert gas. This is known as isobaric counter diffusion, and presents a problem for very deep dives. For example, after using a very helium-rich trimix at the deepest part of the dive, a diver will switch to mixtures containing progressively less helium and more oxygen and nitrogen during the ascent. Nitrogen diffuses into tissues 2.65 times slower than helium, but is about 4.5 times more soluble. Switching between gas mixtures that have very different fractions of nitrogen and helium can result in "fast" tissues (those tissues that have a good blood supply) increasing their total inert gas loading. This is often found to provoke inner ear decompression sickness, as the ear seems particularly sensitive to this effect.

Stroke

A stroke (either ischemic or hemorrhagic) involving the posterior fossa is a cause of central vertigo. Risk factors for a stroke as a cause of vertigo include increasing age and known vascular risk factors. Presentation may more often involve headache or neck pain, additionally, those who have had multiple episodes of dizziness in the months leading up to presentation are suggestive of stroke with prodromal TIAs. The HINTS exam as well as imaging studies of the brain (CT, CT angiogram, MRI) are helpful in diagnosis of posterior fossa stroke.

Management

Definitive treatment depends on the underlying cause of vertigo. People with Ménière's disease have a variety of treatment options to consider when receiving treatment for vertigo and tinnitus including: a low-salt diet and intratympanic injections of the antibiotic gentamicin or surgical measures such as a shunt or ablation of the labyrinth in refractory cases. Common drug treatment options for vertigo may include the following:
- Anticholinergics such as hyoscine hydrobromide (scopolamine)
- Anticonvulsants such as topiramate or valproic acid for vestibular migraines
- Antihistamines such as betahistine, dimenhydrinate, or meclizine, which may have antiemetic properties
- Beta blockers such as metoprolol for vestibular migraine
- Corticosteroids such as methylprednisolone for inflammatory conditions such as vestibular neuritis or dexamethasone as a second-line agent for Ménière's disease

All cases of decompression sickness should be treated initially with 100%

oxygen until hyperbaric oxygen therapy (100% oxygen delivered in a high-pressure chamber) can be provided. Several treatments may be necessary, and treatment will generally be repeated until either all symptoms resolve, or no further improvement is apparent.

A. Translate the following sentences into Chinese.

1. Benign paroxysmal positional vertigo is more likely in someone who gets repeated episodes of vertigo with movement and is otherwise normal between these episodes. The episodes of vertigo should last less than one minute. The Dix-Hallpike test typically produces a period of rapid eye movements known as nystagmus in this condition. In Ménière's disease there is often ringing in the ears, hearing loss, and the attacks of vertigo last more than twenty minutes. In labyrinthitis the onset of vertigo is sudden and the nystagmus occurs without movement. In this condition vertigo can last for days. More severe causes should also be considered. This is especially true if other problems such as weakness, headache, double vision, or numbness occur.

2. Vertigo can also be classified into objective, subjective, and pseudo vertigo. Objective vertigo describes when the person has the sensation that stationary objects in the environment are moving. Subjective vertigo refers to when the person feels as if they are moving. The third type is known as pseudo vertigo, an intensive sensation of rotation inside the person's head. While this classification appears in textbooks, it is unclear what relation it has to the pathophysiology or treatment of vertigo.

3. A number of conditions that involve the central nervous system may lead to vertigo including: lesions caused by infarctions or hemorrhage, tumors present in the cerebellopontine angle such as a vestibular schwannoma or cerebellar tumors, epilepsy, cervical spine disorders such as cervical spondylosis, degenerative ataxia disorders, migraine headaches, lateral medullary syndrome, Chiari malformation, multiple sclerosis, parkinsonism, as well as cerebral dysfunction. Central vertigo may not improve or may do so more slowly than vertigo caused by disturbance to peripheral structures. Alcohol can result in positional alcohol nystagmus (PAN).

4. Ménière's disease is an inner ear disorder of unknown origin, but is thought to be caused by an increase in the amount of endolymphatic fluid present in the inner ear (endolymphatic hydrops). However, this idea has not been directly confirmed with histopathologic studies, but electrophysiologic studies have been suggestive of this mechanism. Ménière's disease frequently presents with recurrent, spontaneous attacks of severe vertigo in combination with ringing in the ears (tinnitus), a feeling of pressure or fullness in the ear (aural fullness), severe nausea or vomiting, imbalance, and hearing loss. As the disease worsens, hearing loss will progress.

5. Definitive treatment depends on the underlying cause of vertigo. People with Ménière's disease have a variety of treatment options to consider when receiving treatment for vertigo and tinnitus including: a low-salt diet and intratympanic injections of the antibiotic gentamicin or surgical measures such as a shunt or ablation of the labyrinth in refractory cases.

B. **Prepare a lecture on vertigo syndrome after doing the further reading above.**

扫码获取
提示

Unit 25

Sexually Transmitted Infections

I Warming-up

A. Match the following words and phrases with their Chinese translations.

A	unprotected	1	难点
B	genome	2	攻击
C	retrovirus	3	复制
D	incredible	4	体液
E	helper T cells	5	污染的
F	replicate	6	无保护的
G	bodily fluids	7	辅助 T 细胞
H	contaminated	8	基因组
I	target	9	逆转录病毒
J	catch	10	难以置信的

B. Complete the sentences with the following words or phrases in their proper forms.

spread through	comeback	hide out	contract
expect to	activate	progress	claim

1. Cytogenetics is very important in the myelodysplastic syndromes' （MDS） diagnosis, _____ , and prognosis.

2. HIV _____ exchanges of bodily fluids by unprotected sex and contaminated needles.

3. Individuals of any age，sexual orientation，gender and race can _____ HIV.

4. With antiretroviral therapy，most HIV-positive people can _____ live long and healthy lives.

5. His _____ fight will be televised on Network TV.

6. But HIV _____ somewhere our current drugs cannot reach it: inside the DNA of healthy T cells.

7. When the researchers looked at a specific set of genes that kill cancer cells，TF-2 was found to _____ the genes.

8. If you are still not satisfied，you may be able to _____ compensation.

C. Watch the video *Why It's So Hard to Cure AIDS* and answer the questions.

扫码获取视频

1. How HIV infects people and progresses into AIDS?

2. Why HIV is called as a retrovirus?

3. What is helper T cells functioned in people's immune system?

4. Can you explain how do AIDS medications work?

5. After watching the video，do you know why it's so hard to cure AIDS?

Ⅱ Dialogue

扫码获取
音频及文本

A. Listen to the dialogue for the first time and try to get the general idea.

B. Listen to the dialogue for the second time and try to answer the following questions.

1. What does AIDS mean?

2. What is the epidemiology of the disease?

3. What symptoms do the AIDS patients have?

4. How do we diagnose the disease?

5. What do you know about the prophylactic measures to AIDS?

C. **Choose the following words and/or expressions to complete the sentences in their proper forms.**

immunodeficiency	免疫缺陷	opportunistic	机会性的
progression	进展	impair	损害
breastfeeding	母乳喂养	develop	发展
involve	涉及	product	产品
transmit	传播	prophylaxis	预防
countermeasure	对策	separate	分离

1. Treatment consists of highly active antiretroviral therapy（HAART）which can slow _____ of the disease and may lead to a near-normal life expectancy, but these medication are expensive and have side effects.

2. The clinical symptoms of AIDS may vary, and not all patients present the said symptoms. When the lungs are _____, dyspnea, thoracalgia, and coughing may present.

3. The use of the condom in sex is one of the most effective _____ to AIDS and many other sexually transmitted infections（STIs）.

4. HIV could also _____ the nervous system and cardiovascular system.

5. Once HIV infection _____ into AIDS, patients may present a number of clinical symptoms, which, at the initial stage, look like a common cold or influenza.

6. AIDS is an abbreviation, standing for Acquired _____ Syndrome(AIDS). It is an infectious disease caused by HIV.

7. Never borrow or share personal care _____, such as toothbrushes, shavers and razors, to name only a few.

8. The virus spreads in mainly 3 ways. The most frequent mode of _____ is through unprotected sexual intercourse.

9. HIV is transmitted from infected mothers to infants and some other ways, for example, _____.

10. The human immunity is thus broken, which leads to a series of _____ infections, such as herpes zoster, fungi infection of the oral cavity, and tuberculosis.

D. **Read the dialogue and try to make a conversation with your classmates.**

扫码获取
提示

E. Translate the following Chinese into English.

T—Teacher   Sa—Student A   Sb—Student B
Sc—Student C

Sc：What is the epidemiology of the disease?

T：The virus spreads in mainly 3 ways. 1. 主要是通过无保护的性交传播，particularly anal sex and oral sex，either heterosexually or homosexually. The second is through blood. 2. 主要包括输血，消毒不严的注射器，甚至器官组织移植传播。Lastly，3. 就是感染的母亲传给婴儿，比如母乳喂养。

1. _____
2. _____

_____
3. _____

_____

Sa：4. 据说，握手、亲吻也能传染，is that true?

　4. _____

T：5. 目前尚无证据表明 HIV transmission involves touch，insects，food，water，sneezing，coughing，toilet，swimming，sweat，tears，shared eating and drinking，therefore，casual person-to-person contact in any setting is safe.

　5. _____

Sc：What symptoms do the patients have?

T：After being infected with HIV，6. HIV 感染后，最开始的数年至 10 余年可无任何临床表现。Once developed into AIDS，patients may present a number of clinical

symptoms，which，7. 一般初期的症状如同普通感冒、流感样。The patient could have fatigue，loss of appetite，fever. 8. 随着病情的加重，症状日见增多，such as the presence of *Candida albicans* in the skin and mucosa，herpes simplex，herpes zoster，purpura，hemophysallis and ecchymosis. Gradually the visceral organs are involved，in which the persistent fever of unknown origin could present，lasting for as long as 3 to 4 months. People with AIDS could also have symptoms like coughing，shortness of breath，dyspnea，recurrent diarrhea，hemafecia，enlargement of the liver and spleen and malignant cancers，and many others. The clinical symptoms vary，and not all patients present with the above mentioned symptoms. When the lungs are involved，dyspnea，thoracalgia and coughing may be present；when gastrointestinal tract is involved，we can see recurrent diarrhea，abdominal pain，emaciation and weakness；it could also impair the nervous system and cardiovascular system.

6. _____

_____
7. _____
8. _____

III Further Reading: HIV/AIDS

Human immunodeficiency virus infection and acquired immunodeficiency syndrome (HIV/AIDS) is a spectrum of conditions caused by infection with the human immunodeficiency virus, a retrovirus. Following initial infection a person may not notice any symptoms, or may experience a brief period of influenza-like illness. Typically, this is followed by a prolonged period with no symptoms. If the infection progresses, it interferes more with the immune system, increasing the risk of developing common infections such as tuberculosis, as well as other opportunistic infections, and tumors which are otherwise rare in people who have normal immune function. These late symptoms of infection are referred to as acquired immunodeficiency syndrome. This stage is often also associated with unintended weight loss.

HIV is spread primarily by unprotected sex (including anal and oral sex), contaminated blood transfusions, hypodermic needles, and from mother to child during pregnancy, delivery, or breastfeeding. Some bodily fluids, such as saliva, sweat and tears, do not transmit the virus.

Methods of prevention include safe sex, needle exchange programs, treating those who are infected, as well as both pre- and post-exposure prophylaxis. Disease in a baby can often be prevented by giving both the mother and child antiretroviral medication. There is no cure or vaccine; however, antiretroviral treatment can slow the course of the disease and may lead to a near-normal life expectancy. Treatment is recommended as soon as the diagnosis is made. Without treatment, the average survival time after infection is 11 years.

In 2019, about 38 million people worldwide were living with HIV and 690,000 deaths had occurred in that year. An estimated 20.6 million of these live in eastern and southern Africa. Between the time that AIDS was identified (in the early 1980s) and 2019, the disease has caused an estimated 32.7 million deaths worldwide. HIV/AIDS is considered a pandemic—a disease outbreak which is present over a large area and is actively spreading.

HIV/AIDS has had a large impact on society, both as an illness and as a source of discrimination. The disease also has large economic impacts. There are many misconceptions about HIV/AIDS, such as the belief that it can be transmitted by casual non-sexual contact. The disease has become subject to many controversies involving religion, including the Catholic Church's position not to support condom use as prevention. It has attracted international medical and political attention as well as large-scale funding since it was identified in the 1980s.

Signs and symptoms

There are three main stages of HIV infection: acute infection, clinical latency, and AIDS.

Acute infection

The initial period following the contraction of HIV is called acute HIV, primary HIV or acute retroviral syndrome. Many individuals develop an influenza-like illness or a mononucleosis-like illness 2—4 weeks after exposure while others have no significant symptoms. Symptoms occur in 40%—90% of cases and most commonly include fever, large tender lymph nodes, throat inflammation, a rash, headache, tiredness, and/or sores of the mouth and genitals. The rash, which occurs in 20%—50% of cases, presents itself on the trunk and is maculopapular, classically. Some people also develop opportunistic infections at this stage. Gastrointestinal symptoms, such as vomiting or diarrhea may occur. Neurological symptoms of peripheral neuropathy or Guillain-Barré syndrome also occurs. The duration of the symptoms varies, but is usually one or two weeks.

Owing to their nonspecific character, these symptoms are not often recognized assigns of HIV infection. Even cases that do get seen by a family doctor or a hospital are often misdiagnosed as one of the many common infectious diseases with overlapping symptoms. Thus, it is recommended that HIV be considered in people presenting with an unexplained fever who may have risk factors for the infection.

Clinical latency

The initial symptoms are followed by a stage called clinical latency, asymptomatic HIV, or chronic HIV. Without treatment, this second stage of the natural history of HIV infection can last from about three years to over 20 years (on average, about eight years). While typically there are few or no symptoms at first, near the end of this stage many people experience fever, weight loss, gastrointestinal problems and muscle pains. Between 50% and 70% of people also develop persistent generalized lymphadenopathy, characterized by unexplained, non-painful enlargement of more than one group of lymph nodes (other than in the groin) for over three to six months.

Although most HIV-1 infected individuals have a detectable viral load and in the absence of treatment will eventually progress to AIDS, a small proportion (about 5%) retain high levels of CD4 + T cells (T helper cells) without antiretroviral therapy for more than five years. These individuals are classified as "HIV controllers" or long-term nonprogressors (LTNP). Another group consists of those who maintain a low or undetectable viral load without anti-retroviral treatment, known as "elite controllers" or "elite suppressors". They represent approximately 1 in 300 infected persons.

Acquired immunodeficiency syndrome

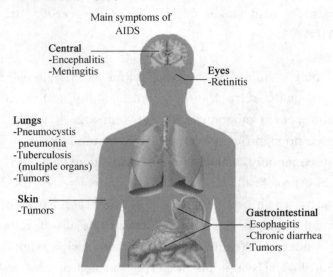

Main symptoms of
AIDS

Central
-Encephalitis
-Meningitis

Eyes
-Retinitis

Lungs
-Pneumocystis
 pneumonia
-Tuberculosis
 (multiple organs)
-Tumors

Skin
-Tumors

Gastrointestinal
-Esophagitis
-Chronic diarrhea
-Tumors

Fig. Main Symptoms of AIDS

Acquired immunodeficiency syndrome (AIDS) is defined as an HIV infection with either a CD4 + T cell count below 200 cells per μL or the occurrence of specific diseases associated with HIV infection. In the absence of specific treatment, around half of people infected with HIV develop AIDS within ten years. The most common initial conditions that alert to the presence of AIDS are pneumocystis pneumonia (40%), cachexia in the form of HIV wasting syndrome (20%), and esophageal candidiasis. Other common signs include recurrent respiratory tract infections.

Opportunistic infections may be caused by bacteria, viruses, fungi, and parasites that are normally controlled by the immune system. Which infections occur depends partly on what organisms are common in the person's environment. These infections may affect nearly every organ system.

People with AIDS have an increased risk of developing various viral-induced cancers, including Kaposi's sarcoma, Burkitt's lymphoma, primary central nervous system lymphoma, and cervical cancer. Kaposi's sarcoma is the most common cancer, occurring in 10% to 20% of people with HIV. The second-most common cancer is lymphoma, which is the cause of death of nearly 16% of people with AIDS and is the initial sign of AIDS in 3% to 4%. Both these cancers are associated with human herpesvirus 8 (HHV-8). Cervical cancer occurs more frequently in those with AIDS because of its association with human papillomavirus (HPV). Conjunctival cancer (of the layer that lines the inner part of eyelids and the white part of the eye) is also more common in those with HIV.

Additionally, people with AIDS frequently have systemic symptoms such as prolonged fevers, sweats (particularly at night), swollen lymph nodes, chills, weakness, and unintended weight loss. Diarrhea is another common symptom, present in about 90% of people with AIDS. They can also be affected by diverse psychiatric and neurological symptoms independent of opportunistic infections and cancers.

Pathophysiology

After the virus enters the body there is a period of rapid viral replication, leading to an abundance of virus in the peripheral blood. During primary infection, the level of HIV may reach several million virus particles per milliliter of blood. This response is accompanied by a marked drop in the number of circulating CD4+ T cells. The acute viremia is almost invariably associated with activation of CD8+ T cells, which kill HIV-infected cells, and subsequently with antibody production, or seroconversion. The CD8+ T cell response is thought to be important in controlling virus levels, which peak and then decline, as the CD4+ T cell counts recover. A good CD8+ T cell response has been linked to slower disease progression and a better prognosis, though it does not eliminate the virus.

Ultimately, HIV causes AIDS by depleting CD4+ T cells. This weakens the immune system and allows opportunistic infections. T cells are essential to the immune response and without them, the body cannot fight infections or kill cancerous cells. The mechanism of CD4+ T cell depletion differs in the acute and chronic phases. During the acute phase, HIV-induced cell lysis and killing of infected cells by CD8+ T cells accounts for CD4+ T cell depletion, although apoptosis may also be a factor. During the chronic phase, the consequences of generalized immune activation coupled with the gradual loss of the ability of the immune system to generate new T cells appear to account for the slow decline in CD4+ T cell numbers.

Although the symptoms of immune deficiency characteristic of AIDS do not appear for years after a person is infected, the bulk of CD4+ T cell loss occurs during the first weeks of infection, especially in the intestinal mucosa, which harbors the majority of the lymphocytes found in the body. The reason for the preferential loss of mucosal CD4+ T cells is that the majority of mucosal CD4+ T cells express the CCR5 protein which HIV uses as a co-receptor to gain access to the cells, whereas only a small fraction of CD4+ T cells in the bloodstream do so. A specific genetic change that alters the CCR5 protein when present in both chromosomes very effectively prevents HIV-1 infection.

HIV seeks out and destroys CCR5 expressing CD4+ T cells during acute infection. A vigorous immune response eventually controls the infection and initiates the clinically latent phase. CD4+ T cells in mucosal tissues remain particularly affected. Continuous HIV replication causes a state of generalized immune activation persisting throughout the chronic phase. Immune activation, which is reflected by the increased activation state of immune cells and release of pro-inflammatory cytokines, results from the activity of several HIV gene products and the immune response to ongoing HIV replication. It is also linked to the breakdown of the immune surveillance system of the gastrointestinal mucosal barrier caused by the depletion of mucosal CD4 + T cells during the acute phase of disease.

Prevention

Sexual contact

Consistent condom use reduces the risk of HIV transmission by approximately 80% over the long term. When condoms are used consistently by a couple in which one person is infected, the rate of HIV infection is less than 1% per year. There is some evidence to suggest that female condoms may provide an equivalent level of protection. Application of a vaginal gel containing tenofovir (a reverse transcriptase inhibitor) immediately before sex seems to reduce infection rates by approximately 40% among African women. By contrast, use of the spermicide nonoxynol-9 may increase the risk of transmission due to its tendency to cause vaginal and rectal irritation.

Comprehensive sexual education provided at school may decrease high-risk behavior. A substantial minority of young people continues to engage in high-risk practices despite knowing about HIV/AIDS, underestimating their own risk of becoming infected with HIV. Voluntary counseling and testing people for HIV does not affect risky behavior in those who test negative but does increase condom use in those who test positive. Enhanced family planning services appear to increase the likelihood of women with HIV using contraception, compared to basic services.

Pre-exposure

Antiretroviral treatment among people with HIV whose CD4 count $\leqslant$ 550 cells/μL is a very effective way to prevent HIV infection of their partner (a strategy known as treatment as prevention, or TASP). TASP is associated with a 10- to 20-fold reduction in transmission risk. Pre-exposure prophylaxis (PrEP) with a daily dose of the medications tenofovir, with or without emtricitabine, is effective in people at high risk including men who have sex with men, couples where one is HIV-positive, and young heterosexuals in Africa. It may also be effective in intravenous drug users, with a study finding a decrease in risk of 0.7 to 0.4 per 100 person years. An institute, in 2019, recommended PrEP in those who are at high risk.

Universal precautions within the health care environment are believed to be effective in decreasing the risk of HIV. Intravenous drug use is an important risk factor, and harm reduction strategies such as needle-exchange programs and opioid substitution therapy appear effective in decreasing this risk.

Post-exposure

A course of antiretrovirals administered within 48 to 72 hours after exposure to HIV-positive blood or genital secretions is referred to as post-exposure prophylaxis (PEP). The use of the single agent zidovudine reduces the risk of a HIV infection five-fold following a needle-stick injury. As of 2013, the prevention regimen recommended consists of three medications—tenofovir, emtricitabine and raltegravir—as this may reduce the risk further.

PEP treatment is recommended after a sexual assault when the perpetrator is known to be HIV-positive, but is controversial when their HIV status is unknown. The duration of treatment is usually four weeks and is frequently associated with adverse effects—where zidovudine is used, about 70% of cases result in adverse effects such as nausea (24%), fatigue (22%), emotional distress (13%) and headaches (9%).

A. Translate the following sentences into Chinese.

1. If the infection progresses, it interferes more with the immune system, increasing the risk of developing common infections such as tuberculosis, as well as other opportunistic infections, and tumors which are otherwise rare in people who have normal immune function.

2. There is no cure or vaccine; however, antiretroviral treatment can slow the course of the disease and may lead to a near-normal life expectancy. Treatment is recommended as soon as the diagnosis is made. Without treatment, the average survival time after infection is 11 years.

3. Owing to their nonspecific character, these symptoms are not often recognized as signs of HIV infection. Even cases that do get seen by a family doctor or a hospital are often misdiagnosed as one of the many common infectious diseases with overlapping symptoms.

4. Additionally，people with AIDS frequently have systemic symptoms such as prolonged fevers，sweats（particularly at night），swollen lymph nodes，chills，weakness，and unintended weight loss. Diarrhea is another common symptom，present in about 90% of people with AIDS. They can also be affected by diverse psychiatric and neurological symptoms independent of opportunistic infections and cancers.

5. The CD8＋T cell response is thought to be important in controlling virus levels，which peak and then decline，as the CD4＋T cell counts recover. A good CD8＋T cell response has been linked to slower disease progression and a better prognosis，though it does not eliminate the virus.

B. Prepare a lecture on HIV/AIDS after doing the further reading above.

扫码获取
提示

Unit 26

Malaria

I Warming-up

A. Match the following words and phrases with their Chinese translations.

A	anopheles mosquito	1	疟原虫
B	malaria	2	氯喹
C	plasmodium	3	青蒿素
D	parasite	4	耐药性
E	tropical zone	5	抗疟药物治疗
F	mosquito-control measures	6	热带
G	antimalarial medications	7	防蚊措施
H	artemisinin	8	疟疾
I	chloroquine	9	寄生虫
J	drug resistance	10	按蚊

B. Complete the sentences with the following words or phrases in their proper forms.

risk	be associated with	available	expose to
recommend	either ... or ...	detect	combination

1. Methods that use the polymerase chain reaction (PCR) to _____ the parasite's DNA have been developed, but are not widely used in areas where malaria is common due to

their cost and complexity.

2. Several medications have already been _____ to prevent malaria in travelers to areas where the disease is common.

3. It is _____ that in areas where malaria is common，malaria is confirmed if possible before treatment is started due to concerns of increasing drug resistance.

4. The second medication may be _____ mefloquine，lumefantrine，_____ sulfadoxine/pyrimethamine.

5. The recommended treatment for malaria is a _____ of antimalarial medications that includes an artemisinin.

6. The _____ of disease can be reduced by preventing mosquito bites by using mosquito nets and insect repellents，or with mosquito-control measures such as spraying insecticides and draining standing water.

7. There is convincing evidence of a link between _____ mosquito bites and malaria.

8. Malaria _____ commonly _____ poverty and has a major negative effect on economic development.

 C. Watch the video _WHO—Key Facts about the Malaria_ and answer the questions.

扫码获取视频

1. What are the causes of malaria?

2. What are the commonly seen symptoms in malaria?

3. What are the recommended measures to prevent the malaria?

4. What medications are recommended to treat the malaria?

5. What do you think are the medical examinations for malaria?

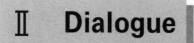 **II Dialogue**

扫码获取
音频及文本

A. Listen to the dialogue for the first time and try to get the general idea.

B. Listen to the dialogue for the second time and try to answer the following questions.

1. What's wrong with this patient?

2. Why this patient is asked to have a plasmodium test?

3. What should we take care of in some abdomen-type malaria cases?

4. What are particularly complained of in Zanzibar by malaria patients?

5. What should be done to prevent or delay anti-malaria drug resistance?

C. Choose the following words and/or expressions to complete the sentences in their proper forms.

upper respiratory tract infection	上呼吸道感染	abdominal tenderness	腹部触痛
heart-lung auscultation	心肺听诊	unbearable	无法忍受的
various	不同的	tell ... from ...	把……区别于……
be different from	不同于	rebound tenderness	反跳痛
be similar to	相似于	gastric-intestinal	胃肠道的
acute abdomen	急腹症	respond to	用……治疗有效

1. They've been living and working peacefully with members of _____ ethnic groups.

2. America's current economic downturn is markedly _____ previous recessions.

3. The basic design of the car is very _____ that of earlier models.

4. Many people find the idea of any kind of invasive surgery _____.

5. Can you _____ American English _____ British English?

6. Even very young premature babies _____ their mother's presence.

7. _____ metaplasia is a common finding in countries with a high prevalence of H. pylori infection.

8. Abdomen was soft，no tenderness and _____. Liver and spleen were impalpable.

9. The acute appendicitis is one of the most common surgical _____, which can take place at any age.

10. Influenza is basically an extreme _____, and，by itself，is rarely fatal.

D. Read the dialogue and try to make a conversation with your classmates.

扫码获取
提示

E. Translate the following Chinese into English.

I—Intern   P—Patient   D—Doctor

I：1. 你哪儿不舒服？

1. _____

P：I have been feeling ill for a week and have

had a bad headache since yesterday. 2. 三天前我因喉咙痛,来医院看病,开了些药,但效果不好。

2. _____

_____

I：Have you caught a fever?

P：Yes. A little.

I：3. 你感到发冷、发抖吗?

3. _____

P：No.

I：Anything else? 4. 你咳嗽吗? 有没有腹泻?

4. _____

P：No. Only a bad headache.

I：5. 你过去有这么严重的头痛现象吗?

5. _____

P：Yes,6. 但没有这一次厉害。过去头痛几乎不用药就好了。

6. _____

_____

I：Let me have a look at your throat. Open your mouth. Say "ah". Right.（Takes blood pressure）OK. 7. 现在躺在床上。（Does auscultation, examines the abdomen）Please get up. 8. 给你这些血常规化验单和胸透单。你去化验室和放射室,I'll wait here for the reports.

7. _____

8. _____

_____

P：Here are the reports.

Ⅲ Further Reading：Malaria and Artemisinin

The term malaria originates from Mediaeval Italian：mala aria—"bad air"; the disease was formerly called ague or marsh fever due to its association with swamps and marshland. The term first appeared in the English literature about 1829. Malaria was once common in most of Europe and North America，where it is no longer endemic，though imported cases do occur.

Malaria is a mosquito-borne infectious disease of humans and other animals caused by Plasmodium. Malaria causes symptoms that typically include fever，fatigue，vomiting and headaches. In severe cases it can cause yellow skin，seizures，coma or death. The disease is transmitted by the biting of mosquitos，and the symptoms usually begin ten to fifteen days after being bitten. If not appropriately treated，people may have recurrences of the disease months later. In those who have recently survived an infection，re-infection typically causes milder symptoms. This partial resistance disappears over months to years if the person has no continuing exposure to malaria.

The disease is transmitted most commonly by an infected female Anopheles mosquito. The mosquito bite introduces the parasites from the mosquito's saliva into a person's blood. The parasites travel to the liver where they mature and reproduce. Five species of Plasmodium can infect and be spread by humans.

Most deaths are caused by P. falciparum because P. vivax, P. ovale, and P. malariae generally cause a milder form of malaria. Malaria is typically diagnosed by the microscopic examination of blood using blood films, or with antigen-based rapid diagnostic tests. Methods that use the polymerase chain reaction (PCR) to detect the parasite's DNA have been developed, but are not widely used in areas where malaria is common due to their cost and complexity.

The risk of disease can be reduced by preventing mosquito bites by using mosquito nets and insect repellents, or with mosquito-control measures such as spraying insecticides and draining standing water. Several medications are available to prevent malaria in travellers to areas where the disease is common. Occasional doses of the medication sulfadoxine/pyrimethamine are recommended in infants and after the first trimester of pregnancy in areas with high rates of malaria. Despite a need, no effective vaccine exists, although efforts to develop one are ongoing. The recommended treatment for malaria is a combination of antimalarial medications that includes an artemisinin. The second medication may be either mefloquine, lumefantrine, or sulfadoxine/pyrimethamine. Quinine along with doxycycline may be used if an artemisinin is not available. It is recommended that in areas where the disease is common, malaria is confirmed if possible before treatment is started due to concerns of increasing drug resistance. Resistance among the parasites has developed to several antimalarial medications; for example, chloroquine-resistant P. falciparum has spread to most malarial areas, and resistance to artemisinin has become a problem in some parts of Southeast Asia.

The disease is widespread in the tropical and subtropical regions that exist in a broad band around the equator. This includes much of Sub-Saharan Africa, Asia, and Latin America. Malaria is commonly associated with poverty and has a major negative effect on economic development. In Africa it is estimated to result in losses of US $ 12 billion a year due to increased healthcare costs, lost ability to work, and effects on tourism. The World Health Organization reports there were 198 million cases of malaria worldwide in 2013. This resulted in an estimated 584,000 to 855,000 deaths, the majority (90%) of which occurred in Africa.

Signs and symptoms

The signs and symptoms of malaria typically begin 8—25 days following infection, but may occur later in those who have taken antimalarial medications as prevention. Initial manifestations of the disease—common to all malaria species—are similar to flu-like symptoms, and can resemble other conditions such as sepsis, gastroenteritis, and viral diseases. The presentation may include headache, fever, shivering, joint pain, vomiting, hemolytic anemia, jaundice, hemoglobin in the urine, retinal damage, and convulsions.

The classic symptom of malaria is paroxysm—a cyclical occurrence of sudden coldness followed by shivering and then fever and sweating, occurring every two days (tertian fever) in P. vivax and P. ovale infections, and every three days (quartan fever) for P. malariae. *P. falciparum* infection can cause recurrent fever every 36—48 hours, or a less pronounced and almost continuous fever.

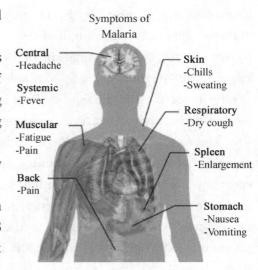

Symptoms of Malaria

Central
-Headache

Systemic
-Fever

Muscular
-Fatigue
-Pain

Back
-Pain

Skin
-Chills
-Sweating

Respiratory
-Dry cough

Spleen
-Enlargement

Stomach
-Nausea
-Vomiting

Severe malaria is usually caused by P. falciparum (often referred to as falciparum malaria). Symptoms of falciparum malaria arise 9—30 days after infection. Individuals with cerebral malaria frequently exhibit neurological symptoms, including abnormal posturing, nystagmus, conjugate gaze palsy (failure of the eyes to turn together in the same direction), opisthotonus, seizures, or coma.

Complications

Malaria has several serious complications. Among these is the development of respiratory distress, which occurs in up to 25% of adults and 40% of children with severe P. falciparum malaria. Possible causes include respiratory compensation of metabolic acidosis, noncardiogenic pulmonary oedema, concomitant pneumonia, and severe anaemia. Although rare in young children with severe malaria, acute respiratory distress syndrome occurs in 5%—25% of adults and up to 29% of pregnant women. Coinfection of HIV with malaria increases mortality. Kidney failure is a feature of blackwater fever, where haemoglobin from lysed red blood cells leaks into the urine.

Infection with P. falciparum may result in cerebral malaria, a form of severe malaria that involves encephalopathy. It is associated with retinal whitening, which may be a useful clinical sign in distinguishing malaria from other causes of fever. An enlarged spleen, enlarged liver or both of these, severe headache, low blood sugar, and haemoglobin in the urine with kidney failure may occur. Complications may include spontaneous bleeding, coagulopathy, and shock.

Malaria in pregnant women is an important cause of stillbirths, infant mortality, miscarriage and low birth weight, particularly in *P. falciparum* infection, but also with *P. vivax.*

Severe and complicated malaria

Cases of severe and complicated malaria are almost always caused by infection with P. falciparum. The other species usually cause only febrile disease. Severe and complicated malaria cases are medical emergencies since mortality rates are high (10% to 50%).

Recommended treatment for severe malaria is the intravenous use of antimalarial drugs. For severe malaria, parenteral artesunate was superior to quinine in both children and adults. In another systematic review, artemisinin derivatives (artemether and arteether) were as efficacious as quinine in the treatment of cerebral malaria inchildren. Treatment of severe malaria involves supportive measures that are best done in a critical care unit. This includes the management of high fevers and the seizures that may result from it. It also includes monitoring for poor breathing effort, low blood sugar, and low blood potassium. Artemisinin derivatives have the same or better efficacy than quinolones in preventing deaths in severe or complicated malaria. Quinine loading dose helps to shorten the duration of fever and increases parasite clearance from the body. There is no difference in effectiveness when using intrarectal quinine compared to intravenous or intramuscular quinine in treating uncomplicated/complicated falciparum malaria. There is insufficient evidence for intramuscular arteether to treat severe malaria. The provision of rectal artesunate before transfer to hospital may reduce the rate of death for children with severe malaria.

Cerebral malaria is the form of severe and complicated malaria with the worst neurological symptoms. There is insufficient data on whether osmotic agents such as mannitol or urea are effective in treating cerebral malaria. Routine phenobarbitone in cerebral malaria is associated with fewer convulsions but possibly more deaths. There is no evidence that steroids would bring treatment benefits for cerebral malaria.

There is insufficient evidence to show that blood transfusion is useful in either reducing deaths for children with severe anaemia or in improving their haematocrit in one month. There is insufficient evidence that iron chelating agents such as deferoxamine and deferiprone improve outcomes of those with malaria falciparum infection.

Mosquito control

Vector control refers to methods used to decrease malaria by reducing the levels of transmission by mosquitoes. For individual protection, the most effective insect repellents are based on DEET or picaridin. However, there is insufficient evidence that mosquito repellents can prevent malaria infection.

Insecticide-treated mosquito nets (ITNs) and indoor residual spraying (IRS) are effective, have been commonly used to prevent malaria, and their use has contributed significantly to the decrease in malaria in the 21st century. ITNs and IRS may not be sufficient to completely eliminate the disease as these interventions depend on how many people use nets, how many gaps in insecticide there are (low coverage areas), if people are not protected when outside of the home, and an increase in mosquitoes that are resistant to insecticides. Modifications to people's houses to prevent mosquito exposure may be an important long term prevention measure.

Mosquito nets help keep mosquitoes away from people and reduce infection rates and transmission of malaria. Nets are not a perfect barrier and are often treated with an insecticide designed to kill the mosquito before it has time to find a way past the net. Insecticide-treated nets are estimated to be twice as effective as untreated nets and offer greater than 70% protection compared with no net. Between 2000 and 2008, the use of ITNs saved the lives of an estimated 250,000 infants in Sub-Saharan Africa. About 13% of households in Sub-Saharan countries owned ITNs in 2007 and 31% of African households were estimated to own at least one ITN in 2008. In 2000, 1.7 million (1.8%) African children living in areas of the world where malaria is common were protected by an ITN. That number increased to 20.3 million (18.5%) African children using ITNs in 2007, leaving 89.6 million children unprotected and to 68% African children using mosquito nets in 2015. Most nets are impregnated with pyrethroids, a class of insecticides with low toxicity. They are most effective when used from dusk to dawn. It is recommended to hang a large "bed net" above the center of a bed and either tuck the edges under the mattress or make sure it is large enough such that it touches the ground. ITN is beneficial towards pregnancy outcomes in malaria-endemic regions in Africa but more data is needed in Asia and Latin America.

In areas of high malaria resistance, piperonyl butoxide combined with pyrethroids in ITN is effective in reducing malaria infection rates.

Other mosquito control methods

People have tried a number of other methods to reduce mosquito bites and slow the spread of malaria. Efforts to decrease mosquito larvae by decreasing the availability of open water where they develop, or by adding substances to decrease their development, are effective in some locations. Electronic mosquito repellent devices, which make very high-frequency sounds that are supposed to keep female mosquitoes away, have no supporting evidence of effectiveness. There is a low certainty evidence that fogging may have an effect on malaria transmission. Larviciding by hand delivery of chemical or microbial insecticides into water bodies containing low larval distribution may reduce malarial transmission. There is insufficient evidence to determine whether larvivorous fish can decrease mosquito density and transmission in the area.

Artemisinin

Artemisinin and its semisynthetic derivatives are a group of drugs used against malaria due to Plasmodium falciparum. It was discovered in 1972 by Tu Youyou, who shared the 2015 Nobel Prize in Physiology or Medicine for her discovery. Treatments containing an artemisinin derivative (artemisinin-combination therapies, ACTs) are now standard treatment worldwide for P. falciparum malaria as well as malaria due to other species of Plasmodium. Artemisinin is isolated from the plant Artemisia annua, sweet wormwood, a herb employed in Chinese traditional medicine. A precursor compound can be produced using a genetically-engineered yeast, which is much more efficient than using the plant.

Chemically, artemisinin is a sesquiterpene lactone containing an unusual peroxide bridge. This endoperoxide 1,2,4-trioxane ring is responsible for the drug's mechanism of action. Few other natural compounds with such a peroxide bridge are known.

Artemisinin and its derivatives have been used for the treatment of malarial and parasitic worm (helminth) infections. They have the advantage over other drugs in having an ability to kill faster and kill all the life cycle stages of the parasites. But low bioavailability, poor pharmacokinetic properties and high cost of the drugs are major drawbacks of their use. Use of the drug by itself as a monotherapy is explicitly discouraged by the World Health Organization, as there have been signs that malarial parasites are developing resistance to the drug. Therapies that combine artemisinin or its derivatives with some other antimalarial drug are the preferred treatment for malaria.

Qinghaosu, it was one of many candidates tested as possible treatments for malaria by Chinese scientists, from a list of nearly 5,000 traditional Chinese medicines. Tu Youyou also discovered that a low-temperature extraction process could be used to isolate an effective antimalarial substance from the plant. Tu says she was influenced by a traditional Chinese herbal medicine source *The Handbook of Prescriptions for Emergency Treatments* written in 340 CE by Ge Hong saying that this herb should be steeped in cold water. This book contained the useful reference to the herb: "A handful of *qinghao* immersed with two litres of water, wring out the juice and drink it all."

Tu's team subsequently isolated a useful extract. Results were published in the *Chinese Medical Journal* in 1979. The extracted substance, once subject to purification, proved to be useful starting point to obtain purified artemisinin. A 2012 review reported that artemisinin-based therapies were the most effective drugs for treatment of malaria at that time; it was also reported to clear malaria parasites from patients' bodies faster than other drugs.

In the late 1990s, Novartis filed a new Chinese patent for a combination treatment with artemether and lumefantrine, providing the first artemisinin-based combination therapies (Coartem) at reduced prices to the World Health Organization. In 2006, after artemisinin had become the treatment of choice for malaria, the WHO called for an immediate halt to single-drug artemisinin preparations in favor of combinations of artemisinin with another malaria drug, to reduce the risk of parasites developing resistance.

A. Translate the following sentences into Chinese.

1. Malaria is a mosquito-borne infectious disease of humans and other animals caused by Plasmodium. Malaria causes symptoms that typically include fever, fatigue, vomiting and headaches. In severe cases it can cause yellow skin, seizures, coma or death.

2. The disease is transmitted most commonly by an infected female Anopheles mosquito. The mosquito bite introduces the parasites from the mosquito's saliva into a person's blood. The parasites travel to the liver where they mature and reproduce.

3. It is recommended that in areas where the disease is common, malaria is confirmed if possible before treatment is started due to concerns of increasing drug resistance.

4. Malaria is commonly associated with poverty and has a major negative effect on economic development. In Africa it is estimated to result in losses of US $ 12 billion a year due to increased healthcare costs, lost ability to work, and effects on tourism.

5. The risk of disease can be reduced by preventing mosquito bites by using mosquito nets and insect repellents, or with mosquito-control measures such as spraying insecticides and draining standing water.

B. Prepare a lecture on malaria after doing the further reading above.

扫码获取
提示

Unit 27

Epidemic Diseases (Typhoid Fever, Dengue Fever, Yellow Fever, and Black Fever)

I Warming-up

A. Match the following words and phrases with their Chinese translations.

A	viral	1	食道
B	descending colon	2	消化系统
C	pancreas	3	出血性的
D	plague	4	创造
E	a bunch of	5	病毒性的
F	create	6	降结肠
G	hemorrhagic	7	胰腺
H	esophagus	8	一群
I	digestive system	9	十二指肠
J	duodenum	10	疫病

B. Complete the sentences with the following words or phrases in their proper forms.

inflame	pop up	occur	estimate
replicate	bleed	take steps to	die from

1. Colds mutate even while they're infecting you, and new strains _____ so often that by the time drug-makers develop a new vaccine against one variation, the serum is already out of date.

2. If flossing hurts or makes your gum _____, keep working at it.

3. Facing the serious environmental pollution problems, we need to _____ solve these problems immediately.

4. International interest in the therapeutic qualities of the Mediterranean diet began back in the late 1950s, when medical researchers started to link the _____ of heart disease with diet.

5. It is also important to avoid asthma triggers—stimuli that irritate and _____ the airways.

6. People living in the most deprived areas are four times more prone to _____ avoidable causes than counterparts in more affluent places.

7. Scientists _____ that smoking reduces life expectancy by around 2 years on average.

8. Nothing has the capacity to _____ itself except DNA.

 C. Watch the video *Yellow Fever* and answer the questions.

扫码获取视频

1. What are the causes of yellow fever?

2. Why yellow fever is called yellow fever?

3. What are the most recommended measure to prevent the yellow fever?

4. How many new cases of yellow fever occur every year?

5. Around the world, how many people are at risk of getting the yellow fever?

II Dialogue

扫码获取
音频及文本

 A. Listen to the dialogue for the first time and try to get the general idea.

B. Listen to the dialogue for the second time and try to answer the following questions.

1. What's wrong with this patient?

2. How do we confirm the typhoid fever?

3. What's dengue fever clinically characterized?

4. What are the clinical manifestations of yellow fever?

5. How can these infectious diseases be differentiated?

C. Choose the following words and/or expressions to complete the sentences in their proper forms.

quarantine	检疫隔离		present	出现
on top of	在……之上		erythema	红斑
characterize	特征		differentiate	鉴别诊断
enlarge	增大		viability	生命力
bradycardia	心动过缓		divide	划分
parasitic	寄生虫性的		resist	耐受

1. Salmonella Typhi has a strong _____ in natural world. In water, it can live as long as 2 to 3 weeks while in feces, it can live up to 1 to 2 months.

2. Visceral Leishmaniasis can be _____ into two types: cutaneous Leishmaniasis and lymphonodus Leishmaniasis.

3. Dengue fever is clinically _____ with sudden onset, high fever, muscle pain, bone marrow pain, joint pain and fatigue.

4. _____ typhoid fever, there are dengue fever, yellow fever and black fever, and many others.

5. Salmonella Typhi is low temperature _____, being able to survive in frozen environment for a number of months, therefore, it is highly infectious.

6. Black fever, which is also called as visceral Leishmaniasis, is a chronic _____ disease caused by Leishmania donovani.

7. The cutaneous Leishmaniasis _____ with skin nodules, papulae and erythema and occasionally with color fading spots on the face, limbs or trunk.

8. You should be _____ in hospital in case of the adverse health impact on your family members or people around you.

9. They can be _____ by their respective epidemiological histories and symptoms, but the diagnosis can be confirmed only when we have detected respective pathogen or specific antibody.

10. In some cases, patients may have rash, bleeding and _____ of lymph nodes.

D. Read the dialogue and try to make a conversation with your classmates.

扫码获取
提示

E. Translate the following Chinese into English.

D—Doctor   I—Intern   P—Patient

D：What have brought you here?

P：I have been feeling ill recently，fatigued and exhausted. 1. 吃饭没胃口、咳嗽，嗓子还疼得厉害。

　　1. _____

D：How long have you been sick? Do you have any other discomforts?

P：2. 发烧快一个星期了，oh yes，I have got some rashes in my body.

　　2. _____

D：Really? Let me examine it ... .

D：3. 我建议你住院治疗，同时我们会进行进一步的检测。

　　3. _____

P：Do I? 4. 能否在门诊治?

　　4. _____

D：You are likely to have the typhoid fever，which is an infectious disease. 5. 必须住院隔离治疗，否则可能会影响你的家人和周围人的健康。

　　5. _____

　　_____

P：OK.

...（Patient Leaves）

I： Professor，is typhoid fever highly infectious? How do we confirm the disease?

D：Yes，it is. Typhoid fever is an infectious disease due to Salmonella Typhi. 6. 伤寒杆菌在自然界中的生命力非常强。In water，it can live as long as 2 to 3 weeks while in feces，it can live up to 1 to 2 months. 7. 耐低温,在冰冻环境中可存活数月，therefore，it is highly infectious. So far as this patient is concerned，he is not only having such typical typhoid symptoms as continuous high fever，he also has roseola on the skin. Surely as it is, typhoid fever can be confirmed if we can do further examination by detecting the Salmonella Typhi from the blood，bone marrow，urine，stool or roseola scrapings.

　　6. _____

　　7. _____

I：Are there any other such infectious diseases in the place where China Medical Team works?

D：Yes. 8. 除了伤寒,还有登革热、黄热病和黑热病等。

　　8. _____

　　_____

Ⅲ　Further Reading: Typhoid Fever, Dengue Fever, Yellow Fever, and Black Fever

Text A　Typhoid fever

Typhoid fever, also known simply as typhoid, is a bacterial infection due to Salmonella typhi that causes symptoms which may vary from mild to severe and usually begin six to thirty days after exposure. The name typhoid means "resembling typhus" due to the similarity in symptoms. Often there is a gradual onset of a high fever over several days. Weakness, abdominal pain, constipation, and headaches also commonly occur. Diarrhea is uncommon and vomiting is not usually severe. Some people develop a skin rash with rose colored spots. In severe cases there may be confusion. Without treatment symptoms may last weeks or months. Other people may carry the bacterium without being affected; however, they are still able to spread the disease to others. Typhoid fever is a type of enteric fever along with paratyphoid fever.

The cause is the bacterium Salmonella typhi, also known as Salmonella enterica serotype Typhi, growing in the intestines and blood. Typhoid is spread by eating or drinking food or water contaminated with the feces of an infected person. Risk factors include poor sanitation and poor hygiene. Those who travel to the developing world are also at risk and only humans can be infected. Diagnosis is by either culturing the bacteria or detecting the bacterium's DNA in the blood, stool, or bone marrow. Culturing the bacterium can be difficult. Bone marrow testing is the most accurate. Symptoms are similar to that of many other infectious diseases. Typhus is a different disease.

A typhoid vaccine can prevent about 30% to 70% of cases during the first two years. The vaccine may have some effect for up to seven years. It is recommended for those at high risk or people traveling to areas where the disease is common. Other efforts to prevent the disease include providing clean drinking water, better sanitation, and better handwashing. Until it has been confirmed that an individual's infection is cleared, the individual should not prepare food for others. Treatment of disease is with antibiotics such as azithromycin, fluoroquinolones or third generation cephalosporins. Resistance to these antibiotics has been developing, which has made treatment of the disease more difficult.

In 2015 there were 12.5 million new cases worldwide. The disease is most common in India. Children are most commonly affected. Rates of disease decreased in the developed world in the 1940s as a result of improved sanitation and use of antibiotics to treat the disease. Each year in the United States about 400 cases are reported and it is estimated that the disease occurs in about 6,000 people. In 2015 it resulted in about 149,000 deaths worldwide—down from 181,000 in 1990 (about 0.3% of the global total). The risk of death may be as high as 20% without treatment. With treatment it is between 1% and 4%.

Treatment

The rediscovery of oral rehydration therapy in the 1960s provided a simple way to prevent many of the deaths of diarrheal diseases in general.

Where resistance is uncommon, the treatment of choice is a fluoroquinolone such as ciprofloxacin. Otherwise, a third-generation cephalosporin such as ceftriaxone or cefotaxime is the first choice. Cefixime is a suitable oral alternative.

Typhoid fever, when properly treated, is not fatal in most cases. Antibiotics, such as ampicillin, chloramphenicol, trimethoprim-sulfamethoxazole, amoxicillin, and ciprofloxacin, have been commonly used to treat typhoid fever in microbiology. Treatment of the disease with antibiotics reduces the case-fatality rate to about 1%.

When untreated, typhoid fever persists for three weeks to a month. Death occurs in 10% to 30% of untreated cases. In some communities, however, case-fatality rates may reach as high as 47%.

Text B Dengue fever

Dengue fever is a mosquito-borne tropical disease caused by the dengue virus. Symptoms typically begin three to fourteen days after infection. These may include a high fever, headache, vomiting, muscle and joint pains, and a characteristic skin rash. Recovery generally takes two to seven days. In a small proportion of cases, the disease develops into severe dengue, also known as dengue hemorrhagic fever, resulting in bleeding, low levels of blood platelets and blood plasma leakage, or into dengue shock syndrome, where dangerously low blood pressure occurs.

Dengue is spread by several species of female mosquitoes of the Aedes genus, principally Aedes aegypti. The virus has five serotypes; infection with one type usually gives lifelong immunity to that type, but only short-term immunity to the others. Subsequent infection with a different type increases the risk of severe complications. A number of tests are available to confirm the diagnosis including detecting antibodies to the virus or its RNA.

A vaccine for dengue fever has been approved and is commercially available in a number of countries. As of 2018, the vaccine is only recommended in individuals who have been previously infected, or in populations with a high rate of prior infection by age nine. Other methods of prevention include reducing mosquito habitat and limiting exposure to bites. This may be done by getting rid of or covering standing water and wearing clothing that covers much of the body. Treatment of acute dengue is supportive and includes giving fluid either by mouth or intravenously for mild or moderate disease. For more severe cases, blood transfusion may be required. About half a

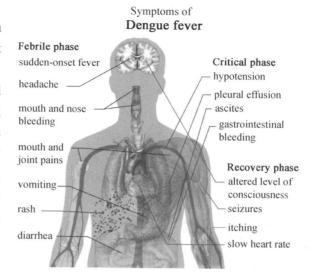

Symptoms of
Dengue fever

Febrile phase
sudden-onset fever
headache
mouth and nose bleeding
mouth and joint pains
vomiting
rash
diarrhea

Critical phase
— hypotension
— pleural effusion
— ascites
— gastrointestinal bleeding

Recovery phase
— altered level of consciousness
— seizures
— itching
— slow heart rate

million people require hospital admission every year. Paracetamol (acetaminophen) is recommended instead of nonsteroidal anti-inflammatory drugs (NSAIDs) for fever reduction and pain relief in dengue due to an increased risk of bleeding from NSAID use.

Dengue has become a global problem since the Second World War and is common in more than 120 countries, mainly in Southeast Asia, South Asia and South America. About 390 million people are infected a year and approximately 40,000 die. In 2019 a significant increase in the number of cases was seen. The earliest descriptions of an outbreak date from 1779. Its viral cause and spread were understood by the early 20th century. Apart from eliminating the mosquitos, work is ongoing for medication targeted directly at the virus. It is classified as a neglected tropical disease.

Management

There are no specific antiviral drugs for dengue; however, maintaining proper fluid balance is important. Treatment depends on the symptoms. Those who can drink, are passing urine, have no "warning signs" and are otherwise healthy can be managed at home with daily follow-up and oral rehydration therapy. Those who have other health problems, have "warning signs", or cannot manage regular follow-up should be cared for in hospital. In those with severe dengue care should be provided in an area where there is access to an intensive care unit.

Intravenous hydration, if required, is typically only needed for one or two days. In children with shock due to dengue a rapid dose of 20 mL/kg is reasonable. The rate of fluid administration is then titrated to a urinary output of 0.5—1 mL/kg/h, stable vitalsigns and normalization of hematocrit. The smallest amount of fluid required to achieve this is recommended.

Invasive medical procedures such as nasogastric intubation, intramuscular injections and arterial punctures are avoided, in view of the bleeding risk. Paracetamol (acetaminophen) is used for fever and discomfort while NSAIDs such as ibuprofen and aspirin are avoided as they might aggravate the risk of bleeding. Blood transfusion is initiated early in people presenting with unstable vital signs in the face a decreasing hematocrit, rather than waiting for the hemoglobin concentration to decrease to some predetermined "transfusion trigger" level. Packed red blood cells or whole blood are recommended, while platelets and fresh frozen plasma are usually not. There is not enough evidence to determine if corticosteroids have a positive or negative effect in dengue fever.

During the recovery phase intravenous fluids are discontinued to prevent a state of fluid overload. If fluid overload occurs and vital signs are stable, stopping further fluid may be all that is needed. If a person is outside of the critical phase, a loop diuretic such as furosemide may be used to eliminate excess fluid from the circulation.

Text C Yellow fever

Yellow fever is a viral disease of typically short duration. In most cases, symptoms include fever, chills, loss of appetite, nausea, muscle pains particularly in the back, and headaches. Symptoms typically improve within five days. In about 15% of people, within a day of improving the fever comes back, abdominal pain occurs, and liver damage begins causing yellow skin. If this occurs, the risk of bleeding and kidney problems is increased.

The disease is caused by yellow fever virus and is spread by the bite of an infected female mosquito. It infects only humans, other primates, and several types of mosquitoes. In cities, it is spread primarily by Aedes aegypti, a type of mosquito found throughout the tropics and subtropics. The virus is an RNA virus of the genus Flavivirus. The disease may be difficult to tell apart from other illnesses, especially in the early stages. To confirm a suspected case, blood-sample testing with polymerase chain reaction (PCR) is required.

A safe and effective vaccine against yellow fever exists, and some countries require vaccinations for travelers. Other efforts to prevent infection include reducing the population of the transmitting mosquitoes. In areas where yellow fever is common, early diagnosis of cases and immunization of large parts of the population are important to prevent outbreaks. Once a person is infected, management is symptomatic; no specific measures are effective against the virus. Death occurs in up to half of those who get severe disease.

In 2013, yellow fever resulted in about 127,000 severe infections and 45,000 deaths worldwide, with nearly 90 percent of these occurring in African nations.

Nearly a billion people live in an area of the world where the disease is common. It is common in tropical areas of the continents of South America and Africa, but not in Asia. Since the 1980s, the number of cases of yellow fever has been increasing. This is believed to be due to fewer people being immune, more people living in cities, people moving frequently, and changing climate increasing the habitat for mosquitoes.

The disease originated in Africa and spread to South America in the 17th century with the Spanish and Portuguese importation of enslaved Africans from sub-Saharan Africa. Since the 17th century, several major outbreaks of the disease have occurred in the Americas, Africa, and Europe. In the 18th and 19th centuries, yellow fever was considered one of the most dangerous infectious diseases; numerous epidemics swept through major cities of the US and in other parts of the world.

In 1927, yellow fever virus was the first human virus to be isolated.

Treatment

As with other Flavivirus infections, no cure is known for yellow fever. Hospitalization is advisable and intensive care may be necessary because of rapid deterioration in some cases. Certain acute treatment methods lack efficacy: passive immunization after the emergence of symptoms is probably without effect; ribavirin and other antiviral drugs, as well as treatment with interferons, are ineffective in yellow fever patients. Symptomatic treatment includes rehydration and pain relief with drugs such as paracetamol (acetaminophen). Acetylsalicylic acid (aspirin) should not be given because of its anticoagulant effect, which can be devastating in the case of internal bleeding that may occur with yellow fever.

Epidemiology in Africa and South America

Yellow fever is common in tropical and subtropical areas of South America and Africa. Worldwide, about 600 million people live in endemic areas. The WHO estimates that 200,000 cases of disease and 30,000 deaths a year occur, but the number of officially reported cases is far lower.

In Africa

An estimated 90% of yellow fever infections occur on the African continent. In 2016, a large outbreak originated in Angola and spread to neighboring countries before being contained by a massive vaccination campaign.

Phylogenetic analysis has identified seven genotypes of yellow fever viruses, and they are assumed to be differently adapted to humans and to the vector A. aegypti. Five genotypes (Angola, Central/East Africa, East Africa, West

Africa I , and West Africa II) occur only in Africa. West Africa genotype I is found in Nigeria and the surrounding region. West Africa genotype I appears to be especially infectious, as it is often associated with major outbreaks. The three genotypes found outside of Nigeria and Angola occur in areas where outbreaks are rare. Two outbreaks, in Kenya (1992—1993) and Sudan (2003 and 2005), involved the East African genotype, which had remained undetected in the previous 40 years.

In South America

In South America, two genotypes have been identified (South American genotypes I and II). Based on phylogenetic analysis these two genotypes appear to have originated in West Africa and were first introduced into Brazil. The date of introduction of the predecessor African genotype which gave rise to the South American genotypes appears to be 1822 (95% confidence interval 1701 to 1911). The historical record shows an outbreak of yellow fever occurred in Recife, Brazil, between 1685 and 1690. The disease seems to have disappeared, with the next outbreak occurring in 1849. It was likely introduced with the importation of slaves through the slave trade from Africa. Genotype I has been divided into five subclades, A through E.

In late 2016, a large outbreak began in Minas Gerais state of Brazil that was characterized as a sylvan or jungle epizootic. It began as an outbreak in brown howler monkeys, which serve as a sentinel species for yellow fever, that then spread to men working in the jungle. No cases had been transmitted between humans by the A. aegypti mosquito, which can sustain urban outbreaks that can spread rapidly. In April 2017, the sylvan outbreak continued moving toward the Brazilian coast, where most people were unvaccinated. By the end of May the outbreak appeared to be declining after more than 3,000 suspected cases, 758 confirmed and 264 deaths confirmed to be yellow fever. The Health Ministry launched a vaccination campaign and was concerned about spread during the Carnival season in February and March. The CDC issued a Level 2 alert (practice enhanced precautions.)

A Bayesian analysis of genotypes I and II has shown that genotype I accounts for virtually all the current infections in Brazil, Colombia, Venezuela, and Trinidad and Tobago, while genotype II accounted for all cases in Peru. Genotype I originated in the northern Brazilian region around 1908 (95% highest posterior density interval [HPD]: 1870—1936). Genotype II originated in Peru in 1920 (95% HPD: 1867—1958). The estimated rate of mutation for both genotypes was about 5×10^{-4} substitutions/site/year, similar to that of other RNA viruses.

Text D Black fever

Black fever, which is also called as visceral Leishmaniasis (VL), is a chronic parasitic disease caused by Leishmania donovani. It is an acute infectious disease of high mortality, characterized by frontal and occipital headache, intense lumbar pain, malaise, a moderately high continuous fever, and a rash on wrists, palms, ankles, and soles from the second to the fifth day, later spreading to all parts of the body.

Causes

Leishmaniasis is transmitted by the bite of infected female phlebotomine sandflies which can transmit the protozoa Leishmania. The sandflies inject the infective stage, metacyclic promastigotes, during blood meals. Metacyclic promastigotes that reach the puncture wound are phagocytized by macrophages and transform into amastigotes. Amastigotes multiply in infected cells and affect different tissues, depending in part on which Leishmania species is involved. These differing tissue specificities cause the differing clinical manifestations of the various forms of leishmaniasis. Sandflies become infected during blood meals on infected hosts when they ingest macrophages infected with amastigotes. In the sandfly's midgut, the parasites differentiate into promastigotes, which multiply, differentiate into metacyclic promastigotes, and migrate to the proboscis.

The genomes of three Leishmania species (L. major, L. infantum, and L. braziliensis) have been sequenced, and this has provided much information about the biology of the parasite. For example, in Leishmania, protein-coding genes are understood to be organized as large polycistronic units in a head-to-head or tail-to-tail manner; RNA polymerase II transcribes long polycistronic messages in the absence of defined RNA pol II promoters, and Leishmania has unique features with respect to the regulation of gene expression in response to changes in the environment. The new knowledge from these studies may help identify new targets for urgently needed drugs and aid the development of vaccines.

Signs and symptoms

The symptoms of leishmaniasis are skin sores which erupt weeks to months after the person is bitten by infected sand flies.

Leishmaniasis may be divided into the following types:

Cutaneous leishmaniasis is the most common form, which causes an open sore at the bite sites, which heals in a few months to a year and half, leaving an unpleasant-looking scar. Diffuse cutaneous leishmaniasis produces widespread skin lesions which resemble leprosy, and may not heal on its own.

Mucocutaneous leishmaniasis causes both skin and mucosal ulcers with damage primarily of the nose and mouth.

Visceral leishmaniasis or kala-azar ("black fever") is the most serious form, and is potentially fatal if untreated. Other consequences, which can occur a few months to years after infection, include fever, damage to the spleen and liver, and anemia.

Leishmaniasis is considered one of the classic causes of a markedly enlarged (and therefore palpable) spleen; the organ, which is not normally felt during examination of the abdomen, may even become larger than the liver in severe cases.

Diagnosis

Leishmaniasis is diagnosed in the hematology laboratory by direct visualization of the amastigotes (Leishman-Donovan bodies). Buffy-coat preparations of peripheral blood or aspirates from marrow, spleen, lymph nodes, or skin lesions should be spread on a slide to make a thin smear and stained with Leishman stain or Giemsa stain (pH 7.2) for 20 minutes. Amastigotes are seen within blood and spleen monocytes or, less commonly, in circulating neutrophils and in aspirated tissue macrophages. They are small, round bodies 2—4 μm in diameter with indistinct cytoplasm, a nucleus, and a small, rod-shaped kinetoplast. Occasionally, amastigotes may be seen lying free between cells. However, the retrieval of tissue samples is often painful for the patient and identification of the infected cells can be difficult. So, other indirect immunological methods of diagnosis are developed, including enzyme-linked immunosorbent assay, antigen-coated dipsticks, and direct agglutination test. Although these tests are readily available, they are not the standard diagnostic tests due to their insufficient sensitivity and specificity.

Several different polymerase chain reaction tests are available for the detection of Leishmania DNA. With this assay, a specific and sensitive diagnostic procedure is finally possible.

Most forms of the disease are transmitted only from nonhuman animals, but some can be spread between humans. Infections in humans are caused by about 21 of 30 species that infect mammals; the different species look the same, but they can be differentiated by isoenzyme analysis, DNA sequence analysis, or monoclonal antibodies.

Treatment

The treatment is determined by where the disease is acquired, the species of Leishmania, and the type of infection. For visceral leishmaniasis in India, South

America, and the Mediterranean, liposomal amphotericin B is the recommended treatment and is often used as a single dose. Rates of cure with a single dose of amphotericin have been reported as 95%. In India, almost all infections are resistant to pentavalent antimonials. In Africa, a combination of pentavalent antimonials and paromomycin is recommended. These, however, can have significant side effects. Miltefosine, an oral medication, is effective against both visceral and cutaneous leishmaniasis. Side effects are generally mild, though it can cause birth defects if taken within 3 months of getting pregnant. It does not appear to work for L. major or L. braziliensis.

The evidence around the treatment of cutaneous leishmaniasis is poor. A number of topical treatments may be used for cutaneous leishmaniasis. Which treatments are effective depends on the strain, with topical paromomycin effective for L. major, L. tropica, L. mexicana, L. panamensis, and L. braziliensis. Pentamidine is effective for L. guyanensis. Oral fluconazole or itraconazole appears effective in L. major and L. tropica.

A. Translate the following sentences into Chinese.

1. A typhoid vaccine can prevent about 30% to 70% of cases during the first two years. The vaccine may have some effect for up to seven years. It is recommended for those at high risk or people traveling to areas where the disease is common. Other efforts to prevent the disease include providing clean drinking water, better sanitation, and better handwashing.

2. Dengue is spread by several species of female mosquitoes of the Aedes genus, principally Aedes aegypti. The virus has five serotypes; infection with one type usually gives lifelong immunity to that type, but only short-term immunity to the others. Subsequent infection with a different type increases the risk of severe complications.

3. Treatment of acute dengue is supportive and includes giving fluid either by mouth or intravenously for mild or moderate disease. For more severe cases, blood transfusion may be required. About half a million people require hospital admission every year. Paracetamol (acetaminophen) is recommended instead of nonsteroidal anti-inflammatory drugs (NSAIDs) for fever reduction and pain relief in dengue due to an increased risk of bleeding from NSAID use.

4. As with other Flavivirus infections, no cure is known for yellow fever. Symptomatic treatment includes rehydration and pain relief with drugs such as paracetamol (acetaminophen). Acetylsalicylic acid (aspirin) should not be given because of its anticoagulant effect, which can be devastating in the case of internal bleeding that may occur with yellow fever.

5. The treatment is determined by where the disease is acquired, the species of Leishmania, and the type of infection. For visceral leishmaniasis in India, South America, and the Mediterranean, liposomal amphotericin B is the recommended treatment and is often used as a single dose. Rates of cure with a single dose of amphotericin have been reported as 95%.

B. Prepare a lecture on epidemic diseases after doing the further reading above.

扫码获取
提示

Unit 28

Blood Tests

I Warming-up

A. Match the following words and phrases with their Chinese translations.

A	protein	1	低血钙症
B	calcium levels	2	钙水平
C	hypercalcemia	3	营养不良
D	constipation	4	荷尔蒙
E	hypocalcemia	5	肾结石
F	poor nutrition	6	蛋白质
G	kidney stone	7	便秘
H	metabolism	8	常规体检
I	hormone	9	新陈代谢
J	routine physical examination	10	血钙过多

B. Complete the sentences with the following words or phrases in their proper forms.

pulmonary function	medium	healthcare	blood sample
hormones	assess	collect blood	regardless of

1. _____ from an artery is more painful than collecting from a vein, but complications are rare and you may have some bleeding, bruising, or soreness at the spot where the

needle was put in.

2. Blood tests are often used in _____ to determine physiological and biochemical states, such as disease, mineral content, pharmaceutical drug effectiveness, and organ function.

3. Blood flows throughout the body, acting as a _____ that provides oxygen and nutrients to tissues and carries waste products back to the excretory systems for disposal.

4. Blood gas analysis of arterial blood is primarily used to monitor carbon dioxide and oxygen levels related to _____, but is also used to measure blood pH and bicarbonate levels for certain metabolic conditions.

5. A complete blood count is performed in several steps. At first, _____ are analyzed using a hematology analyzer to estimate concentration of hemoglobin, and to count erythrocytes, leukocytes and thrombocytes and other parameters.

6. A bone marrow examination is also used when the clinical picture and results of blood tests are inconclusive to make the diagnosis, and to _____ a possible spreading of lymphoma when there are no abnormal cells in the blood.

7. _____ why you're having a blood test, it's important to remember that while blood tests help providers diagnose health issues, they aren't diagnoses. An abnormal blood test result may not mean you have a serious medical condition.

8. There are many different blood tests. Some tests focus on your blood cells and platelets. Some evaluate substances in your blood such as electrolytes, proteins and _____. Others measure certain minerals in your blood.

 C. Watch the video about *Blood Tests* and answer the questions.

扫码获取视频

1. What's being tested in calcium test and why is calcium test important?

2. Why is calcium requested as a part of investigation?

3. What are the symptoms of hypercalcemia and hypocalcemia?

4. Who need calcium monitoring as a part of regular lab test?

5. What is the cause of hypercalcemia and hypocalcemia?

扫码获取
音频及文本

Ⅱ Dialogue

A. Listen to the dialogue for the first time and try to get the general idea.

B. Listen to the dialogue for the second time and try to answer the following questions.

1. Which part do you think should be better for capillary blood sampling?

2. What kind of patient should take a direct lymphocyte count?

3. Which do you think is the best way for Plasmodium detection?

4. How can we detect sickle cells 30 minutes later without waiting for 1 to 3 hour later?

5. Why must we set the test tubes upright while doing the blood sedimentation tests?

C. Choose the following words and/or expressions to complete the sentences in their proper forms.

anemia	贫血	dilution	稀释
bone marrow aspiration	骨髓穿刺	essential	基本的,必不可少的
myeloma	骨髓瘤	pallor	脸色苍白
enzyme	酶	peripheral smear	外周涂层
genetic mutation	基因突变	sedimentation	沉淀,沉积
hemolysis	溶血	capillary	毛细血管

1. When the liver is damaged, it releases substances called _____ into the blood. Levels of proteins produced by the liver begin to drop.

2. The best place for _____ blood sampling is in the ring finger or at the heels in case of a child.

3. It may result from several facts, like which part you take the sample, whether the diluent is clean, whether the counting chamber is cleared and how long the sample has been kept after _____.

4. According to the experiments, when the test tube tilts 3°, the _____ will be 30% faster. So it is important to keep the test tube straight, or the findings will not be correct.

5. You may have inherited certain _____ that cause medical conditions. Your provider may take blood samples for genetic analysis so you know if you're at risk of developing a specific condition.

6. It's probably fair to say blood tests are last on most people's list of fun things to do. But blood tests are an _____ tool healthcare providers use to monitor your overall health or diagnose medical conditions.

7. A complete physical examination in anemia is necessary. Signs of anemia itself are neither sensitive nor specific; however, _____ is common with severe anemia.

8. The _____ is highly sensitive to excessive RBC production and hemolysis. It is more accurate than automated technologies for recognition of altered RBC structure, thrombocytopenia, nucleated RBCs, or immature granulocytes.

9. _____ and biopsy are usually not indicated in the evaluation of anemia and are only done when one of the following conditions is present: unexplained anemia; more than one cell lineage abnormality.

10. If _____ is suspected or there is severe osteoporosis, an ultrasound-guided biopsy is done because it is the safest to avoid penetrating the pelvis.

D. Read the dialogue and try to make a conversation with your classmates.

扫码获取
提示

E. Translate the following Chinese into English.

S—Student   D—Doctor

S: Good morning, Dr. Wang, 1. 您说用毛细血管采血法应该采集哪个部位更好？
   1. _____
   _____

D: The left ring finger ventromedial part or at the heels in case of a child.

S: Why is it so?

D: 2. 因为这些部位血液循环好，检验结果比较接近静脉血，能较准确反映病人的真实情况，而且也容易消毒。
   2. _____
   _____
   _____

Oh, I see. May I ask some other questions?

D: Yes.

S: 3. 今天上午我为同一个病人做了二次红细胞计数. Why was there such a large difference?
   3. _____
   _____

D: 4. 你用的吸管法还是试管法？

4. _____

S: A pipet.

D: 5. 影响结果的因素很多, like which part you take the sample, whether the diluent is clean, whether the counting chamber is cleared and how long the sample has been kept after dilution. For example, 6. 采血部位有渗血,结果可偏高;7. 渗血导致吸管外有余血,采血部位有水肿,结果可偏低。
   5. _____
   6. _____
   7. _____

S: Perhaps it was caused by the different length of time after the second dilution.

D: That's possible.

S: Dr. Wang, 8. 什么时候病人需要做淋巴细胞直接计数？

8. _____

D: Those patients who suffer from AIDS, agammaglobulinemia, and thymus hypoplasia.

S: I see.

Ⅲ Further Reading: Blood Tests

A blood test is one of the most common tests healthcare providers use to monitor your overall health or help diagnose medical conditions. You may have a blood test as part of a routine physical examination or because you have certain symptoms.

There are many different blood tests. Some tests focus on your blood cells and platelets. Some evaluate substances in your blood such as electrolytes, proteins and hormones. Others measure certain minerals in your blood.

Regardless of why you're having a blood test, it's important to remember that blood tests help healthcare providers diagnose health issues. But blood test results aren't diagnoses. An abnormal blood test result may not mean you have a serious medical condition.

Your blood plays a big role in your overall health and contains a lot of information about what may be going on in your body. That's one reason why blood tests are a common medical test. A healthcare provider may do a blood test because:

• It's time for your regular physical. During a checkup, your provider may order blood tests to check on your overall health. They may order a blood test that evaluates many parts of your blood, such as a complete blood count (CBC), basic metabolic panel (BMP) or a comprehensive metabolic panel.

• Your provider recommends screening tests. Screening tests are done before you have any symptoms. They may recommend screening tests if you're at risk of developing certain conditions, such as cancer. For example, if you're at risk for developing coronary artery disease, your healthcare provider may order several blood tests to evaluate that risk.

• You don't feel well. If you have specific symptoms, your provider may order blood tests to determine what's causing them. For example, if you have symptoms that may be signs you're pregnant, your provider will do a pregnancy test. The blood test looks for a specific hormone your body only ever makes when you're pregnant.

• You have a medical condition that happens when certain genes change (mutate). Depending on your situation, your blood cells and platelets may show information about the specific changes. Understanding which genes changed may help your provider plan your treatment.

• You're receiving treatment for a medical condition. Your provider may use regular blood tests to see if treatment is working.

• You may have inherited certain genetic mutations that cause medical conditions. Your provider may take blood samples for genetic analysis so you know if you're at risk of developing a specific condition.

In a broad sense, a blood test shows changes in your body. Blood test results don't show a complete picture. Instead, they're a kind of snapshot. After seeing that snapshot, your provider may do other blood tests to get a closer view. Here's a glimpse of what your healthcare provider may see with blood tests:

- The tests show if your blood is working as it should. For example, your red blood cells carry oxygen throughout your body. A blood test may show you have low red blood cell levels (anemia). If healthcare providers look at your cells under a microscope, they may see your red blood cells are larger than normal or shaped differently than normal red blood cells. These differences may be signs of blood disorders or blood cancers.
- They show if you have normal levels of enzymes and electrolytes. Enzymes are proteins that help speed up the chemical reactions that build up and break down substances in your body. Electrolytes do several things, such as helping your body regulate chemical reactions and maintaining the balance between fluids inside and outside your cells.

There are many different blood tests. Some tests—such as complete blood count tests, basic metabolic panels, complete metabolic panels and electrolyte panels—check on several different elements in your blood at the same time. Other blood tests look for very specific elements in your blood.

The most common blood test that includes several specialized tests. CBC tests:

- Count and measure your red blood cells, white blood cells and your platelets. A CBC test includes a hematocrit test that measures the percentage of red blood cells in your blood.
- Measure your hemoglobin levels.
- Measure variations in your red blood cells' size and volume with an RDW blood test (RDW stands for "red blood cell distribution width").
- Measure the average size of your red blood cells with a mean corpuscular volume (MCV) test.

A basic metabolic panel (BMP) measures several substances in your blood. Healthcare providers use BMPs to evaluate your overall health and screen for or monitor health issues. A BMP may include a:

- Blood glucose test: Screens for diabetes.
- Calcium blood test: Checks to make sure you have appropriate levels of calcium, a mineral that helps with many of your body's functions.
- Blood urea nitrogen (BUN) test: Measures the amount of urea, a waste product that passes through your kidneys. BUN tests show the amount of urea nitrogen in your kidneys.

- Creatine kinase (CK) test: Screens for a waste product your muscles produce. High CK levels may be a sign of injured or damaged muscles.
- Sodium levels.
- CO_2 blood test: Measures the amount of bicarbonate in your blood. This test detects carbon dioxide.
- Serum potassium test: Measures potassium levels. Potassium supports your heart, nerve and muscle function and your metabolism.
- Chloride blood test: Checks on chloride, an electrolyte that helps keep your body fluids and acids balanced.
- Globulin blood test: Measures how much of this protein your liver produces.

What does a comprehensive metabolic panel show?

Comprehensive metabolic panels (CMP) include all the blood tests done as part of a basic metabolic panel. Additional blood tests include:
- Albumin blood test: Albumin is a protein in your blood plasma. This test checks on kidney and liver function.
- Alanine transaminase (ALT): Healthcare providers use this test to assess liver health.
- Alkaline phosphatase (ALP): High levels of this enzyme may indicate liver disease or certain bone disorders.
- Ammonia levels: Blood tests will show the amount of ammonia in your blood. High ammonia levels may be a sign of liver and kidney damage.
- Bilirubin blood test: Bilirubin is a substance in your liver's bile. Too much bile in your blood may be a sign of liver issues.
- Aspartate transferase: Sometimes called AST, this test measures the amount of the enzyme aspartate transferase in your blood. Providers use this test to assess liver health.

Electrolytes are minerals in your blood. Imbalance with electrolytes may be a sign of issues with your heart, kidneys or your lungs. An electrolyte panel includes all electrolyte tests in BMPs and CMPs. Additional electrolyte levels tested include magnesium and anion gap. Magnesium supports your brain, heart and muscles. Anion gap tests check the acid-base balance in your blood.

What blood tests do healthcare providers use to help diagnose specific conditions?

While the various blood and electrolyte panel tests provide a lot of information, there are disease-specific blood tests that help providers diagnose and treat specific conditions.

Allergies

An allergy blood test checks your blood for increased levels of immunoglobulin E (IgE) antibodies. The test can help detect allergies to foods, pets, pollen or other irritating substances.

Autoimmune diseases

Autoimmune diseases happen when your immune system accidentally attacks your body instead of protecting it from intruders like viruses, parasites and cancer. Your provider may order the following blood tests:

• Antinuclear antibody test: Antinuclear antibodies (ANA) are antibodies that mistakenly attack your immune system. Large amounts of ANA in your blood may be a sign of certain autoimmune disorders.

• CE complement blood test: Providers may use this test to diagnose and monitor autoimmune disorders like rheumatoid arthritis or lupus.

• C-reactive protein (CRP) test: Your liver makes and releases this protein. High C-reactive protein levels may be a sign of inflammatory conditions, including some autoimmune diseases.

• Erythrocyte sedimentation rate (ESR): ESR tests help detect inflammation.

• Peripheral blood smear (PBS): This is a technique healthcare providers use to examine your red and white blood cells and your platelets under a microscope.

Cancer/Noncancerous blood disorders

Healthcare providers may use several different tests to diagnose and treat cancer, blood cancer and noncancerous blood disorders.

Blood tests for cancer fall into four basic categories—complete blood count, tumor markers, blood protein testing and circulating tumor tests. CBC, tumor markers and circulating tumor tests may help detect some solid tumors. Blood in your poop (stool) or pee (urine) may also be a sign of cancer.

Complete blood count (CBC)

A CBC measures red and white blood cell and platelet levels. Abnormally high or low blood cell or platelet levels may be a sign of some types of cancer.

Tumor markers

Tumor markers are substances made by cancerous cells or your body's normal cells in response to cancer. Tumor marker blood tests include:

• Alpha-fetoprotein (AFP) for liver cancer.

• CA-125 blood test for ovarian cancer.

• Calcitonin for thyroid cancer.

• Cancer antigens 15-3 and 27-29 for breast cancer.

• Carcinoembryonic antigen (CEA) for a range of cancers.

• Human chorionic gonadotropin (HCG) for testicular cancer and ovarian cancer.

• Prostate-specific antigen (PSA) for prostate cancer.

Circulating tumor test

The circulating tumor test is a relatively new blood test for cancer. This test looks for cancerous cells that have broken away from a tumor and into your bloodstream. Currently, it can help monitor certain types of cancer, such as breast, prostate and colorectal cancers. Scientists are still developing the technology.

Healthcare providers may use the same tests to diagnose blood cancer or noncancerous blood disorders:

• D-dimer test: Healthcare providers use this test to diagnose blood clotting disorders.

• Fibrinogen test: Fibrinogen is a protein that helps with blood clotting.

• Kappa or Lambda free light chain: This test detects high protein levels in your blood plasma. Healthcare providers may use this test to diagnose amyloidosis, which is a noncancerous blood disorder, or to diagnose blood cancers such as multiple myeloma.

• Prothrombin time test (PTT): Healthcare providers may use this test to diagnose blood clotting disorders.

• Reticulocyte count: This test checks to see if your bone marrow is producing enough healthy red blood cells.

Some blood tests don't involve providing blood samples, such as:

• Fecal occult blood test (FOBT): FOBTs screen for colorectal cancer by looking for blood in your poop (stool).

• Urinalysis: Healthcare providers may use this test to detect blood cells in your pee (urine).

Your endocrine system is made of organs called glands. Glands produce hormones. Healthcare providers may use blood tests to diagnosis conditions affecting parts of your endocrine system. Common blood tests include:

• Blood glucose test: This test measures your blood glucose level. It's used to diagnose diabetes. Another diabetes blood test is A1C, which measures blood glucose over time.

• Thyroid stimulating hormone test (TSH): There are several blood tests to diagnose thyroid disorders.

• Pancreas blood tests: Your pancreas produces enzymes. These tests check lipase and amylase levels.

Some blood tests evaluate your risk of developing heart disease:

• Cardiac blood tests: Your healthcare provider may order these tests if you're at risk of having a heart attack or developing heart disease.

• Arterial blood gas (ABG) test: This test measures oxygen levels and carbon dioxide levels, among other things. Healthcare providers may do this test to diagnose acute heart failure and cardiac arrest.

Your healthcare provider may recommend specialized blood tests, including:

• Ammonia levels: Blood tests will show the amount of ammonia in your blood. High ammonia levels may be a sign of liver and kidney damage.

• Blood alcohol content (BAC): This test measures the amount of alcohol in your system.

• Ferritin: You may have a ferritin test if your CBC tests show you don't have enough iron.

What should I do to prepare for my blood test?

That depends on the kind of test you're having. For example, some blood tests require you to fast for several hours before the test. You may be asked not to drink any liquids apart from a few sips of water. Most blood tests don't require fasting, but it's a good idea to ask your healthcare provider what to avoid before your blood test. Other steps may include:

• If you don't need to fast before your blood test and you're able to drink water, try to drink as much as you can before your test. Being well-hydrated may make it easier for healthcare providers to obtain blood.

• Use moisturizer on your arms. It may make it easier for your provider to insert the needle and obtain blood.

• Boost your blood pressure right before your blood test by doing some gentle exercise while waiting to be called in for your test.

Phlebotomists—healthcare providers with special training in drawing blood—do blood tests. During the blood test process:

• You'll sit in a chair with an armrest where you can stretch your arm out in front of you.

• If you're wearing a long-sleeve shirt, you'll roll up your sleeve past your elbow.

• The phlebotomist will wipe an antiseptic liquid in the bend of your arm (on the other side of your elbow) and put an elastic band around your arm (above your elbow).

• They may ask you to make a fist to encourage blood flow.

• They'll insert a needle into your arm. This typically happens very quickly. You may feel the needle go into your skin. This is called venipuncture.

• The blood flows into a tube that's sealed and sent to a lab for analysis. The phlebotomist may need to take several samples of your blood, depending on the blood tests your healthcare provider ordered.

• Once the phlebotomist has obtained enough blood, they'll remove the stretchy band that's strapped around your arm and removes the needle.

• Then, they'll put a bandage on the area where the needle went into your skin.

Are there different ways to do blood tests?

All blood tests involve obtaining blood samples. Venipuncture (from a vein) is the most common procedure. Other procedures are:

• Finger stick: Your provider pricks one of your fingers with a needle to collect a tiny amount of blood. The blood sample is saved on a special strip of paper that's sent to a lab for analysis.

• Heel stick: All babies born in the U.S. have blood tests by pricking their heel with a needle to obtain a blood sample.

• Arterial blood gas test: In this test, providers take blood from one of your arteries instead of a vein.

How much blood is taken during blood tests?

That depends on the kind of blood test. On average, a complete blood count (CBC) test may take as much as 30 milliliters (mL) of blood. It may sound like a lot of blood, particularly if you're watching your blood flow into several sample tubes. But it's not—the average adult has 4,500 to 5,700 milliliters of blood in their body.

Do blood tests hurt?

They can, depending on the kind of blood test you have. It's important to remember that phlebotomists receive training on how to obtain blood samples quickly and without causing pain.

That said, tests that take blood from an artery tend to hurt more than tests that take blood from a vein. And with venipuncture, taking blood from a vein may hurt a bit if the phlebotomist has trouble inserting the needle into your vein. Let your phlebotomist know if you have any discomfort. They'll try different ways to obtain samples of your blood.

I'm always anxious about having blood tests. What can I do to relax?

Many people feel anxious about blood tests. Some ways to cope include:
• Understanding why you're having specific blood tests.
• Taking deep breaths as the needle goes into your arm.
• Looking away so you don't see the needle enter your arm.
• Finding a way to distract your attention, such as silently counting to 10.

What happens after my blood test?

Your provider will put a bandage on the spot where the needle went in. Depending on the blood test, they may recommend you rest for a minute or so before standing up and leaving.

When will I know my test results?

That depends on the blood test and your provider's preferences. Your provider likely will explain how you'll receive results. Some blood test results are available within a few hours. Others, like genetic test results, typically take longer.

Some healthcare organizations offer online access to test results. But your provider may prefer to discuss your results in a telephone conversation or in person.

My healthcare provider wants to talk to me about my test results. Does that mean something's wrong?

Not necessarily. If your tests were part of your routine medical checkup, your healthcare provider may want to review results with you. They may have recommendations about ways you can improve your health. If you've received treatment for a medical condition, your provider may want to discuss your test results in detail and put the results in context.

A. Translate the following sentences into Chinese.

1. There are many different blood tests. Some tests focus on your blood cells and platelets. Some evaluate substances in your blood such as electrolytes, proteins and hormones. Others measure certain minerals in your blood.

2. Your blood plays a big role in your overall health and contains a lot of information about what may be going on in your body. That's one reason why blood tests are a common medical test.

3. There are many different blood tests. Some tests—such as complete blood count tests, basic metabolic panels, complete metabolic panels and electrolyte panels.

4. Blood tests for cancer fall into four basic categories—complete blood count, tumor markers, blood protein testing and circulating tumor tests. CBC, tumor markers and circulating tumor tests may help detect some solid tumors.

5. An abnormal blood test result may not mean you have a serious medical condition. If your healthcare provider recommends blood tests, they'll be glad to explain why they recommend the test and what the test may show.

B. Prepare a lecture on blood tests after doing the further reading above.

扫码获取
提示

Interpretation of Radiograph

Ⅰ Warming-up

A. Match the following words and phrases with their Chinese translations.

A	medial	1	氟脱氧葡萄糖
B	malignancy	2	下方的
C	metastatic	3	腋下的
D	consolidation	4	钼靶摄影
E	low-density	5	单发的
F	fluorodeoxyglucose	6	内侧的
G	mammography	7	恶性肿瘤
H	axillary	8	转移的
I	solitary	9	低密度影
J	inferior	10	实变影

B. Complete the sentences with the following words or phrases in their proper forms.

visualize	workup	detect	confuse
demonstrate	reconstruct	avidity	turn out

1. Here's an example of a patient with lymphoma and there's an FDG _____ large lymphomatous mass in the pelvis.

2. It will not be seen on neither the FDG PET nor the CT component of an FDG PET CT，but rather be easily _____ on mammography as well as breast MRI or ultrasound.

3. So it is known that the FDG PET CT is not sensitive for _____ of the primary breast malignancy.

4. Certain inflammatory states should not be _____ with breast cancer.

5. These results _____ convincingly that our campaign is working.

6. These results provide support for researchers' prediction that naltrexone will _____ to be toxic to certain types of bacteria.

7. Cardiovascular magnetic resonance imaging（CMR）is becoming an integral part of the diagnostic _____ and is one of the preferred techniques for evaluating patients with ischemic heart disease.

8. Probe into the value of the spiral CT 3-dimensional image _____ used in the diagnosis of the complicated membrum minor articulus trauma.

扫码获取视频

 C. **Watch the video** *Clinical Impact of PET CT on Breast Cancer* **and answer the questions.**

1. What are more sensitive and specific in diagnostic imaging for smaller but clinically important primary breast cancer?

2. What is Ax LND? Why should it be done?

3. How can we differentiate post-surgical inflammation from breast malignancy in imaging manifestations?

4. How can we differentiate post-mastectomy fat necrosis from breast tumor in imaging manifestations?

5. What do you think is the diagnostic value of PET CT?

II Dialogue

扫码获取
音频及文本

A. **Listen to the dialogue for the first time and try to get the general idea.**

1. What does the CT scan show about the patient?

2. Why does the PG think that osteoid osteoma should be considered first?

3. What are the imaging manifestations for osteoid osteoma?

4. What is the diagnostic value of CT scan in this case?

5. What is the diagnostic value of MRI scan in this case?

C. Choose the following words and/or expressions to complete the sentences in their proper forms.

correspond	对应	locate	位于
signal	信号	exclude	排除
manifest	表现	valuable	有价值的
stage	阶段	to be related to	与……相关
support	支持	consider	考虑
consist of	组成	undergo	进行

1. In the early _____ of the lesion, the tumor nest is relatively small, composed of hyperplastic osteoblasts.

2. The lesion of this patient is mainly _____ as focal bone destruction of the medial bone cortex of the lower end of the right femur.

3. The pain was obvious at night. The skin of the _____ part had no redness, heat, and tenderness.

4. In addition, the patient's clinical symptoms (no local redness, swelling, heat, pain) and laboratory findings (no leukocytosis) do not _____ a bone abscess.

5. In mature lesions, the nest _____ highly calcified atypical trabecular bone, while the nest appears dense.

6. After admission, the patient _____ X-ray, CT and MRI examinations of the left thigh in our department.

7. MRI is less clear than CT for nests, but MRI is more _____ for subperiosteal osteoid osteomas.

8. According to the imaging characteristics and clinical manifestations of the lesion, I believe that osteoid osteoma should be _____ first.

9. The lesion is mainly _____ in the cortical area, and the surrounding cancellous bone density is increased.

10. T1WI on MRI showed that the focal bone destruction area on the medial side of the

femur was nodular and had slightly lower _____.

D. Read the dialogue and try to make a conversation with your classmates.

扫码获取
提示

E. Translate the following Chinese into English.

PG—Postgraduate   Dir—Director

PG：

Good morning! 1. 我先向大家汇报一下病例。

1. _____

The patient was an 11-year-old girl. 2. 感觉左大腿内下方肿胀、疼痛一个多月。The pain was obvious at night. The skin of the corresponding part had no redness，heat，and tenderness. There was no history of trauma，and the laboratory examination was normal. 3. 患者入院后在我科进行了左大腿的 X 光片、CT 和 MRI 检查。

2. _____

3. _____

_____

4. 在 X 线平片（图1）上可以看到左股骨内下侧局灶性低密度灶。The lesion is mainly located in the cortical area，and the surrounding cancellous bone density is increased. Lamellar periosteal reaction can be seen adjacent to the cortex of the lesion（arrow）. Swelling of the surrounding soft tissues.

4. _____

_____

5. CT 图像显示股骨内侧皮质内局灶性骨质破坏区，reactive osteosclerosis in the adjacent cancellous bone，obvious periosteal reaction in the surrounding area，and dense periosteal reaction near the lesion side（Figure 2，white arrow）.

5. _____

6. MRI 的 T_1 WI 显示股骨内侧的局灶性骨质破坏区呈结节状稍低信号（图 2，白箭），the peripheral lamellar periosteum reaction was also low signal，7. 冠状位及横断位 T_2 WI 示局灶性骨质破坏区呈高信号（图 3D、F，白箭），hyperintense edema shadow in and surrounding soft tissues in the medullary cavity（Figure 3D，white arrow），and significantly strengthened focal bone destruction area after enhancement（Fig. 3E，G，black arrow），and the periosteum around the lesion was thickened and strengthened. The lesion of this patient is mainly manifested as focal bone destruction of the medial bone cortex of the lower end of the right femur，and 8. 根据病变的影像学特点及临床表现，我认为应首先考虑骨样骨瘤，and chronic bone abscess can not be excluded. The Director was requested to conduct further analysis.

6. _____

7. _____

_____

8. _____

III Further Reading: Medical Imaging

Medical imaging is the technique and process of imaging the interior of a body for clinical analysis and medical intervention, as well as visual representation of the function of some organs or tissues (physiology). Medical imaging seeks to reveal internal structures hidden by the skin and bones, as well as to diagnose and treat disease. Medical imaging also establishes a database of normal anatomy and physiology to make it possible to identify abnormalities.

As a discipline and in its widest sense, it is part of biological imaging and incorporates radiology, which uses the imaging technologies of X-ray radiography, magnetic resonance imaging, ultrasound, endoscopy, elastography, tactile imaging, thermography, medical photography, nuclear medicine functional imaging techniques as positron emission tomography (PET) and single-photon emission computed tomography (SPECT).

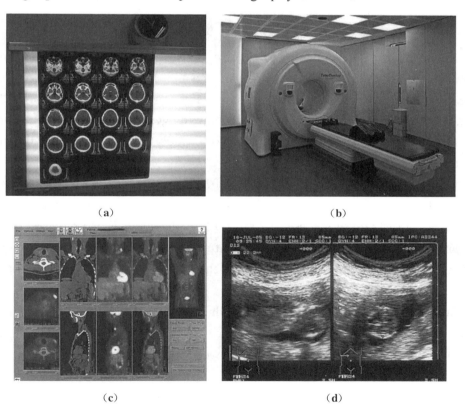

(a)　　　　　　　　　　　　　　(b)

(c)　　　　　　　　　　　　　　(d)

(a) The results of a CT scan of the head are shown as successive transverse sections. (b) An MRI machine generates a magnetic field around a patient. (c) PET scans use radiopharmaceuticals to create images of active blood flow and physiologic activity of the organ or organs being targeted. (d) Ultrasound technology is used to monitor pregnancies because it is the least invasive of imaging techniques and uses no electromagnetic radiation.

CT scan

A CT scan or computed tomography scan (formerly known as a computed axial tomography or CAT scan) is a medical imaging technique that uses computer-processed combinations of multiple X-ray measurements taken from different angles to produce tomographic (cross-sectional) images (virtual "slices") of a body, allowing the user to see inside the body without cutting. The personnel that perform CT scans are called radiographers or radiologic technologists.

Since its introduction in the 1970s, CT has become an important tool in medical imaging to supplement X-rays and medical ultrasonography. It has more recently been used for preventive medicine or screening for disease, for example CT colonography for people with a high risk of colon cancer, or full-motion heart scans for people with high risk of heart disease. A number of institutions offer full-body scans for the general population although this practice goes against the advice and official position of many professional organizations in the field primarily due to the radiation dose applied.

Initially, the images generated in CT scans were in the transverse (axial) anatomical plane, perpendicular to the long axis of the body. Modern scanners allow the scan data to be reformatted as images in other planes. Digital geometry processing can generate a three-dimensional image of an object inside the body from a series of two-dimensional radiographic images taken by rotation around a fixed axis. These cross-sectional images are widely used for medical diagnosis and therapy.

One study estimated that as many as 0.4% of cancers in the United States resulted from CT scans, and that this may have increased to as much as 1.5% to 2% based on the rate of CT use in 2007. Others dispute this estimate, as there is no consensus that the low levels of radiation used in CT scans cause damage. Lower radiation doses are used in many cases, such as in the investigation of renal colic.

Side effects from contrast agents, administered intravenously in some CT scans, might impair kidney performance in patients with kidney disease, although this risk is now believed to be lower than previously thought.

Head

CT scanning of the head is typically used to detect infarction, tumors, calcifications, haemorrhage, and bone trauma. Of the above, hypodense (dark) structures can indicate edema and infarction, hyperdense (bright) structures indicate calcifications and haemorrhage and bone trauma can be seen as disjunction in bone windows. Tumors can be detected by the swelling and anatomical distortion they cause, or by surrounding edema. Ambulances equipped with small bore multi-slice CT scanners respond to cases involving stroke or head trauma. CT scanning of the head is also used in CT-guided stereotactic surgery and radiosurgery for treatment of intracranial tumors, arteriovenous malformations, and other surgically treatable conditions using a device known as the N-localizer.

Lungs

A CT scan can be used for detecting both acute and chronic changes in the lung parenchyma, the tissue of the lungs. It is particularly relevant here because normal two-dimensional X-rays do not show such defects. A variety of techniques are used, depending on the suspected abnormality. For evaluation of chronic interstitial processes such as emphysema, and fibrosis, thin sections with high spatial frequency reconstructions are used; often scans are performed both on inspiration and expiration. This special technique is called high resolution CT that produces a sampling of the lung, and not continuous images.

An incidentally found nodule in the absence of symptoms (sometimes referred to as an incidentaloma) may raise concerns that it might represent a tumor, either benign or malignant. Perhaps persuaded by fear, patients and doctors sometimes agree to an intensive schedule of CT scans, sometimes up to every three months and beyond the recommended guidelines, in an attempt to do surveillance on the nodules. However, established guidelines advise that patients without a prior history of cancer and whose solid nodules have not grown over a two-year period are unlikely to have any malignant cancer. For this reason, and because no research provides supporting evidence that intensive surveillance gives better outcomes, and because of risks associated with having CT scans, patients should not receive CT screening in excess of those recommended by established guidelines.

Cardiac

A CT scan of the heart is performed to gain knowledge about cardiac or coronary anatomy. Traditionally, cardiac CT scans are used to detect, diagnose, or follow up coronary artery disease. More recently CT has played a key role in the fast evolving field of transcatheter structural heart interventions, more specifically in the transcatheter repair and replacement of heart valves.

The main forms of cardiac CT scanning are:

Coronary CT angiography (CTA): the use of CT to assess the coronary arteries of the heart. The subject receives an intravenous injection of radiocontrast, and then the heart is scanned using a high-speed CT scanner, allowing radiologists to assess the extent of occlusion in the coronary arteries, usually in order to diagnose coronary artery disease.

Coronary CT calcium scan: also used for the assessment of severity of coronary artery disease. Specifically, it looks for calcium deposits in the coronary arteries that can narrow arteries and increase the risk of heart attack. A typical coronary CT calcium scan is done without the use of radiocontrast, but it can possibly be done from contrast-enhanced images as well.

To better visualize the anatomy, post-processing of the images is common. Most common are multiplanar reconstructions (MPR) and volume rendering. For more complex anatomies and procedures, such as heart valve interventions, a true 3D reconstruction or a 3D print is created based on these CT images to gain a deeper understanding.

Magnetic resonance imaging (MRI)

A magnetic resonance imaging instrument (MRI scanner), or "nuclear magnetic resonance (NMR) imaging" scanner as it was originally known, uses powerful magnets to polarize and excite hydrogen nuclei (i.e., single protons) of water molecules in human tissue, producing a detectable signal which is spatially encoded, resulting in images of the body. The MRI machine emits a radio frequency (RF) pulse at the resonant frequency of the hydrogen atoms on water molecules. Radio frequency antennas ("RF coils") send the pulse to the area of the body to be examined. The RF pulse is absorbed by protons, causing their direction with respect to the primary magnetic field to change. When the RF pulse is turned off, the protons "relax" back to alignment with the primary magnet and emit radio-waves in the process. This radio-frequency emission from the hydrogen-atoms on water is what is detected and reconstructed into an image. The resonant frequency of a spinning magnetic dipole (of which protons are one example) is called the Larmor frequency and is determined by the strength of the main magnetic field and the chemical environment of the nuclei of interest. MRI uses three electromagnetic fields: a very strong (typically 1.5 to 3 teslas) static magnetic field to polarize the hydrogen nuclei, called the primary field; gradient fields that can be modified to vary in space and time (on the order of 1 kHz) for spatial encoding, often simply called gradients; and a spatially homogeneous radio-frequency (RF) field for manipulation of the hydrogen nuclei to produce measurable signals, collected through an RF antenna.

Like CT, MRI traditionally creates a two-dimensional image of a thin "slice" of the body and is therefore considered a tomographic imaging technique. Modern MRI instruments are capable of producing images in the form of 3D blocks, which may be considered a generalization of the single-slice, tomographic, concept. Unlike CT, MRI does not involve the use of ionizing radiation and is therefore not associated with the same health hazards. For example, because MRI has only been in use since the early 1980s, there are no known long-term effects of exposure to strong static fields (this is the subject of some debate; see "Safety" in MRI) and therefore there is no limit to the number of scans to which an individual can be subjected, in contrast with X-ray and CT. However, there are well-identified health risks associated with tissue heating from exposure to the RF field and the presence of implanted devices in the body, such as pacemakers. These risks are strictly controlled as part of the design of the instrument and the scanning protocols used.

Because CT and MRI are sensitive to different tissue properties, the appearances of the images obtained with the two techniques differ markedly. In CT, X-rays must be blocked by some form of dense tissue to create an image, so the image quality when looking at soft tissues will be poor. In MRI, while any nucleus with a net nuclear spin can be used, the proton of the hydrogen atom remains the most widely used, especially in the clinical setting, because it is so ubiquitous and returns a large signal. This nucleus, present in water molecules, allows the excellent soft-tissue contrast achievable with MRI.

A number of different pulse sequences can be used for specific MRI diagnostic imaging (multiparametric MRI or mpMRI). It is possible to differentiate tissue characteristics by combining two or more of the following imaging sequences, depending on the information being sought: T1-weighted (T1-MRI), T2-weighted (T2-MRI), diffusion weighted imaging (DWI-MRI), dynamic contrast enhancement (DCE-MRI), and spectroscopy (MRI-S). For example, imaging of prostate tumors is better accomplished using T2-MRI and DWI-MRI than T2-weighted imaging alone. The number of applications of mpMRI for detecting disease in various organs continues to expand, including liver studies, breast tumors, pancreatic tumors, and assessing the effects of vascular disruption agents on cancer tumors.

Nuclear medicine

Nuclear medicine encompasses both diagnostic imaging and treatment of disease, and may also be referred to as molecular medicine or molecular imaging and therapeutics. Nuclear medicine uses certain properties of isotopes and the energetic particles emitted from radioactive material to diagnose or treat various pathology. Different from the typical concept of anatomic radiology, nuclear medicine enables assessment of physiology. This function-based approach to medical evaluation has useful applications in most subspecialties, notably oncology, neurology, and cardiology. Gamma cameras and PET scanners are used in e.g. scintigraphy, SPECT and PET to detect regions of biologic activity that may be associated with a disease. Relatively short-lived isotope, such as 99mTc is administered to the patient. Isotopes are often preferentially absorbed by biologically active tissue in the body, and can be used to identify tumors or fracture points in bone. Images are acquired after collimated photons are detected by a crystal that gives off a light signal, which is in turn amplified and converted into count data.

SPECT is a 3D tomographic technique that uses gamma camera data from many projections and can be reconstructed in different planes. A dual detector head gamma camera combined with a CT scanner, which provides localization of functional SPECT data, is termed a SPECT-CT camera, and has shown utility in advancing the field of molecular imaging. In most other medical imaging modalities, energy is passed through the body and the reaction or result is read by detectors. In SPECT imaging, the patient is injected with a radioisotope, most commonly Thallium 201TI, Technetium 99mTC, Iodine 123I, and Gallium 67Ga. The radioactive gamma rays are emitted through the body as the natural decaying process of these isotopes takes place. The emissions of the gamma rays are captured by detectors that surround the body. This essentially means that the human is now the source of the radioactivity, rather than the medical imaging devices such as X-ray or CT.

Positron emission tomography (PET) uses coincidence detection to image functional processes. Short-lived positron emitting isotope, such as 18F, is incorporated with an organic substance such as glucose, creating F18-fluorodeoxyglucose, which can be used as a marker of metabolic utilization. Images of activity distribution throughout the body can show rapidly growing tissue, like tumor, metastasis, or infection. PET images can be viewed in comparison to computed tomography scans to determine an anatomic correlate. Modern scanners may integrate PET, allowing PET-CT, or PET-MRI to optimize the image reconstruction involved with positron imaging. This is performed on the same equipment without physically moving the patient off of the gantry. The resultant hybrid of functional and anatomic imaging information is a useful tool in non-invasive diagnosis and patient management.

Ultrasound

Medical ultrasound uses high frequency broadband sound waves in the megahertz range that are reflected by tissue to varying degrees to produce (up to 3D) images. This is commonly associated with imaging the fetus in pregnant women. Uses of ultrasound are much broader, however. Other important uses include imaging the abdominal organs, heart, breast, muscles, tendons, arteries and veins. While it may provide less anatomical detail than techniques such as CT or MRI, it has several advantages which make it ideal in numerous situations, in particular that it studies the function of moving structures in real-time, emits no ionizing radiation, and contains speckle that can be used in elastography. Ultrasound is also used as a popular research tool for capturing raw data, that can be made available through an ultrasound research interface, for the purpose of tissue characterization and implementation of new image processing techniques. The concepts of ultrasound differ from other medical imaging modalities in the fact that it is operated by the transmission and receipt of sound waves. The high frequency sound waves are sent into the tissue and depending on the composition of the different tissues, the signal will be attenuated and returned at separate intervals. A path of reflected sound waves in a multilayered structure can be defined by an input acoustic impedance (ultrasound sound wave) and the Reflection and transmission coefficients of the relative structures. It is very safe to use and does not appear to cause any adverse effects. It is also relatively inexpensive and quick to perform. Ultrasound scanners can be taken to critically ill patients in intensive care units, avoiding the danger caused while moving the patient to the radiology department. The real-time moving image obtained can be used to guide drainage and biopsy procedures. Doppler capabilities on modern scanners allow the blood flow in arteries and veins to be assessed.

A. Translate the following sentences into Chinese.

1. Medical imaging is the technique and process of imaging the interior of a body for clinical analysis and medical intervention, as well as visual representation of the function of some organs or tissues (physiology).

2. A CT scan or computed tomography scan (formerly known as a computed axial tomography or CAT scan) is a medical imaging technique that uses computer-processed combinations of multiple X-ray measurements taken from different angles to produce tomographic (cross-sectional) images (virtual "slices") of a body, allowing the user to see inside the body without cutting.

3. One study estimated that as many as 0.4% of cancers in the United States resulted from CT scans, and that this may have increased to as much as 1.5% to 2% based on the rate of CT use in 2007. Others dispute this estimate, as there is no consensus that the low levels of radiation used in CT scans cause damage.

4. To better visualize the anatomy, post-processing of the images is common. Most common are multiplanar reconstructions（MPR）and volume rendering. For more complex anatomies and procedures, such as heart valve interventions, a true 3D reconstruction or a 3D print is created based on these CT images to gain a deeper understanding.

5. A magnetic resonance imaging instrument（MRI scanner）, or "nuclear magnetic resonance（NMR）imaging" scanner as it was originally known, uses powerful magnets to polarize and excite hydrogen nuclei（i. e., single protons）of water molecules in human tissue, producing a detectable signal which is spatially encoded, resulting in images of the body.

B. Prepare a lecture on the diagnostic value of CT after doing the further reading above.

扫码获取
提示

Unit 30

Lumbago

I **Warming-up**

A. Match the following words and phrases with their Chinese translations.

A degenerative disc disease
B lumbago
C swab and sterilize
D scoliosis
E herniated disk
F acupuncture physician
G chiropractic care
H organ meridian
I spondylosis
J spinal stenosis

1 腰痛
2 椎间盘突出
3 针灸医生
4 按摩保健
5 器官经络
6 椎管狭窄
7 椎间盘退变性疾病
8 擦拭和消毒
9 颈椎病
10 脊柱侧弯

B. Complete the sentences with the following words or phrases in their proper forms.

restrict	sedentary	afflict	acupuncture
degenerative	overload	susceptible	refer to

1. A large review of studies published in 2015 in the *Annals of Internal Medicine* found that even after adjusting for physical activity, sitting for long periods was associated with

worse health outcomes including heart disease, Type 2 diabetes and cancer. _____ behavior can also increase your risk of dying, either from heart disease or other medical problems.

2. "Women are particularly _____ to developing depression and anxiety disorders in response to stress compared to men," according to Dr. Yehuda, chief psychiatrist at New York's Veteran's Administration Hospital.

3. Because of advances in imaging technology, genetics, biochemistry, and cell biology, scientists have been able to identify similarities among many _____ diseases.

4. On top of that, most of the 3D food printers now are _____ to dry ingredients, because meat and milk products may easily go bad. Some experts are skeptical about 3D food printers, believing they are better suited for fast food restaurants than homes and high-end restaurants.

5. Eating disorders _____ women across the lifespan with peak onset during critical or sensitive developmental periods of reproductive hormone change, such as puberty.

6. Acupuncture points are believed to stimulate the central nervous system. This, in turn, releases chemicals into the muscles, spinal cord, and brain. These biochemical changes may stimulate the body's natural healing abilities and promote physical and emotional well-being. National Institute of Health (NIH) studies have shown that _____ is an effective treatment alone or in combination with conventional therapies to treat various kinds of diseases.

7. The term "society" is the most fundamental one in sociology. Society is a web of social relationship and networking between individuals. Society _____ the people who interact in a specific territory and share culture based on limited social norms and values.

8. Stress and anxiety have become very prevalent in this era of fast-paced living and environmental _____. Acupuncture treatment for stress and anxiety helps patients to restore balance to their bodies and their daily lives.

C. **Watch the video *Acupuncture as Treatment for Back Pain* and answer the questions.**

扫码获取视频

1. What is Bob Lindy going to talk about in the video?

2. Do acupuncture physicians take the same approaches and use points in the same locations?

3. What can acupuncture physicians do once they have swabbed and sterilized the areas?

4. Does Bob Lindy do it with the Guide tubes or free handing when he finds it's a little bit more pain free?

5. In order to help with your chronic or acute lower back pain, what are you suggested to do?

扫码获取
音频及文本

II Dialogue

 A. Listen to the dialogue for the first time and try to get the general idea.

 B. Listen to the dialogue for the second time and try to answer the following questions.

1. What's wrong with the patient?

2. Does the patient feel numbness in his legs or feet?

3. Under what circumstances does the patient feel the pain getting worse?

4. What makes him feel better?

5. Besides some medication，what suggestions does the doctor give to the patient?

C. Choose the following words and/or expressions to complete the sentences in their proper forms.

get worse	变得更糟糕	incurable	不能治愈的
prescribe	开药方	under the circumstances of	
take time	需要时间		在……的情况下
lie on the abdomen	俯卧	medium-to-hard bed	中度到硬度床
discomfort	不适	pick up	捡起
bend over	附身	feel numbness	感觉麻木
leg-raising test	抬腿试验		

1. Physicians who have been on the job for several hours，for example，are more likely to _____ antibiotics to patients when it's unwise to do so. This phenomenon partly accounts for the overuse of antibiotics in some countries.

2. It _____ but she found something she was good at. Now，Nicole teaches girls and women alike how to box.

3. John had suffered from a severe disease for over two years. He stood _____，with his hands pressed against his kidneys.

4. Early one summer morning in 2022，I arrived at the office and _____ in my hands，which I dismissed as mere morning grogginess.

5. This new drug usually causes only minor _____，such as a skin rash，headache or sleepiness.

6. She suffered from a stroke when I was currently living away in Leeds, and gradually her health _____ very quickly over a 3-month period.

7. The idea is that a person who dies from a presently _____ disease could be thawed and revived in the future when a cure has been found.

8. High blood pressure is _____ less often in people who smoke, despite them being at higher risk of heart disease, research suggests.

9. Life expectancy need not be curtailed _____ good nutrition, a reasonable amount of exercise and a decrease in the wear and tear of stressful events.

10. In contrast, performing a passive _____ has been proved as valuable for this purpose.

D. Read the dialogue and try to make a conversation with your classmates.

扫码获取
提示

E. Translate the following Chinese into English.

P—Patient   D—Doctor

D: What's wrong with you, please?

P: I have had a pain in my lower back for more than two months. It has been so bad for the last week that I can't get out of bed and walk. 1. 吃止痛片也没用。

　　1. _____

D: Do you have any other discomforts?

P: Yes. In the leg, and the lateral side of the right calf, it hurts. I have no strength in my legs and I am afraid of the cold.

D: Oh, does the pain run up your leg? What kind of pain is it? Burning pain? Stinging?

P: Yes, it went to the outside of the calf of the right leg. There was no strength in the leg.

D: 2. 腰扭过吗?

　　2. _____

P: Before the illness, I carried a heavy piece of luggage. I think I sprained it then.

D: Where do you feel the pain in your waist? In the middle, or on both sides?

P: Just in the middle.

D: OK, now please lie down in bed and I'll do a physical examination for you.

D: Based on your symptoms, you probably have a herniated lumbar disc. 3. 你需要做个 CT 检查以确诊。Please take the checklist to the CT room and then you'll come back with the result.

　　3. _____

D: Well, it turned out to be a herniated lumbar disc, consistent with your clinical symptoms. These symptoms are mainly caused by compression of the sciatic nerve caused by herniation of the lumbar disc after weight bearing. 4. 我将给你针灸治疗,缓解你的疼痛。

　　4. _____

P: Does acupuncture hurt?

D: 5. 别担心,只有轻微疼痛,还可能有点麻、胀的感觉。You need to be treated once a day for 10 days. Can we start now?

　　5. _____

　　　_____

P: OK.

D: 6. 我还要给你拔几个火罐,局部会有点发紧。

　　6. _____

P: How do you feel?

P: 7. 太神奇了,我的疼痛轻多了。

7. _____

D: All right. After you go back, you'll need full bed rest and avoid bearing weight and

alcohol. 8. 劳累和饮酒都会加重病情。Bye.

8. _____

P: Good-bye. I'll follow your advice.

III Further Reading: Acupuncture and Chinese Herbs for Lumbago

Every year, more than 8% of the global population experiences lumbago. Many people also experience pain in the upper back and neck, making back pain one of the most common medical problems. Lumbago occurs for many reasons, including auto accidents, slip-and-fall accidents, participation in contact sports, and degenerative conditions affecting the bones, discs and nerves of the spine.

Regardless of why you have lumbago, it's important to consult a healthcare professional. Although back pain intensity sometimes improves with rest, you may need treatment before you can return to your normal activities. Acupuncture is an effective treatment involving the insertion of needles, helping reduce pain without addictive medications or surgical procedures that can take you out of commission for several months.

Lumbago is an old term that refers to lower back discomfort due to various causes. It refers to lower back pain that could be caused by anomalies in the spine, joints, muscles, or nerves around the lower back region. Lumbago affects a substantial percentage of adults around the world and can be acute or chronic, causing either a persistent, agonizing pain or a sudden, sharp pain. It can cause restrictions in mobility ranging from mild to severe.

What is lumbago? Lumbago is an acute or persistent discomfort in the lower back that can afflict anyone. The causes for lumbago include but are not restricted to—back injury, herniated (slipped) disk, obesity, weak back muscles, spasms, and tumors (both benign and malignant) in the spinal area.

Many patients with lower back pain tend to be individuals who work for long hours at occupations that require a lot of bending and heavy lifting. Patients who live a sedentary lifestyle, maintain bad posture, and do not exercise regularly are also susceptible to lumbago. Lumbago can also be caused by an underlying ailment, such as degenerative disc disease or arthritis.

What are the common symptoms of lumbago? Here is a checklist of common symptoms such as sharp and acute pain, dull and persistent pain, stabbing pain, burning pain and on specific pain, exhibited by patients suffering from lumbago. Lumbago is essentially a term which covers an umbrella of painful sensations that afflict the lower back area.

When should you seek medical attention? Most cases of back pain should improve over time with self-care and home treatment, possibly within a range of a few days to a couple of weeks.

However, if your back pain persists for longer periods, or if you're suffering from the symptoms mentioned below, it is highly recommended that you consult your Apollo doctor without delay. You are experiencing stabbing pain with no decrease in the intensity of the pain even after sufficient rest. The discomfort radiates down to hips or one or both legs, and especially if the pain spreads below the knee. Your pain medication no longer provides sufficient relief. The pain worsens with the passage of time. The lower back pain is followed by an inexplicable reduction in your weight.

What are the causes of lumbago? Lumbago can be caused by a variety of reasons, the most common of which are strenuous activities which overload the back muscles, improper lifting techniques wherein you lift heavy loads with an improper body posture. Osteoarthritis and spondylosis (spinal arthritis) can also be factors which result in lumbago.

A slipped or herniated disc, osteoporosis, spinal stenosis or nerve compression, scoliosis, and malignant or benign or malignant spinal tumors are all possible reasons why you might be suffering from lumbago.

What are the common risk factors that can lead to lumbago? Lumbago can affect anyone, including children and teenagers. The following factors such as age, lack of exercise, obesity, diseases, incorrect techniques used when lifting, psychological problems and smoking may increase your chances of having lumbago.

Back discomfort becomes increasingly common as you age. You become even more susceptible to back pain as you age over 30 years. Risk of lumbago increases if the patient has weak, unused muscles in the back and abdomen due to lack of physical exercise. In case of obese patients, the lower back is put under additional strain along with weakening of back muscles due to limited physical activity. This makes them prone to lower back pain. Patients are at a higher risk of lumbago if they are suffering from certain types of arthritis and cancer. People who employ incorrect lifting techniques such as using their back instead of legs to lift heavy loads are more prone to lumbago. Back pain also appears to be more common in people who suffer from depression and anxiety. Back pain is more common among smokers. Smoking reduces blood flow to the spine, increasing the risk of osteoporosis.

What are the treatment options available? Lumbago treatment differs depending on several factors, including the patient's age, weight, fitness level, symptoms, severity of pain and more. Treatment options include the hot or cold compresses for brief lower back pain alleviation, anti-inflammatory medication, mild stretches and exercises as suggested by your doctor, spinal manipulation and chiropractic care, surgical procedures, usage of external devices such as back supports, weight-loss and acupuncture and yoga.

How can you prevent lumbago? By improving your physical condition, leading a healthy lifestyle, and practicing good body posture and mechanics, you may be able to avoid or prevent back discomfort.

You can follow these easy tips to keep your back healthy and strong. Exercises tend to be essential. Low-impact aerobics, or exercises that don't strain or jolt your back, can help you build back strength and endurance, as well as improve muscle tone. Swimming and walking are both excellent options to maintain a resilient and strengthened back. Strengthen and stretch your muscles. Exercises that build your core, such as those which focus on abdominal and back muscle strengthening, prepare the muscles around the spine to operate together like a natural corset or support for your back. It is important to maintain a healthy body mass index (BMI). Obesity puts a burden on the spinal muscles. If you're overweight, losing weight can help you avoid lower back pain.

Stop smoking is always suggested. Smoking raises your chances of developing low back discomfort.

At the same time, you are advised to avoid activities that involve sudden twisting or bending or lifting heavy loads manually. Maintain proper posture. Do not slouch. Try and keep the pelvis in a neutral position. Choose the right chair. For those with a desk job, choose a seat with a swivel base, armrests, and good lower back support, if possible. Maintain a level posture with your knees and hips. Alter the positions at least once every half-hour. Lift with caution. Use your legs and maintain a straight posture when lifting heavy items.

Acupuncture is a form of traditional Chinese medicine based on the idea that opposing forces—*yin* and *yang*—need to be balanced. When there's an imbalance in your body's energy flow, you may experience pain, illness and reduced function. Acupuncture, as a medical treatment, addresses this type of imbalance, restoring the normal flow of energy.

Acupuncture is considered to be one of the world's oldest treatments and is part of Traditional Chinese Medicine (TCM). The principle for Chinese medicine is that the body consists of many energy meridians. When *qi* (the Chinese word for vital energy) does not freely flow through these meridians, it can cause pain. The aim of acupuncture is to stimulate the blood flow and the energy flow through these meridians in order to reduce or eliminate pain.

During an acupuncture procedure, the practitioner inserts needles at specific points on the body. This stimulates the central nervous system, prompting the release of pain-relieving chemicals. Traditional acupuncture also rewires the brain by releasing neurotransmitters, which are hormones that carry messages throughout the nervous system. Some neurotransmitters, such as endorphins, block the nerve cells responsible for receiving pain signals. When these cells are blocked, pain signals can't get through, relieving discomfort.

In the use of acupuncture for lumbago, the needles are inserted at various points on the back, concentrating on the lower back and hips. In the case of nerve based pain, some needles are also inserted down the legs. Once the needles are in place, the patient is left for approximately ten minutes, after which the acupuncturist will stimulate the needles by slowly rotating them and leaving them in the skin for another ten minutes.

Because the needles are so thin, very little pain or discomfort is experienced while inserting the needles. However, on sensitive areas on the body, such as around the feet, back of the knee, one does feel a slight prick when the needle is put in place or stimulated.

Once the needles have been in place for around twenty minutes, they are removed, one at a time and the acupuncturist whom is usually educated in Chinese massage therapy will follow the treatment with a relaxing massage, focusing on the painful areas. This massage will further promote blood flow and toxin release in the affected area and ease the tension in the surrounding tissue. The result is usually a very calm, relaxed and fairly pain fee individual.

As the use of acupuncture seems to focus mainly on soft tissue, the pain relief that is experienced could only last for 12 to 48 hours afterwards, especially if the cause of the back pain is structural and not due to tissue damage. When using acupuncture for lumbago, if the spine is out of alignment and is considered to be the main cause of pain, the treatment of surrounding muscles and ligaments are only part of fixing the problem. In the case of a herniated disc, the body needs a lot of time, sometimes even months, for the protrusion in the disc to retract. Due to this, one should consider acupuncture as a complimentary treatment in addition to other medical treatments such as physiotherapy or chiropractic treatment. If you deal with the structural and soft tissue issues at the same time, your chances of a quicker recovery are greatly increased.

Expert acupuncturists do everything they can to make acupuncture safe and pain-free, so adverse side effects are rare. For example, a reputable, licensed acupuncturist follows FDA regulations by targeting energy points with single-use needles and sanitizing everything thoroughly before each session. Before trying acupuncture therapy, consult your doctor, especially if you're pregnant, under the age of 20, have a pacemaker or have a chronic health condition.

Acupuncture is most effective when it's combined with other noninvasive treatment methods, such as chiropractic care and physical therapy. Ask your care team for recommendations regarding treatment options and timing to receive the full benefits of acupuncture.

When researchers from Penn Medicine examined a group of systematic reviews, they discovered that acupuncture provides clinically relevant benefits for people with chronic lower back pain, such as pain relief and improved function.

Cho et al. conducted a multicenter study on the use of acupuncture needles for chronic lower back pain. As part of the study, they recruited participants between the ages of 18 and 65 who experienced non-specific lower back pain for at least three months before the study began. About half of the participants received sham acupuncture (placebo acupuncture), and the other half received individualized acupuncture treatments with single-use needles. They reported that individualized acupuncture is much more effective than sham acupuncture for reducing bothersome lower back pain. Participants who received real acupuncture also reported that their chronic pain was less intense after the treatments.

The western world is more and more considering the benefits of eastern medicine such as acupuncture as we start to see the body holistically. Having used acupuncture myself for the treatment of lower back pain, I can recommend it as part of your "package" to treat chronic pain. Acupuncture for lumbago is generally very successful. It is a great step towards avoiding too much chemicals to rid yourself of pain.

If you seek Chinese medicine treatments, an integral part of your holistic treatment plan will be Chinese herbs. There is no single herb or collection of herbs that is always used for uterine fibroids. It always depends on your specific constitution and root cause.

Of the many types of herbal formulas that can be used to shrink fibroids, one of the most common formulas are Cinnamon & Poria Pills. Much research has been done on this formula and its effect on uterine tumors over the years. A 2019 research article explored the pharmacological effects of this formula on fibroids and discovered that the possible mechanism by which it works is that it induces apoptosis (the death of cells) within the fibroid tumor. Other studies purport its usefulness in treating fibroids because of its anti-tumor and anti-inflammatory effect.

Lumbago is common among people of different ages. However, if we understand its causes, we can prevent it from afflicting us.

A. Translate the following sentences into Chinese.

1. Lumbago is an acute or persistent discomfort in the lower back that can afflict anyone. The causes for lumbago include but are not restricted to—back injury, herniated (slipped) disk, obesity, weak back muscles, spasms, and tumors (both benign and malignant) in the spinal area.

2. Lumbago can be caused by a variety of reasons, the most common of which are strenuous activities which overload the back muscles, improper lifting techniques wherein you lift heavy loads with an improper body posture. Osteoarthritis and spondylosis (spinal arthritis) can also be factors which result in lumbago.

3. Risk of lumbago increases if the patient has weak, unused muscles in the back and abdomen due to lack of physical exercise. In case of obese patients, the lower back is put under additional strain along with weakening of back muscles due to limited physical activity.

4. Treatment options include the hot or cold compresses for brief lower back pain alleviation, anti-inflammatory medication, mild stretches and exercises as suggested by your doctor, spinal manipulation and chiropractic care, surgical procedures, usage of external devices such as back supports, weight-loss and acupuncture and yoga.

5. Acupuncture is considered to be one of the world's oldest treatments and is part of Traditional Chinese Medicine (TCM). The principle for Chinese medicine is that the body consists of many energy meridians. When *qi* (the Chinese word for vital energy) does not freely flow through these meridians, it can cause pain. The aim of acupuncture is to stimulate the blood flow and the energy flow through these meridians in order to reduce or eliminate pain.

B. Prepare a lecture on lumbago after doing the further reading above.

扫码获取
提示

图书在版编目(CIP)数据

临床诊疗英语 / 胡涛主编. —— 南京 : 南京大学出版社,2023.6
ISBN 978 - 7 - 305 - 26950 - 9

Ⅰ. ①临… Ⅱ. ①胡… Ⅲ. ①临床医学 - 英语 Ⅳ.
①R4

中国国家版本馆 CIP 数据核字(2023)第 076981 号

出版发行　南京大学出版社
社　　址　南京市汉口路 22 号　　　　邮　编　210093
出 版 人　金鑫荣
书　　名　临床诊疗英语
主　　编　胡　涛
责任编辑　裴维维　　　　　　　编辑热线　025 - 83592123
照　　排　南京南琳图文制作有限公司
印　　刷　南京玉河印刷厂
开　　本　880×1230　1/16　印张 21.75　字数 750 千
版　　次　2023 年 6 月第 1 版　2023 年 6 月第 1 次印刷
ISBN 978 - 7 - 305 - 26950 - 9
定　　价　69.00 元

网址:http://www.njupco.com
官方微博:http://weibo.com/njupco
官方微信号:njupress
销售咨询热线:(025)83594756